Non-Obstructive Azoospermia

Wael Zohdy • Murat Gül • Rupin Shah
Ashok Agarwal
Editors

Non-Obstructive Azoospermia

A Comprehensive Guide to Causes, Diagnosis, and Treatment

Springer

Editors
Wael Zohdy
Department of Andrology
Cairo University
Giza, Egypt

Rupin Shah
Department of Urology
Lilavati Hospital and Research Centre
Mumbai, Maharashtra, India

Murat Gül
Department of Urology
Selçuk University School of Medicine
Konya, Türkiye

Department of Andrology
Selçuk University School of Medicine
Konya, Türkiye

Ashok Agarwal
Global Andrology Forum
Moreland Hills, OH, USA

ISBN 978-3-031-99430-2 ISBN 978-3-031-99431-9 (eBook)
https://doi.org/10.1007/978-3-031-99431-9

This Springer imprint is published by the registered company Springer Nature Switzerland AG
The registered company address is: Gewerbestrasse 11, 6330 Cham, Switzerland

Foreword

This publication is timely. Our understanding of the aetiology of nonobstructive azoospermia (NOA) is about to change. We are beginning to explore some candidate genes responsible for failed spermatogenesis, and whole-exome and whole-genome sequencing will provide vital diagnostic and therefore prognostic information. Artificial intelligence is already beginning to refine the prediction of spermatogenesis and sperm retrieval, whilst similar technology applied to image analysis is already improving sperm retrieval rates during and after microtesticular dissection.

The editors and authors are to be congratulated, because this book breaks the usual mode of medical reviews and updates. Most reviews reflect the previous publications of a 'campus' or a 'society', or even a continent, but seldom do International senior authors collaborate to provide a truly global overview, particularly of a condition which often defies both proper diagnosis and treatment. Although there is inevitably some overlap in the issues covered, this is not problematic, as there must be room for 'opinions'.

Murat Guls's introduction sets the tone, recognising the wider health outcomes of nonobstructive azoospermia and the importance of diagnosis rather than 'solutions'. Sadek and colleagues (Chap. 15) further explore the psychological aspects of NOA, particularly after failed micro-TESE. In Chap. 14, Logan highlights the difficult decisions we face when separating the chance of finding sperm in a salvage micro-TESE with the chance of real success – a live birth. Urologists are not best placed to understand that the journey of couples after testicular sperm retrieval is often fraught and ultimately disappointing. Another area difficult for many of us to accept is the variability in technical competence, both surgically and embryologically, both of which affect the prediction of success. This is highlighted by Balasingham in Chap. 12.

Rosas further explores and explains laboratory techniques and testicular sperm identification and preservation. I suspect few of us are aware of the range of processes currently available in the laboratory.

Narino's important contribution, broadly addressing the testicular dysgenesis syndrome and its hormonal effects, is an unusual and interesting contribution for andrological readers. We also read Wyn's chapter about fertility restoration in pubertal boys; this is helpful to urologists to gain a perspective about how our adult patients might have reached an azoospermic endpoint.

Although we currently find few headline chromosomal abnormalities in NOA, Tan Lee's Chap. 3 gives a lucid description of what we do know and therefore what we can say to patients who desperately seek reasons for their situation.

Elsewhere, Kavoussi and colleagues should be congratulated on the comprehensive review of the importance of varicocele, a subject which somewhat inexplicably still causes some division of opinion. The review of current guidelines, also by Kavoussi, is extremely helpful, placed at the end of this excellent book. I urge all readers to read Chap. 16 only after reading Chaps. 1 to 15. The current guidelines probably do not reflect our current knowledge.

There is an evident gap between the 'state of the art' and the 'state of the guidelines' which seek to define our practice, and this comprehensive publication goes some way to exploring that gap where necessary, and reinforcing those guidelines when they are equally important.

I commend this excellent book to urologists, andrologists and indeed to endocrinologists, who have an increasingly important role in the management of our patients with nonobstructive azoospermia.

London, UK
Oct 2025

Jonathan Ramsay, MS, FRCF, FRCS (Urol)

Preface

Non-obstructive azoospermia (NOA) is the most challenging problem in male infertility. Affecting a significant proportion of men, NOA represents a complex and heterogeneous entity that interweaves endocrinological, genetic, developmental, and environmental influences. Over the past decades, remarkable progress has been made in unraveling its underlying mechanisms and refining diagnostic and therapeutic strategies. Yet, for many patients and clinicians, NOA poses profound clinical, emotional, social, and ethical challenges.

This book was envisioned to provide a comprehensive, multidisciplinary, and clinically relevant resource for urologists, andrologists, reproductive physicians, and researchers encountering NOA patients. The 16 chapters are carefully structured to progress from fundamental concepts to applied clinical practices and future directions. Beginning with an introduction to NOA, the text explores hormonal aberrations and the genetic spectrum that shape its pathophysiology, followed by strategies to differentiate obstructive from non-obstructive causes of azoospermia. Dedicated chapters illustrate the role of imaging modalities, the management of hypogonadism, and cryopreservation of sperm. The discussion further extends to adolescent care, testicular dysgenesis syndrome, and the role of varicocele repair in selected cases.

Surgical procedures and laboratory techniques for sperm retrieval and processing in NOA are presented in detail, alongside predictors of success and considerations for patients who have undergone prior failed surgical sperm retrieval. Recognizing that infertility poses social, emotional, and financial stress on the affected couples, the book also addresses the emotional and psychological impact of NOA, an often-overlooked but crucial dimension of patient care. To ensure practical applicability, the text integrates current international guidelines while offering perspectives on emerging research, technologies, and the future landscape of NOA management.

We extend our deepest gratitude to the outstanding team of contributors—we have 43 authors from 20 countries—whose dedication, scholarship, and commitment have shaped this book into a comprehensive and authoritative resource. Their collective expertise and tireless efforts brought this project to life. We are also grateful for the exceptional guidance of Lillie Mae Gaurano, Springer Editor, Clinical Medicine (Books), and the meticulous coordination of Dhanapal Palanisamy, Production Editor, whose support ensured the smooth completion of this volume.

This book is lovingly dedicated to our families, mentors, and patients, whose encouragement, wisdom, and resilience continue to inspire our pursuit of progress in the field of male infertility.

Cairo, Egypt — Wael Zohdy, MD, PhD
Konya, Turkey — Murat Gül, MD, FEBU
Mumbai, Maharashtra, India — Rupin Shah, MS, MCh
Moreland Hills, OH, USA — Ashok Agarwal, PhD, HCLD

Contents

Chapter 1
Introduction to NOA

Murat Gül, Nguyen Ho Vinh Phuoc, and Taha Abo-Almagd Abdel-Meguid Hamoda

Key Points

- Nonobstructive azoospermia (NOA) is characterized by the absence of sperm in the ejaculate due to impaired spermatogenesis, affecting approximately 60% of azoospermic men.
- The causes include genetic, endocrine, and iatrogenic factors, with conditions like Klinefelter syndrome and hormonal imbalances playing significant roles.
- Diagnosis involves a microscopic examination of the centrifuged pellet of semen sample.
- Sperm can be detected in 35% of men suspected to have NOA.
- Treatment primarily relies on advanced reproductive techniques, with varying success rates based on the underlying causes.
- Prognosis varies by the underlying condition, with testicular diseases often irreparable. Males with NOA face increased risks of additional health conditions and malignancies.
- Future directions include genetic research to enhance diagnostics and reduce reliance on assisted reproductive technologies (ARTs). Targeted therapy advancements could potentially mitigate the need for costly and invasive treatments.

M. Gül (✉)
Department of Urology, Selçuk University School of Medicine, Konya, Türkiye

Department of Andrology, Selçuk University School of Medicine, Konya, Türkiye

N. H. V. Phuoc
Department of Andrology, Binh Dan Hospital, Ho Chi Minh City, Vietnam

T. A.-A. A.-M. Hamoda
Department of Urology, King Abdulaziz University, Jeddah, Saudi Arabia

W. Zohdy et al. (eds.), *Non-Obstructive Azoospermia*,
https://doi.org/10.1007/978-3-031-99431-9_1

Definition of Nonobstructive Azoospermia (NOA)

Nonobstructive azoospermia (NOA) is a condition characterized by the inability to detect sperm in the ejaculate due to impairment of spermatogenesis rather than a physical blockage in the reproductive tract [1]. Historically, NOA has been recognized as a significant cause of male infertility, with early observations often leading to misunderstandings about its etiology and implications, and, therefore, men with azoospermia were perceived as lacking reproductive capabilities [2]. However, the emergence of testicular sperm extraction (TESE), coupled with in vitro fertilization/intracytoplasmic sperm injection (IVF/ICSI), has enabled men with NOA to engage in biological fatherhood.

Epidemiology of NOA

Infertility affects approximately 15% of all couples. Male azoospermia impacts approximately 1% of the male population and approximately 10–15% of all males experiencing infertility [3]. Approximately 60% of males with azoospermia will experience NOA, which is the most prevalent form of azoospermia. Around 600,000 males of reproductive age in the United States were reported as azoospermic, with the majority of them having NOA [4].

Azoospermic males exhibit a heightened susceptibility to cancer in comparison to the broader populace. The prevalence of azoospermia in males diagnosed with testicular cancer ranges from 5% to 8% [5, 6]. Nevertheless, the precise prevalence of azoospermia is uncertain and is likely to be underreported in underdeveloped countries where modern treatment is either prohibitively expensive or not accessible [7].

Etiology of NOA

Azoospermia can be caused by several factors; however, it can be broadly classified into three main categories: pretesticular, testicular, and post-testicular. Azoospermia can be attributed to endocrine disorders that have a detrimental impact on spermatogenesis. The etiologies of testicular conditions encompass inherent abnormalities in the process of spermatogenesis within the testes. Azoospermia can also be attributed to post-testicular factors, such as the occlusion of the ductal system at any point within the male reproductive canal (obstructive azoospermia), which is out of the scope of this chapter. Table 1.1 provides a comprehensive overview of the several conditions associated with NOA.

Table 1.1 Different etiologies of NOA [3, 8, 9]

Congenital causes
Klinefelter syndrome (47 XXY)
Y-chromosome microdeletions
Cryptorchidism
Kallmann syndrome
Congenital adrenal hyperplasia
Endocrinological causes
Hypogonadotropic hypogonadism
Hyperprolactinemia (pituitary tumors)
Thyroid dysfunction
Iatrogenic conditions
Drugs or medications
Gonadotoxic exposure (chemotherapy or radiotherapy)
Exogenous testosterone or anabolic steroids use
Testicular causes
Varicocele
Testicular torsion
Testicular trauma
Testicular tumors
Epididiymo-orchitis

Diagnosis of NOA

The term "azoospermia" refers to the total lack of sperm in the ejaculate. The confirmation of this diagnosis necessitates the centrifugation of a semen sample at a minimum speed of 3000 g [10] for 15 min at ambient temperature, followed by a high-powered microscopic analysis of the resulting pellet. Ron-El et al. demonstrated that sperm can be detected in 35% of men suspected to have NOA through a thorough investigation of a centrifuged semen sample [11]. The significance of these findings lies in the fact that patients frequently undergo semen analysis, which was previously conducted without employing standardized centrifugation techniques. Thus, clinicians are required to consistently confirm the diagnosis of azoospermia by routinely doing seminal analysis with centrifugation. The presence of even rare sperm in the centrifuged sample indicates the absence of full ductal obstruction and presents the possibility of promptly preserving sperm for in vitro fertilization/intracytoplasmic sperm injection (IVF/ICSI) procedures [12, 13].

The examination of semen should be conducted in accordance with the standards set forth by the World Health Organization. It is recommended that a minimum of two semen samples, taken with a time interval of more than 2 weeks, be evaluated [9, 10].

Management of NOA

Most people with NOA necessitate advanced assisted reproductive techniques (ARTs). Both microscopic TESE (micro-TESE) and ICSI have the potential to provide benefits to these individuals [1]. The rate of unsuccessful sperm retrieval in NOA is elevated and fluctuates depending on the underlying cause. According to reports, the overall success rate for sperm retrieval in these individuals can reach up to 75%, with an average of approximately 50% [12]. Testicular sperm aspiration (TESA), involving the percutaneous insertion of a needle into the testicular parenchyma, has less successful sperm retrieval than micro-TESE among NOA men. Additionally, there exists a notable potential for vascular damage. Furthermore, it has been shown that patients with NOA exhibit a relatively high occurrence of chromosomal abnormalities and DNA damage in their sperm [14]. Additionally, there is a possibility that infertility-related genes that can be inherited by male offspring may be transmitted [15]. If deemed required, it is possible to effectively conduct repeat micro-TESE treatments in order to recover sperm [16].

It is crucial to have a precise diagnosis of the cause of azoospermia whenever feasible prior to initiating the proper treatment. Urologists must establish close collaboration with reproductive specialists due to the potential impact of care timing and coordination on the attainment of optimal outcomes and the enhanced management of azoospermia, hence optimizing sperm quality in affected individuals. Further details on the management of NOA are discussed elsewhere in this book.

Prognosis

Each cause of azoospermia is linked to a distinct prognosis, which can vary from restoring sperm production to the mere detection of sperm in the reproductive system. Azoospermia, a condition characterized by wide variability, can sometimes be effectively treated, leading to the potential restoration of fertility [3]. On the other hand, testicular diseases are typically not able to be reversed, and the effectiveness of therapies for intrinsic testicular abnormalities is considerably lower [3].

Males diagnosed with NOA exhibit a greater prevalence of additional health-related conditions, such as pituitary prolactinomas, diverse testicular neoplasms (including germ cell, Sertoli cell, and Leydig cell tumors), and face a threefold increase in overall risk of developing a future malignancy in comparison to infertile males without NOA [5]. Approximately 30% of males with NOA also experience testosterone insufficiency, typically caused by a malfunction in the Leydig cells [17, 18].

Moreover, a frequent presentation of NOA, Klinefelter syndrome, is associated with increased morbidity and mortality risks. The main conditions linked with these increased risks are the compromised metabolic risk profiles marked by a higher occurrence of type 2 diabetes and a tendency to experience blood clots or embolism, both of which are risk factors for cardiovascular disease [18]. Osteoporosis and bone fractures, along with a heightened incidence of some forms of cancer, autoimmune illnesses, viral diseases, and epilepsy, are other factors that contribute to the increased morbidity observed in individuals with Klinefelter syndrome [19].

Overall, the prognosis of NOA extends beyond infertility, encompassing implications for other health conditions such as metabolic and cardiovascular function. Recognizing and addressing these broader health concerns are essential for optimizing the overall well-being of individuals with NOA.

Future Perspective

Investigating the impact of lifestyle factors such as diet, exercise, and environmental exposures on male fertility could provide valuable insights into preventive measures and adjunctive therapies for NOA [20]. Also, there has been a resurgence of interest in genetic research aimed at identifying the root reasons for idiopathic male infertility. In addition, ongoing research into stem cell technology holds promise for regenerating sperm-producing cells in men with NOA. Utilizing stem cells to replenish spermatogenesis may offer a novel therapeutic avenue for infertility treatment [21]. However, the prevailing tendency has been to bypass advancements in diagnostic assessment in favor of a costlier yet more effective alternative, specifically ART. In an optimal scenario, implementing targeted therapy for male-factor infertility would reduce the reliance on ART, thus circumventing the expenses, hazards, problems, and medical care required for the unaffected female partner [22]. Furthermore, AI-driven algorithms can analyze big data to identify patterns and predict treatment responses. Incorporating AI into clinical decision-making processes could optimize treatment strategies for NOA and enhance patient outcomes [23].

References

1. Sharma M, Leslie SW. Azoospermia. In: StatPearls. Treasure Island: StatPearls; 2024.
2. Esteves SC. Clinical management of infertile men with nonobstructive azoospermia. Asian J Androl. 2015;17(3):459–70.
3. Cocuzza M, Alvarenga C, Pagani R. The epidemiology and etiology of azoospermia. Clinics (Sao Paulo, Brazil). 2013;68(Suppl 1):15–26.
4. Chandra A, Copen CE, Stephen EH. Infertility service use in the United States: data from the national survey of family growth, 1982-2010. Natl Health Stat Rep. 2014;73:1–21.
5. Eisenberg ML, Betts P, Herder D, Lamb DJ, Lipshultz LI. Increased risk of cancer among azoospermic men. Fertil Steril. 2013;100(3):681–5.
6. Petersen PM, Skakkebaek NE, Vistisen K, Rørth M, Giwercman A. Semen quality and reproductive hormones before orchiectomy in men with testicular cancer. J Clin Oncol. 1999;17(3):941–7.
7. Cates W, Farley TM, Rowe PJ. Worldwide patterns of infertility: is Africa different? Lancet. 1985;2(8455):596–8.

8. Cioppi F, Rosta V, Krausz C. Genetics of azoospermia. Int J Mol Sci. 2021;22(6)
9. Schlegel PN. Causes of azoospermia and their management. Reprod Fertil Dev. 2004;16(5):561–72.
10. WHO. WHO laboratory manual for the examination and processing of human semen. In: Organization WH, HRP editors. 6th ed.; 2021.
11. Ron-El R, Strassburger D, Friedler S, Komarovski D, Bern O, Soffer Y, et al. Extended sperm preparation: an alternative to testicular sperm extraction in non-obstructive azoospermia. Hum Reprod. 1997;12(6):1222–6.
12. Corona G, Minhas S, Giwercman A, Bettocchi C, Dinkelman-Smit M, Dohle G, et al. Sperm recovery and ICSI outcomes in men with non-obstructive azoospermia: a systematic review and meta-analysis. Hum Reprod Update. 2019;25(6):733–57.
13. Andrade DL, Viana MC, Esteves SC. Differential diagnosis of azoospermia in men with infertility. J Clin Med. 2021;10(14) https://doi.org/10.3390/jcm10143144.
14. Krausz C, Cioppi F. Genetic factors of non-obstructive azoospermia: consequences on patients' and offspring health. J Clin Med. 2021;10(17)
15. Zhang F, Lu C, Li Z, Xie P, Xia Y, Zhu X, et al. Partial deletions are associated with an increased risk of complete deletion in AZFc: a new insight into the role of partial AZFc deletions in male infertility. J Med Genet. 2007;44(7):437–44.
16. Ghalayini IF, Alazab R, Halalsheh O, Al-Mohtaseb AH, Al-Ghazo MA. Repeated microdissection testicular sperm extraction in patients with non-obstructive azoospermia: outcome and predictive factors. Arab J Urol. 2022;20(3):137–43.
17. Bobjer J, Naumovska M, Giwercman YL, Giwercman A. High prevalence of androgen deficiency and abnormal lipid profile in infertile men with non-obstructive azoospermia. Int J Androl. 2012;35(5):688–94.
18. Patel DP, Brant WO, Myers JB, Zhang C, Presson AP, Johnstone EB, et al. Sperm concentration is poorly associated with hypoandrogenism in infertile men. Urology. 2015;85(5):1062–7.
19. Kanakis GA, Nieschlag E. Klinefelter syndrome: more than hypogonadism. Metabolism. 2018;86:135–44.
20. Balawender K, Orkisz S. The impact of selected modifiable lifestyle factors on male fertility in the modern world. Cent Eur J Urol. 2020;73(4):563–8.
21. Adriansyah RF, Margiana R, Supardi S, Narulita P. Current progress in stem cell therapy for male infertility. Stem Cell Rev Rep. 2023;19(7):2073–93.
22. Tournaye H. Male factor infertility and ART. Asian J Androl. 2012;14(1):103–8.
23. Ghayda RA, Cannarella R, Calogero AE, Shah R, Rambhatla A, Zohdy W, et al. Artificial intelligence in andrology: from semen analysis to image diagnostics. World J Men's Health. 2024;42(1):39–61.

Chapter 2
Endocrine Aberrations of NOA

Fahmi Bahar, Ryan P. Smith, and Fotios Dimitriadis

Introduction

Azoospermia is a laboratory diagnosis where no spermatozoa are found in centrifuged seminal fluid. To establish the diagnosis of azoospermia, at least 2–3 examinations are required [1]. This condition of azoospermia can indeed be quite concerning for couples who wish to have children biologically, leading to feelings of despair and loss of hope for the future [2].

Based on its causes, azoospermia is divided into two types: obstructive azoospermia (OA) and nonobstructive azoospermia (NOA). The prevalence of NOA cases is higher than OA, even though the chances of having children, through ART are much greater in OA cases compared to NOA. In cases of NOA where sperm cannot be obtained through biopsy, the only chance of having children is through sperm donation or adoption. Unfortunately, the option of sperm donation may not be universally applicable due to ethical, and religious reasons [3].

The condition of NOA is closely related to various hormone parameters in the male body. Hormone tests can serve as diagnostic guides and prognostic factors in determining the next steps for patients. Hormones involved in this condition include gonadotropin-releasing hormone (GNRH), FSH, LH, testosterone, estradiol, prolactin, SHB, inhibin B, anti-Mullerian hormone (AMH), and also leptin. The roles

F. Bahar
Faculty of Medicine, Muhammadiyah Palembang University, Palembang, Indonesia

Andrology Section, Siloam Sriwjaya Palembang Hospital, Palembang, Indonesia

R. P. Smith (✉)
Department of Urology, University of Virginia, Charlottesville, VA, USA
e-mail: rps2k@virginia.edu

F. Dimitriadis
Urology Department, Aristotle University Thessaloniki, Thessaloniki, Greece

W. Zohdy et al. (eds.), *Non-Obstructive Azoospermia*,
https://doi.org/10.1007/978-3-031-99431-9_2

of these hormones in NOA cases and their therapeutic management will be discussed in this chapter.

HPG Axis

The essential contributions of the hypothalamic–pituitary–gonadal (HPG) axis to human spermatogenesis cannot be overstated. The pulsatile secretion of gonadotropin-releasing hormone (GnRH) begins at the onset of puberty and exerts its effects on the anterior portion of the pituitary gland to stimulate follicle-stimulating hormone (FSH) and luteinizing hormone (LH). FSH enters the testes and stimulates spermatogenesis via the Sertoli cells' action, and LH conversely stimulates the Leydig cells to produce testosterone.

Endocrine disruption of the HPG axis can result in disrupted spermatogenesis and contribute to the pathogenesis of nonobstructive azoospermia (NOA). The endocrine evaluation of the infertile male is a cornerstone of the fertility assessment, but a primary hormonal cause is found in less than 3% of men. Conversely, 30–70% of infertile men have concurrent endocrine dysfunction with another established diagnostic etiology [4, 5].

Gonadotropin-Releasing Hormone

The hypothalamus produces GnRH in a pulsatile manner. GnRH exists in two isoforms, GnRH1 and GnRH2, with GnRH1 being the predominant isoform. It is a central neuroendocrine regulator of human reproductive function and may be influenced by several neuroendocrine and metabolic factors [5]. It has been reported that the pulsatile secretion of LH and FSH can be dissociated [6] [7]. GnRH has also been identified in human semen, and mature sperm express the GnRH receptor, suggesting that autocrine and paracrine roles may further regular spermatogenesis [8, 5]. GnRH regulation of spermatogenesis manifests in its roles in spermatogonia proliferation, spermatogenesis progression, and germ cell apoptosis [5].

Disruption of GnRH secretion or biosynthesis can result in impaired or absent spermatogenesis. Endocrine profiles of NOA can include eugonadism, hypogonadotropic hypogonadism (HH), and hypergonadotropic hypogonadism. Forty five percent on men with NOA are found to have HH but only in 1–2% of cases of male factor infertility overall [9]. Congenital hypogonadism can be the result of mutations in *KAL1*, *FGFR1,* and *GNRHR*. FSH and LH values of less than 2.5 mIU/mL with concomitant hypogonadism are generally accepted endocrine definitions of hypogonadotropic hypogonadism; however, definitions vary [4, 5, 10].

Kallmann's syndrome is a recognized form of HH due to the failed migration of GnRH neurons from the nasal placode into the brain [4]. In addition to Kallmann's syndrome, congenital or idiopathic HH may also be identified.

Kallmann's syndrome may present with delayed puberty and is inherited as an X-linked autosomal-dominant or -recessive disorder [11]. However, HH predominance is idiopathic, accounting for approximately 70% of patients [12]. Patients with idiopathic HH can present with azoo- or oligospermia as some patients may still have differentiation of gonocytes [13]. Conversely, hypergonadotropic hypogonadism can be seen in the setting of testicular failure of varying etiologies, including late-onset hypogonadism, Klinefelter syndrome, chemotherapy, Y-chromosome microdeletion, toxin exposure, idiopathic, and others [4, 5].

GnRH replacement can be an effective treatment for HH. Pulsatile GnRH administered via a portable pump in two men with HH and azoospermia showed improved spermatogenesis after 42 and 78 days [14, 15]. Separately, the authors demonstrated that GnRH treatment was superior to subcutaneous GnRH treatment and to combination therapy with human menopausal gonadotropin (hMG) and human chorionic gonadotropin (hCG) [15]. Conversely, a study in monkeys showed that GnRH antagonist treatment induced azoospermia after a 9-week continuous infusion, highlighting the critical role of GnRH's influence on spermatogenesis. Cessation of treatment showed normalization of gonadotropins at 2 weeks and normal semen parameters 14–18 weeks post treatment [5, 16].

Gonadotropins

Luteinizing Hormone

Intratesticular testosterone levels are 40–100 times those of serum levels, and high levels are vital to supporting spermatogenesis. Testosterone is produced primarily by the Leydig cells existing in the interstitium of the testes [4]. It is carefully calibrated and influenced by LH, secreted from the anterior pituitary gland. LH binding to its receptor initiates a cyclic adenosine monophosphate-mediated pathway, resulting in testosterone release from the mitochondrial and smooth endoplasmic reticulum membranes [4]. Testosterone and estradiol feedback further regulate LH production [4, 5].

LH levels in normozoospermic men range from 1.8 to 8.6 IU/mL [17]. Several studies have examined the differences between LH levels in OA and NOA. LH levels tend to increase with age in patients with idiopathic NOA [5]. Schoor et al. found that FSH levels and testicular volume were better predictors of OA versus NOA, with 96% of men having an FSH of less than 7.6 mIU/mL or a testicular long axis of greater than 4.6 cm in the setting of OA [18].

Klinefelter syndrome, recognized as a 47 XXY karyotype, will present with increased LH and FSH levels, as well as seminiferous tubule sclerosis [17]. While LH levels are increased, hypogonadism will be present in 50–60% of Klinefelter patients [19]. Isolated LH deficiency has been described as a rare condition leading to enuchoid body habitus, large testes, normal FSH, and small volume ejaculates that may contain low levels of sperm [20, 4]. Testicular replacement therapy will result in the suppression of LH, with recovery prompted by discontinuation of androgen therapy [21, 22].

In the setting of NOA and HH, hCG and hMG can be utilized to support LH and FSH function. hCG is an LH homolog, and doses of 2000 IU subcutaneous or IM three times per week can generally induce appropriate serum improvements in testosterone [23]. Dosing may require titration depending on the underlying etiology. While LH monotherapy has been described as being sufficient to induce spermatogenesis in some forms of hypogonadotropic hypogonadism, FSH is often added at 6 months. This can be accomplished through recombinant FSH or hMG, an FSH analog [24, 25]. Typical dosing is 37.5 IU or 75 IU three times per week. Combination therapy with hCG/FSH is generally more effective than hCG alone in establishing spermatogenesis [26]. Side effects of hCG may include headache, swelling, weight gain, mood changes, and blood clots. rFSH and hMG conversely may result in headache, gynecomastia, hair loss, mood changes, and fatigue. hCG may be used concurrently with testosterone replacement therapy in hopes of preserving spermatogenesis [22].

Follicle-Stimulating Hormone

FSH targets the Sertoli cells in the seminiferous tubules of the testis. *FSH is not strictly required for spermatogenesis in humans but supports Sertoli cell function* [27]. FSH is regulated by inhibin B and activin. Inhibin B, produced by the Sertoli cells, suppresses FSH production, whereas activin stimulates its production. Normal serum FSH levels range from 2 to 7 IU/mL in normospermic men and are frequently elevated in the setting of NOA compared to fertile men [17]. Schoor and Niderberger reported that men with an elevated serum FSH (>7.6 mIU/mL) or a testicular long axis of 4.6 cm or less maybe considered to have NOA [18]. These men are best treated with microdissection testicular sperm extraction for use in in vitro fertilization and intracytoplasmic sperm injection.

FSH levels are often markedly increased in the setting of testicular failure and may be identified in NOA of varying underlying etiologies [4, 5]. Ramasamy et al. reported that FSH groups (<15, 15–30, 31–45, and > 45 mIU/mL) may be predictive of the overall SRR at the time of microTESE. Men with FSH values greater than 15 mIU/mL had higher sperm retrieval rates compared to those with values <15 mIU/mL. FSH patterns may also differ based on histology, including Sertoli cell only, maturation arrest, and hypospermatogenesis [28]. Other authors found that FSH had a moderate value in independently predicting sperm retrieval rates in men with NOA (area under the curve >0.7) [29].

Testosterone replacement therapy will naturally result in the suppression of FSH. Increased serum testosterone levels will lead to direct inhibition of the HPG axis and indirect inhibition through estradiol. Isolated FSH deficiency leads to normal virilization and testosterone levels and may present with oligo- or azoospermia

[30, 31]. While isolated FSH deficiency is rare, it has been described as a result of idiopathic, excess inhibin B, or in the setting of granulosa cell tumors. Patients may also present with an inherent FSH B-subunit deficiency or idiopathic genetic defect [30, 31]. Gonadotoxic therapies or environment toxin exposures may also result in damage to the germinal epithelium reflected in FSH elevation.

Clomiphene citrate and tamoxifen are selective estrogen receptor modulators (SERMs) that are commonly used to treat endocrine dysfunction in male infertility. The selective inhibition of estradiol at the level of the pituitary results in subsequent increases in LH and FSH. Rises in LH hope to improve the intratesticular and serum testosterone levels, creating a more favorable environment for sperm production and treating subsequent hypogonadism. In the setting of NOA, LH and FSH levels may be elevated; however, clomiphene citrate has still been utilized. Hussein et al. demonstrated that treatment with clomiphene citrate in the setting of NOA resulted in 64.3% of men demonstrating sperm in the ejaculate. Sufficient sperm for ICSI were retrieved in all patients despite 35.7% remaining azoospermic [32]. Spermatogenesis response is challenging to predict, and many studies have failed to show similar improvements in spermatogenesis in NOA patients. Sharma et al. found that patient characteristics, pretreatment hormone profile, and degree of impaired spermatogenesis did not predict treatment response. SERMs may result in hypertension, blurry vision, blood clots, low libido, and headache [33, 34]. Clomiphene citrate's safety and efficacy profile, however, is well established, even in men beyond 3 years of treatment [33, 35].

In the setting of NOA with elevated FSH levels and hypogonadism or hypogonadism associated with elevated estradiol (i.e., low testosterone to estradiol ratio, 10:1), aromatase inhibitors (AIs) may be preferred [32, 36, 37, 38]. AIs reduce serum estradiol levels, which results in lower serum levels and limits estrogen feedback at the level of the pituitary. The result is in an increase in the production of FSH and LH. In appropriately selected patients, this will result in improved serum testosterone and spermatogenesis and may improve sperm retrieval rates at the time of microTESE [32, 38]. Patients with NOA and normal baseline total testosterone have been reported to have higher sperm retrieval rates than men with hypogonadism. Men who respond to treatment for hypogonadism may have higher sperm retrieval rates than those who fail to respond [39, 38].

FSH therapy can be accomplished with recombinant FSH or the FSH analog human menopausal gonadotropin. Importantly, the American Urological Association and European Association of Urology guidelines caution that there are no randomized, controlled trials specifically analyzing the benefits of hormone therapy in men with NOA and sperm retrieval rates at the time of microTESE. There are also potential side effects to be considered and a lack of consensus as to the most suitable hormone stimulation regimen. The use of hormone stimulation therapy is still common practice. Guidelines caution that patients with NOA should be informed of the limited data supporting pharmacological manipulation with SERMs, AIs, and gonadotropins prior to surgical intervention. Patients should also be cautioned that this is off-label treatment of hypogonadism ([40, 41]. Patients attempting empiric medical therapy, in the setting of idiopathic infertility and eugonadism, in hopes of improving spermatogenesis should also be advised that the use of SERMs has limited benefits relative to the results of assisted reproductive techniques. FSH analogs can be considered with the aim of improving sperm concentration, pregnancy rate, and live birth rate in men with idiopathic infertility [42, 40, 41].

Testosterone

Testosterone is the primary hormone in the male reproductive system. It is produced by Leydig cells located in the testes under the command of the anterior pituitary gland, which sends LH signals. One of the testosterone receptors is found on Sertoli cells, where testosterone plays a crucial role in spermatogenesis. In cases of azoospermia, total testosterone levels can be used as an indicator to determine whether the cause is obstructive or nonobstructive. Typically, NOA cases exhibit significantly lower testosterone levels compared to infertile men with OA. This is closely related to the larger testis volume in men with OA compared to NOA [43].

In cases of NOA with below-normal testosterone levels, such as in congenital hypogonadotropic hypogonadism (CHH), idiopathic hypogonadotropic hypogonadism (IHH), or Kallmann's syndrome, this condition can still be improved with gonadotropin therapy until spermatozoa can be obtained in the semen. Conversely, in cases of NOA suspected to be due to testicular failure, typically characterized by increased FSH/LH with or without a decrease in testosterone levels, the condition becomes quite complex to manage. Some literature suggests directly proceeding with surgical sperm retrieval using conventional testicular sperm extraction (TESE) or microscopic testicular sperm extraction (microTESE). In contrast, others recommend optimizing hormone levels first, especially increasing testosterone levels because of its close association with success in obtaining spermatozoa during SSR [39].

If the second option is chosen, the possible therapeutic options that may be given include gonadotropin, human chorionic gonadotropin (HCG), human menopausal gonadotropin (HMG), selective estrogen receptor modulators (SERM) such as clomiphene citrate or a combination of these treatments [44, 45, 46, 47, 32, 48, 38, 49, 50].

Estradiol

Unlike the roles of testosterone and gonadotropins in the process of spermatogenesis, which have been extensively studied, the role of estradiol in male infertility has not been widely researched [51]. Estradiol is derived from the aromatization of testosterone, which mainly occurs in adipose tissue by the enzyme aromatase [52]. Additionally, estradiol is synthesized by germ cells in the testes, which is beneficial for the survival of germ cells. Moreover, in mature spermatozoa, this plays a role in capacitation and acrosome reaction [53, 54, 55].

Increased estradiol levels in men can disrupt spermatogenesis processes ranging from oligozoospermia to azoospermia, the latter being classified as NOA. This occurs because estradiol suppresses pituitary levels, thereby reducing testosterone secretion [51]. On the other hand, decreased estradiol levels are also reported to affect germ cell development [56]. The extent to which estradiol levels can lead to azoospermia is still not fully determined. A study by Salam & Blgozah in 2020 involving 166 men with NOAfound that most actually had normal estradiol levels (71.1%), while 10.2% had low estradiol levels, and the remaining 18.7% experienced a significant increase in estradiol levels (mean 60.12 ± 91.34 pg/ml) [51].

There are at least two ways to assess increased estradiol in men, either directly by measuring estradiol levels in the body or indirectly by comparing estradiol and testosterone levels, known as the T/E ratio (an abnormal testosterone/estradiol ratio is typically <10) [57].

Pharmacotherapy for increased estradiol levels in men commonly involves the use of aromatase inhibitors. This option is typically used when testosterone levels are normal, but the T/E ratio is <10. These inhibitors work by blocking the action of the aromatase enzyme, which converts testosterone into estradiol [57]. The most commonly used class of aromatase inhibitors in daily clinical practice are letrozole and anastrozole, both of which are third-generation nonsteroidal aromatase inhibitors [58].

Prolactin

Prolactin is a hormone produced by lactotropic cells in the pituitary gland and plays a crucial role in physiological processes in the human body. For example, in women, prolactin plays a role in milk production during the preparation for breastfeeding [59]. Prolactin receptors are also found in the testes, particularly in Leydig cells, Sertoli cells, and germinal cells. Therefore, spermatogenesis can also be directly influenced by prolactin [60].

In the reproductive system of both females and males, prolactin also plays a significant role, where an increase in this hormone typically decreases fertility in both sexes. In men, high levels of prolactin in the body can lead to hormonal imbalances that can result in disrupted spermatogenesis and may even cause NOA. High levels of prolactin in the body can result in decreased secretion of GnRH from the hypothalamus, which in turn leads to reduced secretion of FSH and LH from the anterior pituitary. These last two hormones are essential for testosterone production and spermatogenesis. Although the occurrence of hyperprolactinemia in male infertility is relatively low (around 1%), it should be taken seriously as it is a condition that can be corrected [61].

Several factors can induce hyperprolactinemia, including pituitary tumors (prolactinoma), the effects of medications such as metoclopramide, risperidone, and phenothiazines, which can increase prolactin levels up to 10 times the normal level [62, 63], or it can also be idiopathic. Besides causing fertility issues, this condition can also lead to sexual dysfunction [64]. In addition to pathological causes, low-level increases in prolactin can also be caused by physiological conditions such as stress or excessive physical exertion [62].

Management and therapy for hyperprolactinemia are customized to its underlying causes. Pharmacotherapy options available for this condition can be found in Table 2.1 [65].

Sex Hormone-Binding Globulin

Once in the circulation, testosterone is bound to proteins, including sex hormone binding globulin (SHBG) and albumin. SHBG is a plasma glycoprotein produced by hepatocytes, and approximately 45–65% of testosterone in the blood is bound to SHBG.

SHBG-bound testosterone decreases the amount of total testosterone available to support spermatogenesis. SHBG increases with age and certain disease states, including liver disease, collagen vascular disease, and chronic illness [5]. This makes serum total testosterone levels less reliable than bioavailable testosterone in some concurrent disease states in the setting of NOA [66, 67]. Estrogen, thyroid hormone, and insulin increase SHBG while SHBG levels fall in the presence of androgens, hypothyroidism, and insulin resistance [5].

Jarecki et al. demonstrated that normal SHBG levels vary between 54.5 and 91.6 nmol/L, with an average of 72.0 nmol/L [68]. Ring et al. found that serum SHBG levels predicted decreased sperm concentration and motility, in a similar manner to FSH [69]. Conversely, Bolufer et al. found no difference in baseline serum SHBG in men with normozoopermia, oligospermia, and azoospermia [70]. In humans, SHBG polymorphisms have been associated with male infertility [71].

Assessment of SHBG may be included in the male fertility evaluation, particularly when comorbid medical conditions may be anticipated to impact SHBG and bioavailable testosterone levels. Clinically, men may present with hypogonadal symptoms of decreased libido, erectile dysfunction, infertility, and low energy, concerning for hypogonadism. Management of hypogonadism may utilize previously described options of SERMs, AIs, or hCG in the setting of fertility preservation [5].

Table 2.1 Pharmacotherapy for hyperprolactinemia

Type	Dose	Side effects
Cabergoline	0.5 mg once weekly, or 0.25 mg twice weekly	Postural hypotension, nausea, constipation, headache, less commonly depression and anxiety
Bromocriptine	1.25 mg–2.5 mg daily	Dizziness, headache, nausea, blurred or double vision,
Quinagolide	0.025 mg–0.075 mg daily	Nausea, headache, loss of appetite

Abnormal SHBG levels may be improved upon by addressing the underlying etiology.

Inhibin B

Inhibins belong to a transforming growth beta superfamily with either a beta A or beta B subunit. Inhibin A is undetectable. Inhibin B is produced by the Sertoli cells in the testis and is involved in spermatogenesis. It is known to suppress FSH production via negative feedback. Conversely, activin stimulates production of inhibin B. Follistatin is also produced by the Sertoli cells and germ cells and regulates germ cell growth and division. It is involved in local inhibition of activin secretion within the testicular parenchyma. A negative correlation between inhibin B and FSH has been demonstrated in infertile patients, with inhibin B decreasing as FSH increases. Inhibin B production depends on FSH, testosterone, and the level of spermatogenesis [4, 5].

Inhibin B levels are lower in men with idiopathic azoospermia compared with severely oligozoospermic patients and normozoospermic men. Pierik et al. found that inhibin B levels negatively correlated with serum FSH levels. The authors found that among NOA patients, patients with Klinefelter syndrome had even lower levels of serum inhibin B [72]. Ballesca et al. reported similar findings in men with NOA and recommended that all azoospermic males have serum inhibin B concentrations determined in addition to FSH prior to undergoing microTESE. Serum inhibin B concentrations were significantly higher among successful microTESE patients [73]. While inhibin B appears to play an important role, Fortesta et al. concluded that it was not specific for discriminating between obstructive and nonobstructive azoospermia. Serum inhibin B was normal in some patients with Sertoli-cell only, of note [74]. Meacham et al. found that inhibin B in combination with FSH is a more sensitive and specific predictor of spermatogenesis compared with inhibin B alone [75].

Inhibin B plays an important role in the regulation of spermatogenesis through its negative feedback mechanism and subsequent control of FSH secretion. NOA patients appear to have reduced levels of inhibin B and elevated levels of FSH with varying inhibin B levels seen depending on the underlying etiology of NOA. The utility of inhibin B as a predictor of successful sperm retrieval during microTESE in the setting of NOA remains to be elucidated [5].

Anti-Mullerian Hormone

Anti-Mullerian hormone (AMH) or Mullerian inhibiting substance (MIS) is a dimeric glycoprotein secreted by the Sertoli cells and is involved in the development of the male genitalia. AMH is a functional marker of Sertoli cells and notably, germ cell number in adults is dependent on the number of Sertoli cells produced in the perinatal period. AMH is structurally similar to inhibin and transforming growth factor beta and high expression perinatally at the critical time period results in regression of the Mũllerian duct [5, 76]. Testosterone downregulates AMH expression and FSH transcriptionally activates AMH production in the absence of androgen signaling [77].

Differentiation of the male genitalia is driven by testosterone and AMH. Disorders of sexual differentiation in males result from aberrations in signaling in one or both of these hormones. For example, mutations in AMH or its receptor AMHRII lead to persistent Mullerian duct syndrome [77]. Patients with persistent Mullerian duct syndrome (PMDS) are 46, XY and retain Mullerian duct derivatives, including a small, underdeveloped uterus [78, 77].

Decreases in AMH have been attributed to impaired Sertoli cell function and the degree of AMH decrease may be related to the severity of infertility, as can be seen in cryptorchidism [79, 80, 81, 77]. Impaired fertility has been found in 30 and 54% of patients with unilateral and bilateral UDT, respectively [82, 83, 84, 85, 77]. A higher degree of serum decline in AMH in boys may suggest a greater risk of adult infertility [76].

AMH, as a marker of Sertoli cell function, can similarly help differentiate between constitutional pubertal delay and congenital HH. A decrease in the number of Sertoli cells corresponds to lower levels of AMH and inhibin B as would be expected in congenital HH [86, 87, 88, 77]. In contrast, delayed puberty would be expected to have normal levels of AMH for the prepubertal state [89, 76].

In patients with NOA increased serum FSH, decreased AMH and inhibin B levels have been described [90, 91, 76]. Patient with NOA may be candidates for microTESE with IVF-ICSI and AMH has been evaluated as a predictor of successful sperm retrieval. As previously noted, there are significant limitations to current predictors of successful microTESE in the setting of NOA. Within the heterogeneity seen in patients with NOA, differences are similarly seen in levels of FSH, inhibin B, AMH, and testosterone. In isolation, these serum markers lack the sensitivity and specificity to guarantee successful sperm retrieval in the setting of NOA [92, 93, 94, 95, 96]. These serum markers, combined with other clinical data, including age, testicular volume, and assessed in a multivariable regression model, may assist with counseling patients regarding sperm retrieval rates [93, 96]. Xu et al. have described that some men with NOA and low or undetectable AMH may undergo successful microTESE with positive pregnancy outcomes [76].

Klinefelter syndrome comprises about 10–12% of NOA patients [97]. In Klinefelter syndrome, AMH levels are within reference ranges until puberty and AMH then declines in adults [98, 99, 100]. Bastida et al. described a phenomenon of an early increase in FSH with low or undetectable AMH and inhibin B in 29 patients with Klinefelter syndrome and in advanced pubertal stages. This may suggest a progressive impairment of fertility and endocrine function during puberty. Xu et al. have described some patients with KS and undetectable serum AMH and testosterone levels who failed to have sperm retrieved at the time of microTESE [77].

While AMH declines in adults with KS, undetectable levels may then portend a poor prognosis in terms of successful sperm retrieval.

In patients with congenital HH, recombinant FSH will result in increased AMH due to proliferation of Sertoli cells. Administration of hCG results in a decline in AMH related to increased testosterone levels that induces inhibition of AMH. The exogenous administration of testosterone replacement therapy does not result in a decline in AMH in patients with congenital HH [76]. The utility of AMH itself, however, may lie in its potential role as a biomarker of infertility. In severe forms of NOA and infertility, undetectable serum AMH levels may portend a poor prognostic indicator for sperm retrieval at the time of microTESE. Its prognostic utility may be higher when combined with other serum markers and clinical data in a multivariable regression model.

Leptin

Leptin is the protein product of the Ob gene and is secreted by adipocytes. Serum levels correlate with adipose tissue mass and is a potent mediator of satiety. It regulates adipose tissue mass, the neuroendocrine system, and it has been suggested that it is involved in signaling the reproductive axis about nutritional status. Hyperleptinemia has been shown to be detrimental to male reproductive function, and it may act at multiple levels of the HPG axis. The molecular mechanisms by which it impacts spermatogenesis remain undefined [101, 102, 5, 103].

It has been proposed that leptin may contribute to the regulation of Leydig and Sertoli cells, and it may play a role in the mechanisms underlying obesity-induced male infertility [104, 5, 105]. Von Sobbe et al. found that semen leptin concentrations were elevated in patients with NOA and were associated with elevated FSH levels. The authors also identified a correlation of semen with serum leptin levels, suggesting that leptin is not actively transported but leaks through the blood–testis barrier [106].

Steinman et al. found that serum leptin concentrations are elevated in about 50% of azoospermic men compared to normozoospermic fertile men. The authors postulated that as the elevation was not gonadotropin dependent, this may indicate a direct effect of leptin on spermatogenesis. They hypothesized that azoospermic men may have a partial leptin insensitivity associated with infertility [102]. Zorn et al. similarly found that serum leptin levels in NOA patients were higher than normozoospermic patients. Among the NOA group, leptin elevations did not differ between Sertoli cell-only syndrome, hypospermatogenesis, or maturation arrest [5, 105].

Investigators have also assessed for differences in seminal leptin levels in fertile and infertile men. Ma et al. sought to improve the prediction accuracy of sperm retrieval in the setting of NOA using leptin and artificial neural networks. The authors found that although the area under the curve for leptin was low, combined use of FSH and leptin improved the prediction accuracy for sperm retrieval in NOA patients, cautioning that further study was needed [107]. Amer et al. recently reported a positive correlation between seminal plasma leptin and microTESE outcomes. The authors evaluated 53 men with NOA and found that seminal plasma leptin levels of 4.05 ng/ml predicted successful sperm retrieval at the time of microTESE with a sensitivity of 73.3% and a specificity of 75%. They suggested that seminal plasma leptin could be used to predict sperm retrieval rates at the time of microTESE in men undergoing the procedure for the first time [108].

The utility of leptin assessment in the serum or semen may lie in its ability to predict sperm retrieval rates in men with NOA. Studies to date indicate that it plays a role in spermatogenesis, with more research needed to identify the molecular mechanisms underlying these associations. Seminal and serum leptin levels may prove to be an adjunct diagnostic marker in NOA.

Special Issues

(a) **Fertility Concerns of Transgender (Transgenders' Azoospermia)**

Transgender is a condition where there is incongruence between gender identity and sex phenotype since birth, with a prevalence of around 0.6% of the population in the United States [109]. Transgender individuals can be divided into two categories: transgender women/transwomen/male to female (MTF) and transgender men/transmen/female to male (FTM). This discussion will focus on the former group. Transgender individuals, specifically transwomen, are at risk of experiencing infertility, such as azoospermia. This risk starts when the individual decides to undergo gender-affirming processes. There are two common gender-affirming processes: medical and surgical. In the medical option (usually involving estrogen hormone), although there is a risk of infertility, there is still a possibility of restoring fertility. Conversely, in the surgical option (orchidectomy), it is irreversible [110].

Gender-affirming hormone therapy (GAHT) for transgender women typically involves estrogen regimens that suppress gonadotropin levels, leading to a decrease in testosterone levels and ultimately causing nonobstructive azoospermia (NOA).

Transgender individuals who are going to undergo gender-affirming hormone therapy (GAHT) should ideally receive counseling beforehand to understand the long-term risks and be provided with options for fertility preservation, such as sperm cryopreservation or embryo cryopreservation (using ova from their partner) [110].

(b) **Oncological-Related Endocrine Aberrations of NOA**.

- **Leydig Cell Tumors**
- Leydig cell tumors (also known as interstitial cell tumors or Leydig cell neoplasms) are a type of tumor that originates from Leydig cells, which are responsible for testosterone synthesis. These cases are rare and can occur at any age, but they are most common in adults aged 30–60 years. They grow

slowly, with the majority being benign, although around 5–10% of them can become malignant [111, 112].

- The signs and symptoms of Leydig cell tumors typically include discomfort in the testis, gynecomastia, infertility, decreased libido, erectile dysfunction, and azoospermia. In prepubertal individuals, patients may present with precock puberty conditions [113].
- The diagnosis is usually made through history taking, physical examination, imaging (ultrasound or MRI), and hormone level tests. Elevated testosterone levels above normal are often found, accompanied by gonadotropin suppression (decreased FSH and LH levels), leading to a condition of nonobstructive azoospermia (NOA). In cases suspected of malignancy, diagnostic tests such as tumor markers AFP, beta HCG, and LDH are necessary. Management depends on the nature of the tumor; if benign, conservative therapy is applied, but if malignant, orchidectomy of the affected testis is necessary, followed by chemotherapy and/or radiotherapy as indicated. Before radical interventions like orchidectomy, patients should be offered the option of sperm banking to preserve their potential for future offspring [114].
- **Seminoma**
- Among other testicular tumors, seminoma is the most common type, accounting for 50% of all testicular tumor cases. Seminoma originates from germ cells. Its exact cause is not fully understood, although genetic factors and environmental exposure are believed to be involved. Additionally, intrauterine estrogen exposure also plays a role [115]. The greatest risk factor is cryptorchidism or undescended testis, which increases the risk of developing seminoma up to four times [116].
- The important thing to note about testicular tumors in relation to NOA is that NOA can occur directly due to the tumor itself and can also result from the treatments given (radical orchidectomy, radiotherapy, chemotherapy).
- **Prolactinoma**
- In the previous subsection, we discussed prolactin and its connection with NOA in general terms. In this subsection, we will specifically discuss prolactinoma, which is a benign tumor of the pituitary gland that produces an excessive amount of prolactin hormone, leading to hyperprolactinemia. Among all types of pituitary tumors, prolactinoma is the most common, with a prevalence of 40–60% [117].
- In men, this condition can lead to a cascade of sexual dysfunction and infertility ranging from oligozoospermia to cryptozoospermia and even azoospermia. Elevated prolactin levels will suppress the secretion of kisspeptin, which in turn weakens GnRH activity, leading to decreased gonadotropin secretion and ultimately resulting in hypogonadism.
- In addition to hypogonadism causing infertility and sexual dysfunction, other signs and symptoms of prolactinoma include gynecomastia, weight gain, galactorrhea, osteopenia/osteoporosis, headaches, and visual disturbances [118].

- The management of prolactinoma is similar to cases of hyperprolactinemia without prolactinoma, involving pharmacotherapy. If therapy with dopamine agonists is deemed inadequate, surgical therapy may be considered as an adjuvant [119].
- **Adrenal Tumors**
- Adrenal tumors are abnormal growths in the adrenal glands, with an average prevalence of 3% and increasing percentages above the age of 50 [120, 121]. In cases like these, two questions need to be answered. First, whether this condition poses a risk of malignancy? Second, whether it causes hormonal imbalance? [122, 123]. If both of these are associated with male infertility, they can be direct or indirect causes. Adrenal tumors that transform from benign to malignant can directly cause NOA. Additionally, the treatment process, which is usually combined with radiotherapy or chemotherapy, can also indirectly contribute to iatrogenic NOA. Although rare, both of these adrenal tumors can lead to hormonal imbalance, specifically an increase in testosterone hormone levels that reduces FSH and LH due to increased negative feedback on the hypothalamus and pituitary gland, thereby decreasing spermatozoa production.

Conclusion

In cases of nonobstructive azoospermia (NOA), hormonal imbalance can serve as the etiology, diagnostic determinant, prognostic factor, therapy success indicator, and predictive factor for the success of surgical sperm retrieval in assisted reproductive technology (ART). Gonadotropin hormones play a primary role because based on these hormones alone (FSH and LH), the cause of azoospermia (obstructive or nonobstructive) can sometimes be established, following history taking, physical examination, and semen analysis. In cases where testosterone levels are normal, but azoospermia is present without other etiologies, it is important to assess estradiol and prolactin hormone levels. An increase in both hormones can potentially lead to nonobstructive azoospermia (NOA) in some cases, and this condition is highly amenable to correction with pharmacotherapy. Because a portion of total testosterone is bound to SHBG, increasing SHBG levels typically lowers testosterone levels and affects spermatogenesis. While most cases of nonobstructive azoospermia (NOA) may require surgical sperm retrieval (SSR), hormone assessment remains necessary to predict SSR success. Moreover, in specific conditions, hormonal therapy is needed to enhance the chances of obtaining spermatozoa during SSR.

References

1. WHO. WHO laboratory manual for the examination and processing of human semen. 6th ed. Geneva: WHO; 2021.
2. Bahar F, Zalika P, Lestari SW, Lunardhi H, I'tishom R, Tanojo TD. Male infertility as a bad news: a review. J Glob Pharm Technol. 2019;11(1s):109–14.
3. Abutari CA, Silalahi AR, Lestari SW, Pramesemara I, Tanojo TD. ART in Indonesia: a current review of ethics. J Glob Pharm Technol. 2019;11(4):408–16.
4. Hotaling JM, Patel Z. Male endocrine dysfunction. Urol Clin North Am. 2014;41(1):39–53. https://doi.org/10.1016/j.ucl.2013.08.010.
5. Tao Y. Endocrine aberrations of human nonobstructive azoospermia. Asian J Androl. 2022;24(3):274–86. https://doi.org/10.4103/aja202181.
6. McCann SM, Kimura M, Walczewska A, Karanth S, Rettori V, Yu WH. Hypothalamic control of gonadotropin secretion by LHRH, FSHRF, NO, cytokines, and leptin. Domest Anim Endocrinol. 1998;15(5):333–44. https://doi.org/10.1016/s0739-7240(98)00029-0.
7. Schneider F, Tomek W, Gründker C. Gonadotropin-releasing hormone (GnRH) and its natural analogues: a review. Theriogenology. 2006;66(4):691–709. https://doi.org/10.1016/j.theriogenology.2006.03.025.
8. Lin J, Mao J, Wang X, Ma W, Hao M, Wu X. Optimal treatment for spermatogenesis in male patients with hypogonadotropic hypogonadism. Medicine (Baltimore). 2019;98(31):e16616. https://doi.org/10.1097/MD.0000000000016616.
9. Sussman EM, Chudnovsky A, Niederberger CS. Hormonal evaluation of the infertile male: has it evolved? Urol Clin North Am. 2008;35(2):147–55., vii. https://doi.org/10.1016/j.ucl.2008.01.010.
10. Trussell JC. Male reproductive endocrinology: when to replace gonadotropins. Semin Reprod Med. 2013;31(4):237–44. https://doi.org/10.1055/s-0033-1345270.
11. Duke VM, Winyard PJ, Thorogood P, Soothill P, Bouloux PM, Woolf AS. KAL, a gene mutated in Kallmann's syndrome, is expressed in the first trimester of human development. Mol Cell Endocrinol. 1995;110(1–2):73–9. https://doi.org/10.1016/0303-7207(95)03518-c.
12. Chiba K, Enatsu N, Fujisawa M. Management of non-obstructive azoospermia. Reprod Med Biol. 2016;15(3):165–73. https://doi.org/10.1007/s12522-016-0234-z.
13. Layman LC, Cohen DP, Xie J, Smith GD. Clinical phenotype and infertility treatment in a male with hypogonadotropic hypogonadism due to mutations Ala129Asp/Arg262Gln of the gonadotropin-releasing hormone receptor. Fertil Steril. 2002;78(6):1317–20. https://doi.org/10.1016/s0015-0282(02)04341-8.
14. Blumenfeld Z, Frisch L, Conn PM. Gonadotropin-releasing hormone (GnRH) antibodies formation in hypogonadotropic azoospermic men treated with pulsatile GnRH–diagnosis and possible alternative treatment. Fertil Steril. 1988a;50(4):622–9. https://doi.org/10.1016/s0015-0282(16)60195-4.
15. Blumenfeld Z, Makler A, Frisch L, Brandes JM. Induction of spermatogenesis and fertility in hypogonadotropic azoospermic men by intravenous pulsatile gonadotropin-releasing hormone (GnRH). Gynecol Endocrinol. 1988b;2(2):151–64. https://doi.org/10.3109/09513598809023623.
16. Weinbauer GF, Surmann FJ, Akhtar FB, Shah GV, Vickery BH, Nieschlag E. Reversible inhibition of testicular function by a gonadotropin hormone-releasing hormone antagonist in monkeys (Macaca fascicularis). Fertil Steril. 1984;42(6):906–14. https://doi.org/10.1016/s0015-0282(16)48264-6.
17. Morley JE, Kaiser FE, Perry HM, Patrick P, Morley PM, Stauber PM, Vellas B, Baumgartner RN, Garry PJ. Longitudinal changes in testosterone, luteinizing hormone, and follicle-stimulating hormone in healthy older men. Metabolism. 1997;46(4):410–3. https://doi.org/10.1016/s0026-0495(97)90057-3.
18. Schoor RA, Elhanbly S, Niederberger CS, Ross LS. The role of testicular biopsy in the modern management of male infertility. J Urol. 2002;167(1):197–200.

19. Okada H, Fujioka H, Tatsumi N, Kanzaki M, Okuda Y, Fujisawa M, Hazama M, Matsumoto O, Gohji K, Arakawa S, Kamidono S. Klinefelter's syndrome in the male infertility clinic. Hum Reprod. 1999;14(4):946–52. https://doi.org/10.1093/humrep/14.4.946.
20. Faiman C, Hoffman DL, Ryan RJ, Albert A. The "fertile eunuch" syndrome: demonstration of isolated luteinizing hormone deficiency by radioimmunoassay technique. Mayo Clin Proc. 1968;43(9):661–7.
21. Ledesma BR, Weber A, Venigalla G, Muthigi A, Thomas J, Narasimman M, White J, Ramasamy R. Fertility outcomes in men with prior history of anabolic steroid use. Fertil Steril. 2023;120(6):1203–9. https://doi.org/10.1016/j.fertnstert.2023.09.016.
22. Wenker EP, Dupree JM, Langille GM, Kovac J, Ramasamy R, Lamb D, Mills JN, Lipshultz LI. The use of HCG-based combination therapy for recovery of spermatogenesis after testosterone use. J Sex Med. 2015;12(6):1334–7. https://doi.org/10.1111/jsm.12890.
23. Vicari E, Mongioì A, Calogero AE, Moncada ML, Sidoti G, Polosa P, D'Agata R. Therapy with human chorionic gonadotrophin alone induces spermatogenesis in men with isolated hypogonadotrophic hypogonadism–long-term follow-up. Int J Androl. 1992;15(4):320–9. https://doi.org/10.1111/j.1365-2605.1992.tb01131.x.
24. Burgués S, Calderón MD. Subcutaneous self-administration of highly purified follicle stimulating hormone and human chorionic gonadotrophin for the treatment of male hypogonadotrophic hypogonadism. Spanish collaborative group on male hypogonadotropic hypogonadism. Hum Reprod. 1997;12(5):980–6. https://doi.org/10.1093/humrep/12.5.980.
25. Kliesch S, Behre HM, Nieschlag E. High efficacy of gonadotropin or pulsatile gonadotropin-releasing hormone treatment in hypogonadotropic hypogonadal men. Eur J Endocrinol. 1994;131(4):347–54. https://doi.org/10.1530/eje.0.1310347.
26. Yang L, Zhang SX, Dong Q, Xiong ZB, Li X. Application of hormonal treatment in hypogonadotropic hypogonadism: more than ten years experience. Int Urol Nephrol. 2012;44(2):393–9. https://doi.org/10.1007/s11255-011-0065-0.
27. Levallet J, Pakarinen P, Huhtaniemi IT. Follicle-stimulating hormone ligand and receptor mutations, and gonadal dysfunction. Arch Med Res. 1999;30(6):486–94. https://doi.org/10.1016/s0188-0128(99)00058-5.
28. Ramasamy R, Lin K, Gosden LV, Rosenwaks Z, Palermo GD, Schlegel PN. High serum FSH levels in men with nonobstructive azoospermia does not affect success of microdissection testicular sperm extraction. Fertil Steril. 2009;92(2):590–3. https://doi.org/10.1016/j.fertnstert.2008.07.1703.
29. Yang Q, Huang Y-P, Wang H-X, Hu K, Wang Y-X, Huang Y-R, Chen B. Follicle-stimulating hormone as a predictor for sperm retrieval rate in patients with nonobstructive azoospermia: a systematic review and meta-analysis. Asian J Androl. 2015;17(2):281–4. https://doi.org/10.4103/1008-682X.139259.
30. Alexiev BA, Alaish SM, Sun C-C. Testicular juvenile granulosa cell tumor in a newborn: case report and review of the literature. Int J Surg Pathol. 2007;15(3):321–5. https://doi.org/10.1177/1066896907302423.
31. Lofrano-Porto A, Casulari LA, Nascimento PP, Giacomini L, Naves LA, da Motta LDC, Layman LC. Effects of follicle-stimulating hormone and human chorionic gonadotropin on gonadal steroidogenesis in two siblings with a follicle-stimulating hormone beta subunit mutation. Fertil Steril. 2008;90(4):1169–74. https://doi.org/10.1016/j.fertnstert.2007.07.1356.
32. Hussein A, Ozgok Y, Ross L, Rao P, Niederberger C. Optimization of spermatogenesis-regulating hormones in patients with non-obstructive azoospermia and its impact on sperm retrieval: a multicentre study. BJU Int. 2013;111(3 Pt B):E110-114. https://doi.org/10.1111/j.1464-410X.2012.11485.x.
33. Krzastek SC, Sharma D, Abdullah N, Sultan M, Machen GL, Wenzel JL, Ells A, Chen X, Kavoussi M, Costabile RA, Smith RP, Kavoussi PK. Long-term safety and efficacy of clomiphene citrate for the treatment of hypogonadism. J Urol. 2019;202(5):1029–35. https://doi.org/10.1097/JU.0000000000000396.

34. Sharma D, Zillioux J, Khourdaji I, Reines K, Wheeler K, Costabile R, Kavoussi P, Smith R. Improvements in semen parameters in men treated with clomiphene citrate-a retrospective analysis. Andrologia. 2019;51(5):e13257. https://doi.org/10.1111/and.13257.
35. Wheeler KM, Smith RP, Kumar RA, Setia S, Costabile RA, Kavoussi PK. A comparison of secondary polycythemia in hypogonadal men treated with clomiphene citrate versus testosterone replacement: a multi-institutional study. J Urol. 2017;197(4):1127–31. https://doi.org/10.1016/j.juro.2016.10.068.
36. Pavlovich CP, King P, Goldstein M, Schlegel PN. Evidence of a treatable endocrinopathy in infertile men. J Urol. 2001;165(3):837–41.
37. Raman JD, Schlegel PN. Aromatase inhibitors for male infertility. J Urol. 2002;167(2 Pt 1):624–9. https://doi.org/10.1016/S0022-5347(01)69099-2.
38. Reifsnyder JE, Ramasamy R, Husseini J, Schlegel PN. Role of optimizing testosterone before microdissection testicular sperm extraction in men with nonobstructive azoospermia. J Urol. 2012;188(2):532–6. https://doi.org/10.1016/j.juro.2012.04.002.
39. Caroppo E, Colpi GM. Hormonal treatment of men with nonobstructive azoospermia: what does the evidence suggest? J Clin Med. 2021;10(3):387. https://doi.org/10.3390/jcm10030387.
40. Schlegel PN, Sigman M, Collura B, De Jonge CJ, Eisenberg ML, Lamb DJ, Mulhall JP, Niederberger C, Sandlow JI, Sokol RZ, Spandorfer SD, Tanrikut C, Treadwell JR, Oristaglio JT, Zini A. Diagnosis and treatment of infertility in men: AUA/ASRM guideline part I. J Urol. 2021a;205(1):36–43. https://doi.org/10.1097/JU.0000000000001521.
41. Schlegel PN, Sigman M, Collura B, De Jonge CJ, Eisenberg ML, Lamb DJ, Mulhall JP, Niederberger C, Sandlow JI, Sokol RZ, Spandorfer SD, Tanrikut C, Treadwell JR, Oristaglio JT, Zini A. Diagnosis and treatment of infertility in men: AUA/ASRM guideline part II. J Urol. 2021b;205(1):44–51. https://doi.org/10.1097/JU.0000000000001520.
42. Minhas S, Bettocchi C, Boeri L, Capogrosso P, Carvalho J, Cilesiz NC, Cocci A, Corona G, Dimitropoulos K, Gül M, Hatzichristodoulou G, Jones TH, Kadioglu A, Martínez Salamanca JI, Milenkovic U, Modgil V, Russo GI, Serefoglu EC, Tharakan T, Verze P, Salonia A, EAU Working Group on Male Sexual and Reproductive Health. European Association of urology guidelines on male sexual and reproductive health: 2021 update on male infertility. Eur Urol. 2021;80(5):603–20. https://doi.org/10.1016/j.eururo.2021.08.014.
43. Huang I-S, Huang WJ, Lin AT. Distinguishing non-obstructive azoospermia from obstructive azoospermia in Taiwanese patients by hormone profile and testis size. J Chin Med Assoc. 2018;81(6):531–5.
44. Amer MK, Ahmed AR, Abdel Hamid AA, GamalEl Din SF. Can spermatozoa be retrieved in non-obstructive azoospermic patients with high FSH level?: A retrospective cohort study. Andrologia. 2019;51(2):e13176.
45. Amer MK, Ahmed HEH, GamalEl Din SF, Fawzy Megawer A, Ahmed AR. Evaluation of neoadjuvant gonadotropin administration with downregulation by testosterone prior to second time microsurgical testicular sperm extraction: a prospective case–control study. Urol J. 2020;87(4):185–90.
46. Aydos K, Ünlü C, Demirel LC, Evirgen O, Tolunay Ö. The effect of pure FSH administration in non-obstructive azoospermic men on testicular sperm retrieval. Eur J Obstet Gynecol Reprod Biol. 2003;108(1):54–8.
47. Hussein A, Ozgok Y, Ross L, Niederberger C. Clomiphene administration for cases of nonobstructive azoospermia: a multicenter study. J Androl. 2005;26(6):787–91.
48. Kato Y, Shiraishi K, Matsuyama H. Expression of testicular androgen receptor in non-obstructive azoospermia and its change after hormonal therapy. Andrology. 2014;2(5):734–40.
49. Shinjo E, Shiraishi K, Matsuyama H. The effect of human chorionic gonadotropin-based hormonal therapy on intratesticular testosterone levels and spermatogonial DNA synthesis in men with non-obstructive azoospermia. Andrology. 2013;1(6):929–35.

50. Shiraishi K, Ohmi C, Shimabukuro T, Matsuyama H. Human chorionic gonadotrophin treatment prior to microdissection testicular sperm extraction in non-obstructive azoospermia. Hum Reprod. 2012;27(2):331–9.
51. Salama N, Blgozah S. Serum estradiol levels in infertile men with non-obstructive azoospermia. Ther Adv Reprod Health. 2020;14:2633494120928342.
52. Phillips KP, Tanphaichitr N. Mechanisms of obesity-induced male infertility. Expert Rev Endocrinol Metab. 2010;5(2):229–51.
53. Carreau S, Bouraima-Lelong H, Delalande C. Role of estrogens in spermatogenesis. Front Biosci Elite. 2012;4(1):1–11.
54. Correia S, Alves MR, Cavaco JE, Oliveira PF, Socorro S. Estrogenic regulation of testicular expression of stem cell factor and c-kit: implications in germ cell survival and male fertility. Fertil Steril. 2014;102(1):299–306.
55. Zanatta AP, Brouard V, Gautier C, Goncalves R, Bouraïma-Lelong H, Mena Barreto Silva FR, Delalande C. Interactions between oestrogen and 1α, 25 (OH) 2-vitamin D 3 signalling and their roles in spermatogenesis and spermatozoa functions. Basic Clin Androl. 2017;27:1–14.
56. Arao Y, Hamilton KJ, Goulding EH, Janardhan KS, Eddy EM, Korach KS. Transactivating function (AF) 2–mediated AF-1 activity of estrogen receptor α is crucial to maintain male reproductive tract function. Proc Natl Acad Sci. 2012;109(51):21140–5.
57. Schlegel PN. Aromatase inhibitors for male infertility. Fertil Steril. 2012;98(6):1359–62.
58. Stephens SM, Polotsky AJ. Big enough for an aromatase inhibitor? How adiposity affects male fertility. Thieme Medical Publishers; 2013. p. 251–7.
59. Freeman MEKB, Lerant A. Prolactin: structure, function, and regulation of secretion. Physiol Rev. 2000;80:1523–631. https://doi.org/10.1152/physrev.2000.80.4.1523.
60. Raut S, Deshpande S, Balasinor NH. Unveiling the role of prolactin and its receptor in male reproduction. Horm Metab Res. 2019;51(04):215–9.
61. Biller B, Luciano A, Crosignani P, Molitch M, Olive D, Rebar R, Sanfilippo J, Webster J, Zacur H. Guidelines for the diagnosis and treatment of hyperprolactinemia. J Reprod Med. 1999;44(12 Suppl):1075–84.
62. Majumdar A, Mangal NS. Hyperprolactinemia. In: Principles and practice of controlled ovarian stimulation in ART; 2015. p. 319–28.
63. Torre DL, Falorni A. Pharmacological causes of hyperprolactinemia. Ther Clin Risk Manag. 2007;3(5):929–51.
64. Buvat J. Hyperprolactinemia and sexual function in men: a short review. Int J Impot Res. 2003;15:373. https://doi.org/10.1038/sj.ijir.3901043.
65. Dabbous Z, Atkin SL. Hyperprolactinaemia in male infertility: clinical case scenarios. Arab J Urol. 2018;16(1):44–52. https://doi.org/10.1016/j.aju.2017.10.002.
66. Ashok S, Sigman M. Bioavailable testosterone should be used for the determination of androgen levels in infertile men. J Urol. 2007;177(4):1443–6.; quiz 1591. https://doi.org/10.1016/j.juro.2006.11.088.
67. Selby C. Sex hormone binding globulin: origin, function and clinical significance. Ann Clin Biochem. 1990;27(Pt 6):532–41. https://doi.org/10.1177/000456329002700603.
68. Jarecki P, Herman WA, Pawliczak E, Lacka K. Can low SHBG serum concentration be a good early marker of male hypogonadism in metabolic syndrome? Diab Metab Syndr Obes. 2019;12:2181–91. https://doi.org/10.2147/DMSO.S218545.
69. Ring J, Welliver C, Parenteau M, Markwell S, Brannigan RE, Köhler TS. The utility of sex hormone-binding globulin in hypogonadism and infertile males. J Urol. 2017;197(5):1326–31. https://doi.org/10.1016/j.juro.2017.01.018.
70. Bolufer P, Rodriguez A, Antonio P, Bosch E, Peiró T. Basal prolactin and the behaviour of the gonadotrophins, testosterone, androstenedione, estradiol, and the sex-hormone-binding globulin during stimulation with clomiphene in subjects with spermatogenic disorders. Exp Clin Endocrinol. 1985;86(2):197–206. https://doi.org/10.1055/s-0029-1210487.
71. Cui Y-R, Guo Y-H, Qiao S-D, Leng L-F, Xie Z-H, Chen H, Wang X-L. Correlation between SHBG gene polymorphism and male infertility in Han population of Henan province of

China: a STROBE-compliant article. Medicine (Baltimore). 2017;96(32):e7753. https://doi.org/10.1097/MD.0000000000007753.

72. Pierik FH, Vreeburg JT, Stijnen T, De Jong FH, Weber RF. Serum inhibin B as a marker of spermatogenesis. J Clin Endocrinol Metab. 1998;83(9):3110–4. https://doi.org/10.1210/jcem.83.9.5121.
73. Ballescá JL, Balasch J, Calafell JM, Alvarez R, Fábregues F, de Osaba MJ, Ascaso C, Vanrell JA. Serum inhibin B determination is predictive of successful testicular sperm extraction in men with non-obstructive azoospermia. Hum Reprod. 2000;15(8):1734–8. https://doi.org/10.1093/humrep/15.8.1734.
74. Foresta C, Bettella A, Petraglia F, Pistorello M, Luisi S, Rossato M. Inhibin B levels in azospermic subjects with cytologically characterized testicular pathology. Clin Endocrinol. 1999;50(6):695–701. https://doi.org/10.1046/j.1365-2265.1999.00659.x.
75. Meachem SJ, Nieschlag E, Simoni M. Inhibin B in male reproduction: pathophysiology and clinical relevance. Eur J Endocrinol. 2001;145(5):561–71. https://doi.org/10.1530/eje.0.1450561.
76. Xu H-Y, Zhang H-X, Xiao Z, Qiao J, Li R. Regulation of anti-Müllerian hormone (AMH) in males and the associations of serum AMH with the disorders of male fertility. Asian J Androl. 2019a;21(2):109–14. https://doi.org/10.4103/aja.aja_83_18.
77. Xu H-Y, Zhang H-X, Xiao Z, Qiao J, Li R. Regulation of anti-Müllerian hormone (AMH) in males and the associations of serum AMH with the disorders of male fertility. Asian J Androl. 2019b;21(2):109–14. https://doi.org/10.4103/aja.aja_83_18.
78. Smith-Harrison LI, Patel MS, Smith RP, Schenkman NS. Persistent Müllerian duct structures presenting as hematuria in an adult: case report of robotic surgical removal and review of the literature. Urol Ann. 2015;7(4):544–6. https://doi.org/10.4103/0974-7796.164859.
79. Demircan M, Akinci A, Mutus M. The effects of orchiopexy on serum anti-Müllerian hormone levels in unilateral cryptorchid infants. Pediatr Surg Int. 2006;22(3):271–3. https://doi.org/10.1007/s00383-006-1646-3.
80. Guibourdenche J, Lucidarme N, Chevenne D, Rigal O, Nicolas M, Luton D, Léger J, Porquet D, Noël M. Anti-Müllerian hormone levels in serum from human foetuses and children: pattern and clinical interest. Mol Cell Endocrinol. 2003;211(1–2):55–63. https://doi.org/10.1016/j.mce.2003.09.011.
81. Matuszczak E, Hermanowicz A, Komarowska M, Debek W. Serum AMH in physiology and pathology of male gonads. Int J Endocrinol. 2013;2013:128907. https://doi.org/10.1155/2013/128907.
82. Cortes D. Cryptorchidism–aspects of pathogenesis, histology and treatment. Scand J Urol Nephrol Suppl. 1998;196:1–54.
83. Engeler DS, Hösli PO, John H, Bannwart F, Sulser T, Amin MB, Heitz PU, Hailemariam S. Early orchiopexy: prepubertal intratubular germ cell neoplasia and fertility outcome. Urology. 2000;56(1):144–8. https://doi.org/10.1016/s0090-4295(00)00560-4.
84. Lee PA, Coughlin MT. Fertility after bilateral cryptorchidism. Evaluation by paternity, hormone, and semen data. Horm Res. 2001;55(1):28–32. https://doi.org/10.1159/000049960.
85. Lee PA, O'Leary LA, Songer NJ, Coughlin MT, Bellinger MF, LaPorte RE. Paternity after unilateral cryptorchidism: a controlled study. Pediatrics. 1996;98(4 Pt 1):676–9.
86. Coutant R, Biette-Demeneix E, Bouvattier C, Bouhours-Nouet N, Gatelais F, Dufresne S, Rouleau S, Lahlou N. Baseline inhibin B and anti-Mullerian hormone measurements for diagnosis of hypogonadotropic hypogonadism (HH) in boys with delayed puberty. J Clin Endocrinol Metab. 2010;95(12):5225–32. https://doi.org/10.1210/jc.2010-1535.
87. Hero M, Tommiska J, Vaaralahti K, Laitinen E-M, Sipilä I, Puhakka L, Dunkel L, Raivio T. Circulating antimüllerian hormone levels in boys decline during early puberty and correlate with inhibin B. Fertil Steril. 2012;97(5):1242–7. https://doi.org/10.1016/j.fertnstert.2012.02.020.
88. Rey RA, Grinspon RP, Gottlieb S, Pasqualini T, Knoblovits P, Aszpis S, Pacenza N, Stewart Usher J, Bergadá I, Campo SM. Male hypogonadism: an extended classification based on a

developmental, endocrine physiology-based approach. Andrology. 2013;1(1):3–16. https://doi.org/10.1111/j.2047-2927.2012.00008.x.
89. Adan L, Lechevalier P, Couto-Silva A-C, Boissan M, Trivin C, Brailly-Tabard S, Brauner R. Plasma inhibin B and antimüllerian hormone concentrations in boys: discriminating between congenital hypogonadotropic hypogonadism and constitutional pubertal delay. Med Sci Monit. 2010;16(11):CR511-517.
90. Esteves SC, Miyaoka R, Agarwal A. An update on the clinical assessment of the infertile male [corrected]. Clinics (Sao Paulo). 2011;66(4):691–700. https://doi.org/10.1590/s1807-59322011000400026.
91. Madani AH, Falahatkar S, Heidarzadeh A, Roshan ZA, Sazgari E, Zareian M. Sensitivity and specificity of serum FSH and testis size in predicting the existence of spermatogenesis in azoospermic infertile men. Andrologia. 2012;44(3):205–9. https://doi.org/10.1111/j.1439-0272.2010.01130.x.
92. Althakafi SA, Mustafa OM, Seyam RM, Al-Hathal N, Kattan S. Serum testosterone levels and other determinants of sperm retrieval in microdissection testicular sperm extraction. Transl Androl Urol. 2017;6(2):282–7. https://doi.org/10.21037/tau.2017.02.04.
93. Cissen M, Meijerink AM, D'Hauwers KW, Meissner A, van der Weide N, Mochtar MH, de Melker AA, Ramos L, Repping S, Braat DDM, Fleischer K, van Wely M. Prediction model for obtaining spermatozoa with testicular sperm extraction in men with non-obstructive azoospermia. Hum Reprod. 2016;31(9):1934–41. https://doi.org/10.1093/humrep/dew147.
94. Isikoglu M, Ozgur K, Oehninger S, Ozdem S, Seleker M. Serum anti-Müllerian hormone levels do not predict the efficiency of testicular sperm retrieval in men with non-obstructive azoospermia. Gynecol Endocrinol. 2006;22(5):256–60. https://doi.org/10.1080/09513590600624366.
95. Li H, Chen L-P, Yang J, Li M-C, Chen R-B, Lan R-Z, Wang S-G, Liu J-H, Wang T. Predictive value of FSH, testicular volume, and histopathological findings for the sperm retrieval rate of microdissection TESE in nonobstructive azoospermia: a meta-analysis. Asian J Androl. 2018;20(1):30–6. https://doi.org/10.4103/aja.aja_5_17.
96. Ramasamy R, Padilla WO, Osterberg EC, Srivastava A, Reifsnyder JE, Niederberger C, Schlegel PN. A comparison of models for predicting sperm retrieval before microdissection testicular sperm extraction in men with nonobstructive azoospermia. J Urol. 2013;189(2):638–42. https://doi.org/10.1016/j.juro.2012.09.038.
97. Forti G, Corona G, Vignozzi L, Krausz C, Maggi M. Klinefelter's syndrome: a clinical and therapeutical update. Sex Dev. 2010;4(4–5):249–58. https://doi.org/10.1159/000316604.
98. Aksglaede L, Juul A. Testicular function and fertility in men with Klinefelter syndrome: a review. Eur J Endocrinol. 2013;168(4):R67–76. https://doi.org/10.1530/EJE-12-0934.
99. Aksglaede L, Christiansen P, Sørensen K, Boas M, Linneberg A, Main KM, Andersson A-M, Skakkebaek NE, Juul A. Serum concentrations of anti-Müllerian hormone (AMH) in 95 patients with Klinefelter syndrome with or without cryptorchidism. Acta Paediatr. 2011;100(6):839–45. https://doi.org/10.1111/j.1651-2227.2011.02148.x.
100. Bastida MG, Rey RA, Bergadá I, Bedecarrás P, Andreone L, del Rey G, Boywitt A, Ropelato MG, Cassinelli H, Arcari A, Campo S, Gottlieb S. Establishment of testicular endocrine function impairment during childhood and puberty in boys with Klinefelter syndrome. Clin Endocrinol. 2007;67(6):863–70. https://doi.org/10.1111/j.1365-2265.2007.02977.x.
101. Khodamoradi K, Parmar M, Khosravizadeh Z, Kuchakulla M, Manoharan M, Arora H. The role of leptin and obesity on male infertility. Curr Opin Urol. 2020;30(3):334–9. https://doi.org/10.1097/MOU.0000000000000762.
102. Steinman N, Gamzu R, Yogev L, Botchan A, Schreiber L, Yavetz H. Serum leptin concentrations are higher in azoospermic than in normozoospermic men. Fertil Steril. 2001;75(4):821–2. https://doi.org/10.1016/s0015-0282(01)01707-1.
103. Zhang J, Gong M. Review of the role of leptin in the regulation of male reproductive function. Andrologia. 2018; https://doi.org/10.1111/and.12965.
104. Martins AD, Moreira AC, Sá R, Monteiro MP, Sousa M, Carvalho RA, Silva BM, Oliveira PF, Alves MG. Leptin modulates human Sertoli cells acetate production and glycolytic

profile: a novel mechanism of obesity-induced male infertility? Biochim Biophys Acta. 2015;1852(9):1824–32. https://doi.org/10.1016/j.bbadis.2015.06.005.
105. Zorn B, Osredkar J, Meden-Vrtovec H, Majdic G. Leptin levels in infertile male patients are correlated with inhibin B, testosterone and SHBG but not with sperm characteristics. Int J Androl. 2007;30(5):439–44. https://doi.org/10.1111/j.1365-2605.2006.00728.x.
106. von Sobbe H-U, Koebnick C, Jenne L, Kiesewetter F. Leptin concentrations in semen are correlated with serum leptin and elevated in hypergonadotrophic hypogonadism. Andrologia. 2003;35(4):233–7. https://doi.org/10.1046/j.1439-0272.2003.00565.x.
107. Ma Y, Chen B, Wang H, Hu K, Huang Y. Prediction of sperm retrieval in men with non-obstructive azoospermia using artificial neural networks: leptin is a good assistant diagnostic marker. Hum Reprod. 2011;26(2):294–8. https://doi.org/10.1093/humrep/deq337.
108. Amer MK, Zohdy W, GamalEl Din SF, Moawad HH, Hasan El Saedy DA, Zaki Gamal EA, Ragab A. Evaluation of the utility of seminal plasma resistin and leptin in predicting successful surgical sperm retrieval in men with non-obstructive azoospermia. J Reprod Infertil. 2023;24(2):108–16. https://doi.org/10.18502/jri.v24i2.12496.
109. Flores AR, Herman J, Gates GJ, Brown TN. How many adults identify as transgender in the United States? Los Angeles: Williams Institute; 2016.
110. Cheng PJ, Pastuszak AW, Myers JB, Goodwin IA, Hotaling JM. Fertility concerns of the transgender patient. Transl Androl Urol. 2019;8(3):209.
111. Jou P, MacLennan GT. Leydig cell tumor of the testis. J Urol. 2009;181(5):2299–300.
112. Mooney KL, Kao C-S. A contemporary review of common adult non–germ cell tumors of the testis and paratestis. Surg Pathol Clin. 2018;11(4):739–58.
113. Hibi H, Yamashita K, Sumitomo M, Asada Y. Leydig cell tumor of the testis, presenting with azoospermia. Reprod Med Biol. 2017;16(4):392–5.
114. Pomajzl A, Siref LE. Leydig cell cancer. 2019
115. Khan O, Protheroe A. Testis cancer. Postgrad Med J. 2007;83(984):624–32.
116. Garner MJ, Turner MC, Ghadirian P, Krewski D. Epidemiology of testicular cancer: an overview. Int J Cancer. 2005;116(3):331–9.
117. Vroonen L, Daly AF, Beckers A. Epidemiology and management challenges in prolactinomas. Neuroendocrinology. 2019;109(1):20–7.
118. Melmed S, Casanueva FF, Hoffman AR, Kleinberg DL, Montori VM, Schlechte JA, Wass JA. Diagnosis and treatment of hyperprolactinemia: an Endocrine Society clinical practice guideline. J Clin Endocrinol Metabol. 2011;96(2):273–88.
119. Wildemberg LE, Fialho C, Gadelha MR. Prolactinomas. Presse Med. 2021;50(4):104080.
120. Russell RP, Masi AT, Richter ED. Adrenal cortical adenomas and hypertension: a clinical pathologic analysis of 690 cases with matched contbols and a review of the literature. Medicine. 1972;51(3):211–25.
121. Weinsaft P. Solitary adrenal cortical adenoma in elderly female; frequency. Arch Pathol. 1964;78:231–3.
122. Ebbehoj A, Li D, Kaur RJ, Zhang C, Singh S, Li T, Atkinson E, Achenbach S, Khosla S, Arlt W. Epidemiology of adrenal tumors-a population-based study in olmsted county. Minn Lancet Diab Endocrinol. 2020;8(11):894.
123. Fassnacht M, Arlt W, Bancos I, Dralle H, Newell-Price J, Sahdev A, Tabarin A, Terzolo M, Tsagarakis S, Dekkers OM. Management of adrenal incidentalomas: European society of endocrinology clinical practice guideline in collaboration with the European network for the study of adrenal tumors. Eur J Endocrinol. 2016;175(2):G1–G34.

Chapter 3
Genetic Spectrum of NOA

Tan V. Le, Asli Metin Mahmutoglu, and Mohamed Arafa

Introduction

Azoospermia is characterized by a total absence of sperm in a man's ejaculate, even after centrifugation. It affects approximately 1% of the male population and roughly 10–15% of infertile men [1]. The majority of azoospermia cases, about two-thirds, are due to significant disruptions in sperm production and are classified as "nonobstructive azoospermia" (NOA). This classification serves to distinguish it from "obstructive azoospermia" (OA), which is caused by blockages in the seminal pathway and accounts for the remaining third of azoospermia cases [1].

A range of secondary conditions, including inflammation of the testes, treatments involving cytotoxic drugs, blockages in the ejaculatory ducts, central nervous system tumors, and various systemic illnesses, can result in azoospermia, representing 35–40% of instances [2]. For hereditary causes, genetic influences are implicated across all aforementioned etiological groups, with certain genetic tests becoming a standard part of the infertility evaluation in men [3]. Genetic assessments are important not only for diagnosis but also for guiding clinical decisions

T. V. Le (✉)
Department of Andrology, Binh Dan Hospital, Ho Chi Minh City, Vietnam

Department of Andrology and Nephro-Urology, Pham Ngoc Thach University of Medicine, Ho Chi Minh City, Vietnam

A. M. Mahmutoglu
Faculty of Medicine, Department of Medical Biology, Yozgat Bozok University, Yozgat, Turkey

M. Arafa
Andrology Department, Cairo University, Cairo, Egypt

Urology Department, Hamad Medical Corporation, Doha, Qatar

Urology Department, Weill Cornell Medicine-Qatar, Doha, Qatar

W. Zohdy et al. (eds.), *Non-Obstructive Azoospermia*,
https://doi.org/10.1007/978-3-031-99431-9_3

and offering precise genetic advice [4]. Chromosomal anomalies and deletions in the azoospermia factor (AZF) regions are commonly investigated in those with azoospermia attributed to primary testicular insufficiency.

NOA manifests as a symptom of various forms of testicular dysfunction, including Sertoli-cell-only syndrome (SCOS), maturation arrest (MA) at numerous stages of germ cell development: spermatogonial and spermatocyte arrest (SGA, SCA), hypospermatogenesis, and mixed types [5]. The clinical presentation of NOA can be quite diverse, as evidenced by the variable histological findings, levels of hormones such as follicle-stimulating hormone (FSH) and luteinizing hormone (LH), testicular volume, and the degree of masculinization in affected individuals [5]. This variation suggests a multitude of both acquired and inherited genetic contributors to the condition. Genetic causes identified thus far—accounting for nearly 30% of NOA instances—primarily involve chromosomal disorders like Klinefelter syndrome (47, XXY), Y-chromosome microdeletions, and single-gene mutations. The increasing scrutiny on NOA stems not only from it representing one of the most challenging male infertility diagnoses but also from epidemiological data indicating a correlation between azoospermia and increased morbidity as well as a reduced lifespan. Considering that roughly half of the men with NOA have a favorable outcome following testicular sperm extraction (TESE), routine genetic testing gains importance for the individual and his potential offspring. Unraveling the genetic foundations of azoospermia promises to enhance patient care by identifying those without spermatogenic potential, flagging individuals at heightened risk for broader health issues, and potentially influencing the well-being of their future generations [5–8].

Genetic Causes of NOA

Klinefelter Syndrome (KS)

KS is the leading cause of NOA, which is characterized by the supernumerary X chromosome in normal male karyotype [9]. The prevalence of this chromosomal abnormality is estimated to be 213:100.000 male fetuses and 1:576 newborn boys, reaching more than 10 men in 100 azoospermic males [10–12]. The karyotype of KS cases is prevailingly represented by 47,XXY, and the remaining part of which is identified by several variants of this aneuploidy and mosaicism (e.g., 48,XXXY, 47,XXY/ 46,XY and 47,XXY/48,XXXY) [10]. The extra chromosome(s) mainly originates from nondisjunction problem of sex chromosomes in parental meiosis (I and/or II) and mitosis of zygote in the early stage. Both parents are almost equally responsible for the nondisjunction problem but in different phases of meiotic division. Maternal nondisjunction can happen during meiosis I or II, whereas paternal ones can occur only in meiosis I [13]. Moreover, maternal age affects the prevalence of KS, raising it four times if the mother's age is more than 40 years via increasing the chance of mitotic errors [10]. The cause(s) of this increase could be the management of early zygotic division by maternal noncoding RNAs and proteins [14].

The clinical phenotypes of KS are relatively diverse; though, gynecomastia, testicular dysfunction, hypergonadotropic hypogonadism, small testis, eunuchoid habitus, tall stature, osteoporosis, and neurocognitive defects are the most common features of KS [15–17]. Mosaicism is the crucial determinant for the clinical manifestations. Men with mosaic KS exhibit milder clinical symptoms than those of nonmosaic ones [18]. Besides mosaicism, certain genetic variants and gene dosage play a role in constituting clinical characteristics, such as tall stature and various anthropometric parameters [19–22]. The copy number of the short-stature homeobox-containing (*SHOX*) gene (up to four copies) located on the pseudoautosomal regions (PAR) of X and Y chromosomes has been linked to tall stature in KS males due to an increase in the sex chromosome number and ultimately in *SHOX* gene dosage [21]. Another variation affecting the height of KS men is the CAG repeat polymorphism of the androgen receptor (AR) gene located on the X chromosome. However, this polymorphism does not affect only tall stature. The shorter or longer CAG repeats are associated with phenotypic and social characteristics of KS, diagnosis time of the disease, and pharmacogenetics of testosterone therapy. The reason behind these effects may be that the androgen action was changed by CAG repeat polymorphism. The origin of the extra X chromosome and the skewed X-chromosome inactivation have not been considered as causes of KS phenotype, including anthropometric features [19, 20, 22]. An investigation of the association between 78 KS comorbidities—which were diagnosed at least 50% more frequently in the KS cases than controls—and molecular factors has also demonstrated that the comorbidities, including infertility, osteoporosis, testicular dysfunction, obesity, and dental caries, result from X-linked gene dosage increase and changes in the protein interactome activity [15]. Moreover, epigenetic modifications have recently drawn attention to KS pathogenesis. KS patients exhibit globally altered DNA methylation profile [23, 24].

A link between KS and spermatogenesis defects is well-known, although the impact of the supernumerary X chromosome on spermatogenesis has not been fully elucidated. Testes of KS individuals are represented by small volume, absence of germ cells, seminiferous tubules with fibrosis and hyalinization, and Leydig cell hyperplasia [16, 25, 26]. However, spermatogenesis can occur in some seminiferous tubules of nonmosaic KS men, originating from euploid germ cells. It can be explained by two hypotheses: gonosomal mosaicism occurring in embryogenesis and testicular mosaicism resulting from loss of extra X chromosome in 47,XXY spermatogonia during mitosis [13, 27]. On the other hand, 47,XXY spermatogonia are also known to complete the spermatogenesis process and form mature spermatozoa [28].

The advancement in the fields of andrology and assisted reproductive technology (ART) has enabled nonmosaic KS males to be fathers of their biological children through the utilization of testicular sperm harvested by SSR. Spermatozoa have been successfully extracted in 20–44% of KS cases who underwent conventional or micro-TESE [29–33]. The pregnancy rate (PR) using these testicular spermatozoa in ICSI is 43%, the same for the live birth rate (LBR). Using fresh or frozen sperm has no impact on PR and LBR [29]. Several factors influence sperm retrieval rate (SRR) positively or negatively; however, this issue remains a matter of debate. A study conducted by Rohayem and colleagues reported that age (≥15–19 years), testosterone (≥7.5 nmol/L), and LH (≤ 17.5 U/ L) were predictive factors for positive SRR. However, a meta-analysis by Corona et al. could not find any significant association between the SRR outcome and factors such as age, testis volume, FSH, LH, and testosterone [29]. Moreover, there is no increased risk of the presence of abnormal karyotype in children of KS males compared to those of other infertile men [34]. Therefore, whether preimplantation genetic diagnosis (PGD) or prenatal genetic analysis is recommendable is still controversial [35].

46,XX Testicular Disorders/Differences of Sex Development

46,XX testicular disorder is a relatively rare condition with an incidence of 1 in 20.000–25.000 newborn males. The clinical findings of this testicular disorder are heterogeneous, notwithstanding that short stature, smaller permanent tooth size, small testis, hypergonadotropic hypogonadism, and azoospermia are involved in the common features of 46,XX individuals [36, 37]. Sex determining region Y (*SRY*) gene is a major influencer for the phenotypic characteristics of 46,XX men [38]. *SRY* located on Yp11.2 encodes a transcription factor, taking part in the determination of testis formation during embryonic development [39]. The majority of the cases with this genetic anomaly have the *SRY* gene in their paternal X chromosome due to the translocation of *SRY*-containing chromosome segment from Y to X chromosome during paternal meiosis. *SRY*$^+$ men are mostly represented by completely reversed male internal and external genitalia. The minority of 46,XX males have no *SRY* gene (SRY$^-$), exhibiting various degrees of virilization [40, 41]. The presented phenotype arising in the absence of *SRY* is caused by loss- or gain-of-function mutations in certain autosomal genes that are involved in testis differentiation and female sex reversal [42]. SRY-related HMG-box-containing gene 9 (*SOX9*) is a target of *SRY* during sex determination. Upregulated *Sox9* plays a role in Sertoli cell proliferation with fibroblast growth factor 9 (*FGF9*) following the initiation of Sertoli cell differentiation. *Sox3* transgenic mice displayed XX male sex reversal, and gonads of which express *Sox9*, resulting in testis differentiation. A duplication in the regulatory regions of *SOX3* gene has also been described in 46,XX males [42]. Moreover, cytogenic and molecular analyses of 46,XX males have demonstrated that a gain-of-function mutation changed copy numbers of *FGF9* gene (duplication) and caused masculinization in these men [43].

Patients of 46,XX testicular disorder are infertile with azoospermia as they do not have AZF regions of Y chromosome that is necessary for spermatogenesis. Therefore, to retrieve spermatozoa through TESE or other methods is not possible. The only chance to be a father for these men is sperm donation or adoption [38].

Chromosomal Translocations

Translocation is rearranging chromosome segments between two or rarely more chromosomes that are usually nonhomologous. Translocation can involve the reciprocal exchange of broken-off segments between chromosomes (reciprocal translocation) or can be due to the fuse of two acrocentric chromosomes close to the centromere region with the missing short arms (Robertsonian translocation) [44]. The frequency of Robertsonian translocation is 0.8% in infertile men, which is ninefold that in newborn males, while for reciprocal translocation, the fold increase is seven [45]. In NOA, the frequency of translocations varies between 1.1% and 2.5% in cases from different countries, such as China, Qatar, Tunisia, Saudi Arabia, and Syria. Reciprocal translocation is mostly seen in NOA men compared to Robertsonian translocations (0.68–1.23% vs 0.3–0.92%). 45,XY,t(14;15), 46,XY,t(7;14), 46,XY,t(14;14–21), 46,XY,t(9;14), 46,XY,t(4;6)(p12;p22), 46,XY,t(7;16)(p11;p13), and 46,XY,t(1;17)(q12;p12) are the common translocation involved in NOA cases [46–49].

The effect of chromosomal translocations on spermatogenesis may differ depending on genes present on the breakpoints or lost chromosome segments. Breakpoints or rearrangements may cause removing promoter or interrupt sequences of genes playing a role in spermatogenesis, resulting in disturbances in this process and infertility [50]. Generally, individuals with autosomal Robertsonian or reciprocal translocations have been characterized by poor semen quality [50, 51]. 1q21, 6p21, 16q21, and 17q11.2 chromosomal regions (breakpoints) have been suggested to be related to poor sperm function. Since genes located on these breakpoints take part in spermatogenesis, or fertility-related processes such as spermiogenesis, spermatogonial proliferation, germ cell apoptosis, sperm capacitation, and sperm motility [51]. Translocation of the X chromosome with certain autosomal chromosomes causes azoospermia in most of the cases [52]. On the other hand, Y-autosome translocations have been rarely reported to be a reason for azoospermia in case reports. 46,X,t(Y;7)(q11.2;p22) translocation was detected in NOA men with spermatogenic arrest, and 46,X,t(Y;1)(q12;q21) was determined in NOA case in a unique combination of inversion of chromosome 9 [inv(9)(p12q13] [53, 54].

The sperm retrieval and pregnancy rates of infertile men with chromosomal abnormalities are lower than those of idiopathic infertile men [48]. Chromosomal abnormalities, including translocation, lead to more unfavorable outcomes of sperm retrieval than KS karyotype in NOA men [55]. In a recent meta-analysis by Mazjoub et al., sperm retrieval rates have been suggested to be 33% for patients with Robertsonian translocations and 50% for men with reciprocal translocations [56]. Besides retrieving spermatozoa, the sperm quality obtained from these patients is also crucial for healthy offspring. Chromosomal rearrangements due to translocations may result in chromosomal malsegregation and the formation of unbalanced spermatozoa during meiosis [51]. The risk of producing unbalanced sperm cells is 5.8–32% in carriers of Robertsonian translocations, increasing the risk of unbalanced embryos, and ultimately miscarriages [57]. For couples, if one of them carries a translocation, genetic counseling is better proposed [44].

Chromosomal Inversions

Inversion is a relatively rare structural chromosomal abnormality in infertile men [44]. Chromosome 9 inversion is found in approximately 4 per 100 infertile men, giving rise to variable phenotypes ranging from poor semen quality to azoospermia

[58]. Pericentric inversion of chromosome 12 [inv(12)(p12q12)] was reported in a Tunisian man with SCOS. Specific genes in this breakpoint region are testis-expressed genes and serve a function in spermatogenesis, inactivation of these genes due to deletion may result in SCOS phenotype [59]. Another inversion related to SCOS is inv.(7)(q22;q31). In this case, successful pregnancy and delivery were achieved by TESE-ICSI [56, 60].

Y Chromosome Microdeletions

The male sex chromosome (Y) is a small acrocentric chromosome, but it is unique in genomic architecture and content due to long palindromes, ampliconic sequences, and segmental duplications [61]. Y chromosome includes pseudoautosomal regions (PARs) in its distal that have sequence similarity with the same region in the X chromosome providing proper pairing of sex chromosomes in meiosis, and male-specific region of Y (MSY) in which nonreciprocal transfer (intrachromosomal gene conversion) occurs. This conversion enables particular genes in Y chromosome to remain at a certain number [62]. Y chromosome contains 147 protein-coding genes, 41 of them are recently added by the Telomere-to-Telomere consortium, most of which are crucial for spermatogenesis. Spermatogenesis-related genes are mostly located in the region named as AZF on Y chromosome [61]. AZF region was first described by Tiepolo and Zuffardi, who found a deletion on Yq11 in six azoospermic men [63]. This region was further mapped to three subregions—AZFa, AZFb, and AZFc—characterized by different spermatogenesis problems [64]. AZFa and AZFb regions partially overlapped [65]. Microdeletions in AZF regions are mostly de novo [64] and result from nonallelic homologous recombination (NAHR) (recombination between nonallelic repeats) owing to ampliconic and palindromic organization of the Y chromosome. There are five fragile sites in Yq causing recurrent deletion of DNA segments in the size of 0.8–7.7 Mb [14]. The most common complete deletion type of Y chromosome is AZFc deletions (~70–80%), which is followed by AZFa (0.5–9%), AZFb (1–7%), and AZFbc (1–20%). AZF deletions are presented by the incidence of 2–10% in azoospermic men [66].

The AZFa region is ~800 kb in length and hosts three genes: ubiquitin-specific peptidase 9 (*USP9Y*), DEAD-box helicase 3 Y-linked (*DDX3Y*), and ubiquitous transcribed Y (*UTY*) [67]. USP9Y encodes a protein involved in the regulation of protein turnover via its ubiquitin C-terminal hydrolase activity. De novo deletion in *USP9Y* gene results in various testicular phenotypes ranging from normozoospermia to azoospermia [68, 69]. DDX3Y, formerly known as DBY, is an ATP-dependent RNA chaperone with a function in group I intron splicing [70]. DDX3Y has recently been suggested as a key factor for spermatogenesis and deletion that causes NOA with SCOS [71]. *UTY,* the recently described gene, is enriched in human germ cells, but its function is not fully known [67]. The reason for complete AZFa deletions has been suggested to be the nonallelic homologous recombination (NAHR) mechanism [66]. The mapping of the breakpoints of the AZFa deletion located in the short arm of the Y chromosome (Yq11) demonstrated that the proximal and the distal breakpoints located in two homologous human endogenous retrovirus 15 (HERV15) sequences (HERV15yq1 and HERV15yq2, respectively) in men with SCOS. HERV15yq1 and HERV15yq2 have identical sequences, and the intrachromosomal recombination events between them have been suggested to culminate in AZFa microdeletion [72].

AZFb region involves 32 genes and transcription units. The complete deletion of AZFb causes the removal of 6.2 Mb region between palindrome 5 (P5) and proximal of P1, caused by NAHR mechanism in individuals with NOA [73]. Deleted genes are mainly expressed in testicular tissue and crucial for germ cell maturation, mutation of which leads to MA [14, 73].

AZFc region hosts 42 genes and transcripts. The deletion breakpoints of complete AZFc deletion are b2 and b4 amplicons in P3 and P1, respectively, and encompass 3.5 Mb. AZFc deletion-related spermatogenic failure is derived from NAHR between b2 and b4 amplicons [73]. The phenotypes of AZFc deletion are variable; spermatozoa may be obtained in the ejaculate but in low concentration (<two million/mL), or azoospermia or cryotozoospermia may be observed in these cases [74]. Even though a spontaneous regression of testicular germ cells over time was reported in a patient with AZFc microdeletion, this could not be successfully validated by other studies [75, 76].

The complete AZFbc deletion can be localized in two different regions: (i) P4 and distal P1 removing 7.0 Mb and 42 genes and transcripts, or (ii) P5 and distal P1 removing interval between P5 and distal P1 (7.7 Mb), deleting 38 genes and transcripts. The reason for this mutation is the same as other AZF region deletions, NAHR [73]. The clinical manifestations of AZFbc deletion are SCOS and MA [66].

Y chromosomal microdeletions screening in men with azoospermia or sperm count less than five million are conducted according to EAA/AMQN guidelines to diagnose AZF deletions [66]. However, this screening is not only important for diagnostic purposes but also is essential for prognosis and therapeutic options such as sperm retrieval techniques as well as ARTs. Individuals with complete AZFa, AZFb, and AZFbc deletions have no chance of retrieval of testicular spermatozoa. In these cases, additional comprehensive analysis of the AZF deletions is necessary to discriminate between complete and partial deletions [14, 66]. Residual spermatogenesis in two nonobstructive azoospermic men without sY127 and sY137—markers of the median and distal part of AZFb region, respectively—has been reported, and extended examination has revealed the presence of the sY1192 in the distal of AZFb region. This finding suggests that the partial deletion of the AZFb region provides the remaining genes, maintaining residual spermatogenesis [77]. AZFc deletion carriers exhibit an increased chance (50–60%) of sperm retrieval by mTESE [78].

Y chromosome microdeletion is presented by high prevalence in individuals with 45,X/46,XY karyotype, suggesting a relation between Yq microdeletions and Y chromosome instability that causes the formation of 45,X0 cell lines. Moreover, 45,X/46,XY mosaicism has been associated with a low SRR rate [79–82]. Genetic counseling to AZF microdeletion carriers except complete AZFa, AZFb, and AZFbc deletions should be recommended about the risk of conceiving a son with spermatogenesis failure [66] (Fig. 3.1).

Monogenic Causes of NOA

Spermatogenesis is a complex and extraordinary process that includes products of more than 2000 genes. Taking into consideration these genetic heterogeneities and the involvement of monogenic causes in all the etiological factors of azoospermia, variability in single gene defects leading to NOA is expected [14, 83].

Congenital Hypogonadotropic Hypogonadism (CHH)

CHH is a rare disease with a male predominance (3.5 to 1), resulting from the deficient production, secretion, or function of gonadotropin-releasing hormone (GnRH). GnRH is a decapeptide and regulates the hypothalamic–pituitary–gonadal (HPG) axis through the GnRH receptor, culminating in the release of gonadotropins. Gonadotropins are crucial hormones for sexual development and fertility [84]. CHH is presented by clinical and genetic heterogeneity. CHH cases manifest by

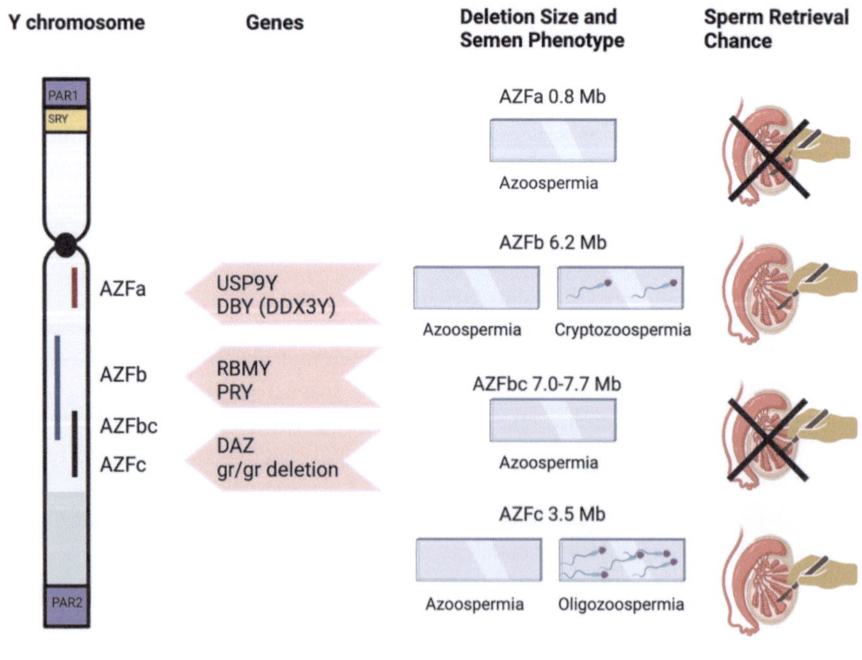

Fig. 3.1 Y chromosome deletions and sperm retrieval chance

reproductive and nonreproductive phenotypes, for example, delay or lack of puberty, micropenis, testis size smaller than 4 mL, cryptorchidism, fertility problems, impaired odor perception (anosmia/hyposmia), synkinesia, renal agenesis, dental impairments, and endocrinal anomalies. Hyposmia or anosmia is identified in nearly half of the CHH patients, and the combination of these hearing problems with CHH is named Kallmann syndrome (KalS) [85]. The prevalence of KalS in men is 1:30.000 [86]. Besides phenotypic heterogeneity, CHH is a genetically complex disease. This complexity resulted from several factors: (i) various inheritance patterns of CHH, including autosomal-dominant, autosomal-recessive, and X-linked-recessive; (ii) incomplete penetrance and variable expressivity; and (iii) oligogenic background of the disease [83, 85].

To date, at least 30 genes have been reported as causes of CHH and/or KalS [87–89]. Anosmin 1 (*ANOS1*) is the first identified gene related to CHH. *ANOS1* (also known as *KAL1*) encodes a protein involved in the regulation of cell junction and neuronal precursor migration. *KAL1* mutation causes X-linked KalS [90]. Several genes are implicated in KalS pathogenesis other than *ANOS1,* including fibroblast growth factor receptor 1 (*FGFR1*, *KAL2*), fibroblast growth factor 8 (*FGF8*, *KAL6*), prokineticin receptor 2 (*PROKR2*, *KAL3*), prokineticin 2 (*PROK2*), semaphorin-3A (*SEMA3A*), and WD repeat-containing protein 11 (*WDR11*). Candidate genes proposed for CHH with normosmia are *GNRHR*, *GNRH1*, kiss-1 metastasis suppressor 1 (*KISS1*), KISS1 receptor (*KISS1R*), tachykinin precursor 3 (*TAC3*), and tachykinin receptor 3 (*TACR3*). However, mutations of the identified genes are responsible for only less than 10% of the cases [84, 90].

Even though the frequency of CHH among NOA cases is very low (~2%), the clinical management of them is well-established [83, 91]. Hormone therapy (e.g., gonadotropins, FSH, and GnRH) is used for the stimulation of virilization and fertility. Fertilization has been reported in almost 50–60% of men with CHH applied TESE-ICSI especially following the improvement of testicular volume [84, 92]. CHH reverse in the ~10–20% of male patients having treatment. The reason behind this reversal, however, remains unexplained [85]. Genetic counseling may be recommended for the patient with an autosomal-dominant form of CHH to eliminate the transmission of the disease to the next generations [84].

Primary Testicular Failure

NOA constituted at least 70% of azoospermia cases, and most of them are characterized by primary testicular failure owing to failed spermatogenesis [93, 94]. NOA men exhibit peculiar testicular phenotypes including but not limited to SCOS, MA, and hypospermatogenesis [14]. Several candidate genes have been proposed for different types of testicular phenotypes; however, some of them are supported by more than two independent studies (established genes), and others are reported in a study that has been validated by in vitro/in vivo study (promising candidate genes), or no precise proof as a causative gene for NOA [83].

- *Candidate Genes for SCOS Phenotype*

  Fanconi anemia complementation group M *(FANCM)* is the only established gene related to SCOS phenotype, while *FANCA*, polo-like kinase 4 (*PLK4*) and WNK lysine-deficient protein kinase 3 (*WNK3*) genes have been reported in only one study and necessitate more studies to connect a causative link to NOA [83]. *FANCM* and *FANCA* are involved in the Fanconi anemia (FA) pathway, but FANCM is not related to FA. *FANCM* plays an important part in maintaining genomic stability through DNA crosslink removal, replication fork repair, and regulation of crossover. The loss-of-function mutation in *FANCM* gene caused an increase in the interstrand crosslink sensitivity in mice spermatogonia and to SCOS. c.1946_1958del (p.P648Lfs*16) homozygous frameshift mutation and bi-allelic loss-of-function mutation have culminated NOA in brothers from Pakistan and Estonia, respectively. Estonian brothers with a loss-of-function variant exhibit SCOS [83, 95]. *FANCA* gene is mostly mutated in FA cases and associated with a syndromic form of NOA. Pathogenic variants of *FANCA* were detected in NOA men with SCOS and indistinct changes in hematological parameters, indicating the possibility of developing FA in these patients in the future [96]. *PLK4*, a member of the polo protein family, is involved in the centriole duplication during the cell cycle. An NOA man with SCOS presented by a heterozygous deletion in the Ser/Thr kinase domain of *PLK4* [97]. Another gene related to SCOS is WNK3 that is highly expressed in the testis and encodes an activator of NKCC1 (also known as solute carrier family 12 member 2, SLC12A2). *NKCC1* is expressed in Sertoli cells and causes spermatogenesis impairments. WNK3 plays a role in the regulation of cation-chloride transporters, and cell signaling, survival, and proliferation. Although the association between NOA and *WNK3* has not been completely elucidated, it has been proposed that *WNK3* illustrated its effects on spermatogenesis through NKCC1. NOA men presenting SCOS were found to be carriers of the pathogenic variant of *WNK3* (p.Glu913Lys) [98].
- *Candidate Genes for MA Phenotype*

  MA is a testicular phenotype in which the largest number of single genes are causatives for this pathology [14]. The majority of the established and nonestablished genes are involved in meiosis and DNA repair [83]. During meiosis, especially in the prophase I stage, certain characteristic events occur. For example, homologous chromosome pairing, synaptonemal complex formation, synapsis, programmed double-strand breaks (DSBs) and repair of them, and crossovers (COs) [99]. Defects in the genes acting in these unique processes via encoded proteins cause spermatogenesis and/or testicular abnormalities [14].

  The initiator of the meiotic double-strand breaks (*SPO11*) gene (promising candidate gene) encoding a specific DNA topoisomerase is responsible for the formation of DSBs in chromosomes, providing recombination in the synaptonemal complex. A causative link between the pathogenic variant of *SPO1* (p.Glu186Lys) and MA has been reported in two brothers [98]. Another gene implicated in both the introduction of DSBs and MA phenotype is meiotic double-stranded break formation protein 1 (*MEI1*), mutation of which has been detected in two brothers with NOA [100]. MEI1 also plays a role in the formation and maintenance of synaptonemal complex and COs, along with synaptonemal complex central element 1 (*SYCE1*), meiosis-specific with OB domain (*MEIOB*), testis expressed 11 (*TEX11*) and *TEX15* [14, 83]. *SYCE1* and *TEX11* are elements of synaptonemal complex but in different locations. Homozygous mutation of *SYCE1* results in MA in not only mice but also in humans, arising from synapsis defects [101, 102]. *TEX11* is mutated in 1% of nonobstructive azoospermic men, and this prevalence reaches 15% in NOA cases with MA [103, 104]. *TEX11* mutations lead to impairments in synapsis and crossover formation. Furthermore, gene dosage of *Tex11* affects recombination levels in meiosis [103–106]. Carriers of *TEX11* loss-of-function mutation have no chance in sperm retrieval [38]. X-linked *TEX15* gene has a function in DSBs repair as well as chromosomal synapsis. TEX15 regulates the recruiting of DNA repair proteins on the damage sites, mutation of which gives rise to meiotic recombination problems. Nonsense mutation of TEX15 gene (c.2130 T > G, p.Y710*) has been suggested to be a reason for progressive spermatogenic failure—oligozoospermia to azoospermia—worsening over time [107]. c.2419A > T (p.Lys807*) and c.3040delT (p.Ser1014Leufs*5) mutations in *TEX15* gene were also found in NOA siblings [108]. *MEIOB* is involved in DNA repair via binding to single-stranded DNA during meiosis and stabilizes the complex of DNA repair protein RAD51/recombinase *DMC1*. This complex is impaired in *MEIOB* mice that are infertile [109, 110]. Different *MEIOB* mutations are presented by infertility with MA in humans, as well [111, 112]. The causative role of meiosis-specific recombinase *DMC1* has been revealed by whole-exome sequencing in both sexes, homozygous missense mutation in *DMC1* contributes to NOA in men and premature ovarian insufficiency in women from a consanguineous family. Male patient displays meiotic arrest at the zygotene stage of prophase I [113].

Movement and cohesion of sister chromatids are crucial for proper meiosis in spermatogenesis. The protein product of the stromal antigen 3 (*STAG3*) gene is necessary for the cohesion of sister chromatids. The meiotic arrest is the pathogenic phenotype of *STAG3* mutation carriers who have decreased sperm retrieval rate [114, 115]. The movement of sister chromatids during meiosis is achieved by dynein-binding protein *CCDC155* (coiled-coil domain containing 155), which is mutated in NOA men [98]. Besides mutations in meiosis-related genes, mutations of genes participating in DNA and RNA processing (*SETX*), repression of transposable elements (*TDRD9*) and transcriptional activator or repressor (*TEF4B*, *ZMYND15*) have also been proposed as the reason of MA phenotype. Genes in NOA pathogenesis have not only impact on the testicular phenotypes of SCOS and MA but also affect more than one phenotype. *TEX14*, *NR5A1*, and *WT1* are involved in them and mutations of them associated with MA and SCOS [83].

- **Gene Candidates Linked to Various Testicular Phenotypes**

  The DMRT1 gene, known for its critical role in the differentiation of testes, has been linked to both syndromic and nonsyndromic types of XY gonadal dysgenesis [116]. Array-CGH investigations revealed deletions within the DMRT1 gene in five individuals from separate groups, all experiencing nonobstructive azoospermia (NOA) independently. It is of particular interest that these deletions in DMRT1 are associated with SCOS and SCA, two specific testicular conditions [117]. Moreover, a notable discovery was a heterozygous deletion impacting exons 1 and 2, which eliminates the entire DM/DNA binding domain, observed in an instance of incomplete SGA, suggesting the significant impact of DMRT1 deletion in NOA cases beyond the scope of XY gonadal dysgenesis [117, 118].

Within the Testis Expressed gene family, TEX14 and TEX15 stand out; TEX14 is crucial for creating and sustaining intercellular connections essential for meiosis and spermatogenesis in vertebrates [119]. This gene's expression is restricted to the testes of humans and mice and shows evolutionary conservation across mammalian species [112]. Recessive mutations in TEX14 have been identified as potent factors for NOA, with affected testicular histology ranging from SCOS to an early MA phenotype, often leading to unsuccessful sperm extraction [98, 112, 118]. TEX15, on the other hand, is vital for the recruitment of DNA repair proteins and has been identified with mutations in NOA and crypto/oligozoospermia cases, marking a significant contrast to TEX14, which is seen as an unfavorable indicator for successful sperm retrieval [106–108, 120].

The NANOS2 gene encodes an RNA-binding protein that plays a role in preserving the spermatogonial stem cell population and preventing premature meiotic initiation [121]. Initial research pinpointed NANOS2 as a likely source of the SCOS phenotype [122], and subsequent findings introduced a homozygous mutation in NANOS2 co-segregating with SCOS in siblings from a consanguineous family. Conversely, an individual case featuring a homozygous start loss mutation exhibited maturation arrest (MA), casting doubt on the straightforward association with SCOS [98].

The genes NR5A1 and WT1 are responsible for encoding Steroidogenic Factor 1 (SF1) and Wilms' tumor protein, respectively, both critical transcription factors involved in the development of gonads across genders. SF1 is specifically regulated by WT1 in a gender-dependent manner [123]. Disturbances in these genes often result in autosomal-dominant conditions linked with nonobstructive azoospermia (NOA), particularly manifesting through Sertoli cell-only syndrome (SCOS) or a halt in maturation (MA) [124–126]. Furthermore, NR5A1 mutations have been identified to trigger autosomal-dominant primary adrenal insufficiency and various 46, XY sexual development disorders (DSD), such as hypospadias, bilateral anorchia, micropenis, and premature ovarian insufficiency (POI) in females [127, 128]. Certain NR5A1 mutations are solely associated with the NOA phenotype, with no overt testicular developmental abnormalities [125, 126, 129]. WT1 alterations, meanwhile, can induce a wide array of congenital anomalies in the kidneys and genital organs, including Denys–Drash syndrome and Wilms' tumor, highlighting the importance of careful clinical oversight for patients, especially those with symptoms indicative of congenital testicular issues [127, 130].

The TDRD9 gene plays a pivotal role in silencing the Line-1 (L1) retrotransposon within the male germ line, crucial for maintaining fertility in both mice and humans [131, 132]. In a significant study, a homozygous frameshift mutation in TDRD9 was identified in individuals from a large Bedouin family with a history of cryptozoospermia/azoospermia due to incomplete MA [132], suggesting that this mutation significantly impairs spermatogenesis, as also seen in TDRD9-deficient mice, though it does not affect female fertility [131, 132].

TAF4B functions as a widespread transcription factor and a selective coactivator of genes, with its homozygous truncating mutations causing NOA/oligozoospermia in a Turkish family with close genetic links. Notably, mice lacking TAF4B suffer from subfertility, attributed to a broad loss of pre-meiotic germ cells, impacting both differentiation and the renewal capabilities of the spermatogonial stem cell pool [133].

Lastly, M1AP is implicated in the progression of meiosis, with new research uncovering mutations in patients with NOA due to MA. Studies across four distinct family groups have demonstrated that biallelic loss-of-function mutations in M1AP correlate with a diverse range of severely compromised spermatogenesis, predominantly characterized by meiotic arrest, leading to azoospermia [134].

- **NOA Candidate Genes with an Unclear Testicular Phenotype**

  Recent discoveries have highlighted PSMC3IP and MCM8 as genes of potential relevance to the condition of NOA. Specifically, PSMC3IP serves an integral function as a coactivator for the proteins DMC1 and RAD51, facilitating meiotic recombination [135, 136], and its association with both NOA and early ovarian failure (POI) has been observed in a family with consanguineous ties to Yemen. A notable discovery was a homozygous mutation in PSMC3IP that results in a stop gain, effectively eliminating the protein's C-terminal end, which segregates alongside both POI and NOA conditions [137]. This mutation in PSMC3IP compromises its ability to bind with the DMC1 and RAD51 proteins, which are crucial for the process of homologous recombination [135].

  Furthermore, the MCM8 gene has been implicated in working with the FA pathway elements to repair crosslinks during DNA replication [138], underscoring its necessity for the proper development and sustenance of gonadal functions across both genders. The presence of homozygous mutations in MCM8, which lead to genomic instability by impairing the repair mechanisms of meiotic DNA, has been identified as a causative factor for NOA in men and POI in women [139] (Table 3.1).

Table 3.1 Genetic causes of NOA

Genetic causes of NOA	Gene													
Klinefelter syndrome (47,XXY)	*47,XXY*			*48,XXXY*				*47,XXY/46,XY*				*47,XXY/48,XXXY*		
46,XX testicular disorders/ differences of sex development	*SOX9*							*SOX3*						
Chromosomal translocations	*45,XY,t (14;15)*	*46,XY,t (7;14)*	*46,XY,t (14;14–21)*	*46,XY,t (9;14)*	*46,XY,t(4;6) (p12;p22)*	*46,XY,t(7;16) (p11;p13)*	*46,XY,t(1;17) (q12;p12)*	*1q21 chromos omal region*	*6p21 chromos omal region*	*16q21 chromos omal region*	*17q11.2 chromos omal region*	*46,X,t(Y;7) (q11.2;p22*	*46,X,t(Y;1) (q12;q21)*	*[inv(9) (p12q13]*
Chromosomal inversions	*inv(9)*				*[inv(12)(p12q12)]*					*inv(7)(q22;q31)*				
Y chromosome Microdeletions	***AZFa***		*USP9Y*		*DDX3Y*		*UTY*		*NAHR*	*HERVyq1*		*HERVyq2*		
	AZFb		*NAHR*											
	AZFc		*NAHR*											
	AZFbc		*NAHR*											
Monogenic causes of nonobstructive azoospermia	*Congenital hypogonadotropic hypogonadism (CHH)*							*ANOS1*						
								FGFR1						
								KAL2						
								FGF8						
								KAL6						
								PROKR2						
								KAL3						
								PROK2						
								SEMA3A						
								WDR11						
								GNRHR						
								GNRH1						
								KISS1						
								KISS1R						
								TAC3						
								TACR3						

	Primary testicular failure	*Candidate genes for SCOS phenotype*	*FANCM*
			FANCA
			PLK4
			WNK3
			*p.P648Lfs*16*
			PLK4
			SLC12A2
			NKCC1
			p.Glu913Lys
		Candidate genes for MA phenotype	*SPO11*
			p.Glu186Lys
			MEI1
			SYCE1
			MEIOB
			TEX11
			TEX15
			DMC1
			STAG3
			CCDC155
			SETX
			TDRD9
			TEF4B
			ZMYND15
			TEX14
			NR5A1
			WT1

(continued)

Table 3.1 (continued)

Genetic causes of NOA	Gene
Gene candidates linked to various testicular phenotypes	*DMRT1*
	TEX14
	TEX15
	NANOS2
	NR5A1
	WT1
	TDRD9
	TAF4B
	M1AP
NOA candidate genes with an unclear testicular phenotype	*PSMC3IP*
	MCM8

TESE Outcome in Individuals with Chromosomal Abnormalities

TESE is acknowledged as the preferred technique for extracting sperm in patients with NOA [140, 141]. Research comparing cTESE and micro-TESE followed by ICSI in NOA patients has been conducted [142–144]. A meta-analysis involving a total of 1890 patients revealed an increased SSR in individuals who underwent micro-TESE compared to cTESE [142–144]. cTESE's SSR varied between 35% and 56% among NOA patients, with micro-TESE offering a 1.5 times higher likelihood of successful sperm recovery, indicating its efficacy over cTESE [1]. Sandro C Esteves reported that the SSR ranged from 16.7% to 45% in the cTESE group and from 42.9% to 63% in the micro-TESE group. This correlation was found to be positively associated with FSH levels and testicular volume [1]. Conversely, another meta-analysis found a 50% SSR in NOA patients via cTESE/micro-TESE, with no significant difference in SSR between the two [145].

Retrospective analysis indicated that no single clinical feature could precisely forecast micro-TESE's sperm recovery success in NOA patients [146]. Moreover, a study found age did not affect micro-TESE's sperm retrieval rates [147], while another indicated better TESE outcomes when performed at a younger age compared to older ages [148]. Factors like testicular size were suggested as prognostic indicators for SSR in NOA cases [149], with testicles larger than 12 ml potentially yielding over 60% SSR accuracy [145]. Thus, testicular volume and age are important SSR predictors in NOA patients. Moreover, heightened testosterone levels emerge as a promising prognosticator for individuals undergoing both micro-TESE and conventional TESE procedures. In contrast, diminished levels of LH and FSH notably correlate with a heightened likelihood of achieving a positive SSR during TESA [56].

Regarding AZF microdeletions, these are categorized into AZFa, AZFb, and AZFc [64]. AZFa and AZFb deletions typically have a poor prognosis with no successful sperm retrieval reported [150], whereas AZFc deletions often lead to successful micro-TESE outcomes [151].

Genetic Counseling Before ICSI in Patients with Genetic Abnormalities

Genetic counseling is essential for couples undergoing infertility treatment, offering crucial insights into the genetic aspects of assisted reproductive technology (ART). Both couples and medical professionals involved in reproductive techniques must understand the potential risks of congenital disabilities and chromosomal abnormalities associated with ART [152]. While genetic experts commonly provide counseling, reproductive staff must have a baseline knowledge of genetics. Before proceeding with ART procedures, patients should receive clear and uniform information about the genetic aspects of the treatment [152].

Chromosomal Abnormalities

Individuals diagnosed with Klinefelter syndrome, characterized by the presence of an extra X chromosome in their genetic makeup (either 47,XXY or a mosaic pattern of 47,XXY/46,XY), experience significant impacts on their reproductive and hormonal functions. This chromosomal variation leads to gonadal failure, which manifests in two primary ways: compromised spermatogenesis resulting in azoospermia, where the semen contains no sperm, and reduced testosterone levels, contributing to less pronounced male secondary sexual characteristics. This dual effect underscores the syndrome's profound influence on both fertility and the expression of male physical traits. Nevertheless, there are reports in the literature documenting the successful retrieval of spermatozoa from some individuals with 47,XXY (Klinefelter syndrome) [78, 153]. These spermatozoa have been subsequently used in ICSI procedures. The corpus of recent studies presents varied findings concerning the risk of aneuploidy in children conceived via intracytoplasmic sperm injection (ICSI) utilizing sperm from individuals with a 47,XXY Klinefelter syndrome. Given this variability in outcomes, it is crucial for couples facing these circumstances to undergo comprehensive genetic counseling. Such counseling should offer an in-depth exploration of the existing evidence, elucidate the potential for fetal aneuploidy, and present the spectrum of options available for early genetic assessment, including preimplantation and prenatal diagnostic techniques.

The counseling should also offer necessary support and reassurance where indicated [78, 153].

Y Chromosome Microdeletions (YCMs)

In addition to chromosomal abnormalities, Y-chromosomal microdeletions (YCMs) represent another genetic factor contributing to male infertility. While men with severe spermatogenic disorders have achieved fatherhood through ICSI, caution is warranted, especially when the spermatogenic disorder is linked to AZF microdeletion. When a boy is conceived through ICSI in such cases, he will inherit the YCMs and similar genetic aberrations. Moreover, there is the potential for the emergence or expansion of microdeletions, broadening the spectrum of inherited genetic anomalies and potentially exacerbating the spermatogenic disorder beyond that of the father. It is crucial to thoroughly communicate these possibilities before engaging in the ART procedure [154].

Preimplantation and Prenatal Genetic Diagnosis

Advancements in genetic analysis and reproductive technologies have paved the way for the innovation of preimplantation genetic testing (PGT). This technique involves a genetic assessment of embryos through a biopsy before they are transferred to the uterus [155]. PGT is categorized into three distinct types: (i) PGT-M, which focuses on detecting single-gene defects; (ii) PGT-SR, aimed at identifying chromosomal structural abnormalities in embryos, particularly in cases with a history of recurrent miscarriages due to translocation carriers; and (iii) PGT-A, which screens for chromosomal numerical abnormalities to select embryos free of such issues for transfer [155]. This selection process aims to enhance implantation success rates and decrease the likelihood of miscarriage. The application and counseling protocols for PGT vary globally, reflecting the diverse regulations and healthcare practices across different regions. The ultimate goal is to ensure equitable access to these sophisticated medical technologies for all individuals requiring them [155].

Embarking on the journey of PGT involves a meticulously structured process that begins with the creation of embryos through IVF or ICSI, techniques that amalgamate sperm and egg outside the human body to initiate conception [155]. The subsequent step in this sophisticated journey involves the careful extraction of cells from the developing embryo, typically from the trophectoderm, which is the layer destined to form the placenta. This biopsy is conducted with precision to ensure the viability of the embryo remains intact while providing the necessary genetic material for analysis [155]. Finally, the essence of PGT culminates in the critical evaluation of these embryonic cells to discern any genetic abnormalities. This assessment is pivotal for the selection of embryos that are free from specific genetic conditions or chromosomal abnormalities. The selected, unaffected embryos are then transferred to the uterus with the hope of achieving a healthy pregnancy. This process not only underscores the advancements in reproductive technology but also highlights the commitment to enhancing the prospects of success in assisted reproductive therapies by minimizing the risk of genetic diseases being passed on to the offspring [155].

While the genetic testing methods employed offer a considerable degree of reliability, there are notable concerns regarding their safety and precision, particularly concerning embryos exhibiting chromosomal mosaicism. Recent studies suggest that although the application of this technique might impact conception rates negatively, it does not appear to elevate the risk of congenital anomalies or developmental delays in children conceived through its use [156, 157].

In counseling sessions, it is important to address the potential limitations of PGT-A, including its inability to match the chromosomal resolution provided by microarray analysis from procedures like chorionic villus sampling (CVS) and amniocentesis. Furthermore, the conversation should extend to the options of CVS and amniocentesis, explaining the minimal risk of miscarriage these procedures carry in comparison to their benefits [158]. In order to manage expectations appropriately, it is essential to communicate upfront the possibility that there may not be any viable embryos for transfer due to potential damage. In cases where the genetic defect is linked to the Y chromosome, considering PGT-A for selecting the female sex might be a reasonable option, a topic that warrants a thorough discussion with the patient or couple involved. Through comprehensive genetic counseling, patients or couples are empowered to make informed decisions that align with their cultural and ethical values. Moreover, the conversation should extend to the options for prenatal diagnosis, including chorionic villus sampling (CVS) and amniocentesis, while also addressing the timing of these procedures and the associated risk of miscarriage [158].

Conclusion

NOA is intricately linked to a range of genetic factors that significantly impact male fertility. As discussed, the recapitulation of these genetic factors is crucial in comprehending the etiology of NOA, including chromosomal abnormalities (Klinefelter syndrome, 46,XX male syndrome, Yq), Y chromosome microdeletions, monogenic causes like congenital hypogonadotropic hypogonadism, primary testicular failure… Understanding these genetic nuances is paramount, serving as the cornerstone for accurate diagnosis and the formulation of tailored treatment approaches. There is a hopeful future for early genetic testing, diagnosis, better therapy, and family planning. The toolkit for identifying genetic factors involved in azoospermia has traditionally been restricted to a handful of conventional methods. These include analysis of the Karyotype, screening for microdeletions in the Y-chromosome, and investigating specific single-gene causes particularly pre-testicular and post-testicular azoospermia instances. Early genetic testing can detect genetic variables that predispose to disease, allowing for earlier interventions and tailored treatment strategies, offering new hope for individuals and couples grappling with NOA-related infertility. ART, PGT, and alternative family-building approaches become viable options, offering a more nuanced and individualized approach to family planning. In essence, the integration of genetic knowledge not only refines NOA management but also guides individuals on their reproductive journey, promising ongoing advancements and improved outcomes in the future.

References

1. Esteves SC. Clinical management of infertile men with nonobstructive azoospermia. Asian J Androl. 2015;17(3):459–70. https://doi.org/10.4103/1008-682x.148719.
2. Rothman CM, Newmark H 3rd, Karson RA. The recurrent varicocele–a poorly recognized problem. Fertil Steril. 1981;35(5):552–6. https://doi.org/10.1016/s0015-0282(16)45500-7.
3. Krausz C, Cioppi F, Riera-Escamilla A. Testing for genetic contributions to infertility: potential clinical impact. Expert Rev Mol Diagn. 2018;18(4):331–46. https://doi.org/10.1080/14737159.2018.1453358.
4. Krausz C, Riera-Escamilla A. Genetics of male infertility. Nat Rev Urol. 2018;15(6):369–84. https://doi.org/10.1038/s41585-018-0003-3.
5. Eisenberg ML, Li S, Behr B, et al. Semen quality, infertility and mortality in the USA. Hum Reprod. 2014;29(7):1567–74. https://doi.org/10.1093/humrep/deu106.
6. Ventimiglia E, Capogrosso P, Boeri L, et al. Infertility as a proxy of general male health: results of a cross-sectional survey. Fertil Steril. 2015;104(1):48–55. https://doi.org/10.1016/j.fertnstert.2015.04.020.

7. Eisenberg ML, Li S, Cullen MR, Baker LC. Increased risk of incident chronic medical conditions in infertile men: analysis of United States claims data. Fertil Steril. 2016;105(3):629–36. https://doi.org/10.1016/j.fertnstert.2015.11.011.
8. Belladelli F, Muncey W, Eisenberg ML. Reproduction as a window for health in men. Fertil Steril. 2023;120(3 Pt 1):429–37. https://doi.org/10.1016/j.fertnstert.2023.01.014.
9. Ghorbel M, Gargouri Baklouti S, Ben Abdallah F, et al. Chromosomal defects in infertile men with poor semen quality. J Assist Reprod Genet. 2012;29(5):451–6. https://doi.org/10.1007/s10815-012-9737-7.
10. Bojesen A, Juul S, Gravholt CH. Prenatal and postnatal prevalence of Klinefelter syndrome: a national registry study. J Clin Endocrinol Metab. 2003;88(2):622–6. https://doi.org/10.1210/jc.2002-021491.
11. Nielsen J, Wohlert M. Chromosome abnormalities found among 34,910 newborn children: results from a 13-year incidence study in Arhus, Denmark. Hum Genet. 1991;87(1):81–3. https://doi.org/10.1007/bf01213097.
12. Van Assche E, Bonduelle M, Tournaye H, et al. Cytogenetics of infertile men. Hum Reprod. 1996;11(Suppl 4):1–24.; discussion 25-6. https://doi.org/10.1093/humrep/11.suppl_4.1.
13. Maiburg M, Repping S, Giltay J. The genetic origin of Klinefelter syndrome and its effect on spermatogenesis. Fertil Steril. 2012;98(2):253–60. https://doi.org/10.1016/j.fertnstert.2012.06.019.
14. Cioppi F, Rosta V, Krausz C. Genetics of azoospermia. Int J Mol Sci. 2021;22(6) https://doi.org/10.3390/ijms22063264.
15. Belling K, Russo F, Jensen AB, et al. Klinefelter syndrome comorbidities linked to increased X chromosome gene dosage and altered protein interactome activity. Hum Mol Genet. 2017;26(7):1219–29. https://doi.org/10.1093/hmg/ddx014.
16. Klinefelter HF Jr, Reifenstein EC Jr, Albright F Jr. Syndrome characterized by gynecomastia, aspermatogenesis without A-Leydigism, and increased excretion of follicle-stimulating hormone. J Clin Endocrinol. 1942;2(11):615–27.
17. Zitzmann M, Aksglaede L, Corona G, et al. European academy of andrology guidelines on Klinefelter syndrome endorsing organization: European Society of Endocrinology. Andrology. 2021;9(1):145–67.
18. Gravholt CH, Chang S, Wallentin M, Fedder J, Moore P, Skakkebæk A. Klinefelter syndrome: integrating genetics, neuropsychology, and endocrinology. Endocr Rev. 2018;39(4):389–423. https://doi.org/10.1210/er.2017-00212.
19. Bojesen A, Hertz JM, Gravholt CH. Genotype and phenotype in Klinefelter syndrome – impact of androgen receptor polymorphism and skewed X inactivation. Int J Androl. 2011;34(6 Pt 2):e642–8. https://doi.org/10.1111/j.1365-2605.2011.01223.x.
20. Chang S, Skakkebæk A, Trolle C, et al. Anthropometry in Klinefelter syndrome–multifactorial influences due to CAG length, testosterone treatment and possibly intrauterine hypogonadism. J Clin Endocrinol Metab. 2015;100(3):E508–17. https://doi.org/10.1210/jc.2014-2834.
21. Ottesen AM, Aksglaede L, Garn I, et al. Increased number of sex chromosomes affects height in a nonlinear fashion: a study of 305 patients with sex chromosome aneuploidy. Am J Med Genet A. 2010;152a(5):1206–12. https://doi.org/10.1002/ajmg.a.33334.
22. Zitzmann M, Depenbusch M, Gromoll J, Nieschlag E. X-chromosome inactivation patterns and androgen receptor functionality influence phenotype and social characteristics as well as pharmacogenetics of testosterone therapy in Klinefelter patients. J Clin Endocrinol Metab. 2004;89(12):6208–17. https://doi.org/10.1210/jc.2004-1424.
23. Sharma A, Jamil MA, Nuesgen N, et al. DNA methylation signature in peripheral blood reveals distinct characteristics of human X chromosome numerical aberrations. Clin Epigenetics. 2015;7(1):76. https://doi.org/10.1186/s13148-015-0112-2.
24. Viana J, Pidsley R, Troakes C, et al. Epigenomic and transcriptomic signatures of a Klinefelter syndrome (47,XXY) karyotype in the brain. Epigenetics. 2014;9(4):587–99. https://doi.org/10.4161/epi.27806.

25. Aksglaede L, Wikström AM, Rajpert-De Meyts E, Dunkel L, Skakkebaek NE, Juul A. Natural history of seminiferous tubule degeneration in Klinefelter syndrome. Hum Reprod Update. 2006;12(1):39–48. https://doi.org/10.1093/humupd/dmi039.
26. Davis SM, Rogol AD, Ross JL. Testis development and fertility potential in boys with Klinefelter Syndrome. Endocrinol Metab Clin N Am. 2015;44(4):843–65. https://doi.org/10.1016/j.ecl.2015.07.008.
27. Sciurano RB, Luna Hisano CV, Rahn MI, et al. Focal spermatogenesis originates in euploid germ cells in classical Klinefelter patients. Hum Reprod. 2009;24(9):2353–60. https://doi.org/10.1093/humrep/dep180.
28. Foresta C, Galeazzi C, Bettella A, et al. Analysis of meiosis in intratesticular germ cells from subjects affected by classic Klinefelter's syndrome. J Clin Endocrinol Metab. 1999;84(10):3807–10. https://doi.org/10.1210/jcem.84.10.6029.
29. Corona G, Pizzocaro A, Lanfranco F, et al. Sperm recovery and ICSI outcomes in Klinefelter syndrome: a systematic review and meta-analysis. Hum Reprod Update. 2017;23(3):265–75. https://doi.org/10.1093/humupd/dmx008.
30. Fullerton G, Hamilton M, Maheshwari A. Should non-mosaic Klinefelter syndrome men be labelled as infertile in 2009? Hum Reprod. 2010;25(3):588–97. https://doi.org/10.1093/humrep/dep431.
31. Levron J, Aviram-Goldring A, Madgar I, Raviv G, Barkai G, Dor J. Sperm chromosome analysis and outcome of IVF in patients with non-mosaic Klinefelter's syndrome. Fertil Steril. 2000;74(5):925–9. https://doi.org/10.1016/s0015-0282(00)01556-9.
32. Ozer C, Caglar Aytac P, Goren MR, Toksoz S, Gul U, Turunc T. Sperm retrieval by microdissection testicular sperm extraction and intracytoplasmic sperm injection outcomes in non-obstructive azoospermic patients with Klinefelter syndrome. Andrologia. 2018; https://doi.org/10.1111/and.12983.
33. Vloeberghs V, Verheyen G, Santos-Ribeiro S, et al. Is genetic fatherhood within reach for all azoospermic Klinefelter men? PLoS One. 2018;13(7):e0200300. https://doi.org/10.1371/journal.pone.0200300.
34. Greco E, Scarselli F, Minasi MG, et al. Birth of 16 healthy children after ICSI in cases of non-mosaic Klinefelter syndrome. Hum Reprod. 2013;28(5):1155–60. https://doi.org/10.1093/humrep/det046.
35. Zitzmann M, Aksglaede L, Corona G, et al. European academy of andrology guidelines on Klinefelter Syndrome Endorsing Organization: European Society of Endocrinology. Andrology. 2021;9(1):145–67. https://doi.org/10.1111/andr.12909.
36. de la Chapelle A. The etiology of maleness in XX men. Hum Genet. 1981;58(1):105–16. https://doi.org/10.1007/bf00284157.
37. Majzoub A, Arafa M, Starks C, Elbardisi H, Al Said S, Sabanegh E. 46 XX karyotype during male fertility evaluation; case series and literature review. Asian J Androl. 2017;19(2):168–72. https://doi.org/10.4103/1008-682x.181224.
38. Krausz C, Cioppi F. Genetic factors of non-obstructive azoospermia: consequences on patients' and offspring health. J Clin Med. 2021;10(17) https://doi.org/10.3390/jcm10174009.
39. Lovell-Badge R, Robertson E. XY female mice resulting from a heritable mutation in the primary testis-determining gene. Tdy Dev. 1990;109(3):635–46. https://doi.org/10.1242/dev.109.3.635.
40. McElreavey K, Vilain E, Abbas N, Herskowitz I, Fellous M. A regulatory cascade hypothesis for mammalian sex determination: SRY represses a negative regulator of male development. Proc Natl Acad Sci USA. 1993;90(8):3368–72. https://doi.org/10.1073/pnas.90.8.3368.
41. Vorona E, Zitzmann M, Gromoll J, Schüring AN, Nieschlag E. Clinical, endocrinological, and epigenetic features of the 46,XX male syndrome, compared with 47,XXY Klinefelter patients. J Clin Endocrinol Metab. 2007;92(9):3458–65. https://doi.org/10.1210/jc.2007-0447.
42. Sutton E, Hughes J, White S, et al. Identification of SOX3 as an XX male sex reversal gene in mice and humans. J Clin Invest. 2011;121(1):328–41. https://doi.org/10.1172/jci42580.

43. Chiang HS, Wu YN, Wu CC, Hwang JL. Cytogenic and molecular analyses of 46,XX male syndrome with clinical comparison to other groups with testicular azoospermia of genetic origin. J Formos Med Assoc. 2013;112(2):72–8. https://doi.org/10.1016/j.jfma.2012.02.009.
44. Okutman O, Rhouma MB, Benkhalifa M, Muller J, Viville S. Genetic evaluation of patients with non-syndromic male infertility. J Assist Reprod Genet. 2018;35(11):1939–51. https://doi.org/10.1007/s10815-018-1301-7.
45. De Braekeleer M, Dao TN. Cytogenetic studies in male infertility: a review. Hum Reprod. 1991;6(2):245–50.
46. Alhalabi M, Kenj M, Monem F, Mahayri Z, Abou Alchamat G, Madania A. High prevalence of genetic abnormalities in Middle Eastern patients with idiopathic non-obstructive azoospermia. J Assist Reprod Genet. 2013;30(6):799–805. https://doi.org/10.1007/s10815-013-9995-z.
47. Amouri A, Hammami W, Kilani O, et al. Chromosomal evaluation in a group of Tunisian patients with non-obstructive azoospermia and severe oligozoospermia attending a Tunisian cytogenetic department. C R Biol. 2014;337(4):223–8. https://doi.org/10.1016/j.crvi.2014.02.006.
48. Arafa MM, Majzoub A, AlSaid SS, et al. Chromosomal abnormalities in infertile men with azoospermia and severe oligozoospermia in Qatar and their association with sperm retrieval intracytoplasmic sperm injection outcomes. Arab J Urol. 2018;16(1):132–9. https://doi.org/10.1016/j.aju.2017.11.009.
49. Xie C, Chen X, Liu Y, Wu Z, Ping P. Multicenter study of genetic abnormalities associated with severe oligospermia and non-obstructive azoospermia. J Int Med Res. 2018;46(1):107–14. https://doi.org/10.1177/0300060517718771.
50. Chen X, Zhou C. Reciprocal translocation and Robertsonian translocation in relation to semen parameters: a retrospective study and systematic review. Andrologia. 2022;54(1):e14262. https://doi.org/10.1111/and.14262.
51. Mayeur A, Ahdad N, Hesters L, et al. Chromosomal translocations and semen quality: a study on 144 male translocation carriers. Reprod Biomed Online. 2019;38(1):46–55. https://doi.org/10.1016/j.rbmo.2018.10.003.
52. Ma S, Yuen BH, Penaherrera M, Koehn D, Ness L, Robinson W. ICSI and the transmission of X-autosomal translocation: a three-generation evaluation of X;20 translocation: case report. Hum Reprod. 2003;18(7):1377–82. https://doi.org/10.1093/humrep/deg247.
53. Barišić A, Buretić Tomljanović A, Starčević Čizmarević N, Ostojić S, Romac P, Vraneković J. A rare Y-autosome translocation found in a patient with nonobstructive azoospermia: case report. Syst Biol Reprod Med. 2021;67(4):307–13. https://doi.org/10.1080/19396368.2021.1898701.
54. Sasagawa I, Nakada T, Adachi Y, et al. Y-autosome translocation associated with azoospermia. Scand J Urol Nephrol. 1993;27(2):285–8. https://doi.org/10.3109/00365599309181269.
55. Takeda T, Iwatsuki S, Hamakawa T, et al. Chromosomal anomalies and sperm retrieval outcomes of patients with non-obstructive azoospermia: a case series. Andrology. 2017;5(3):473–6. https://doi.org/10.1111/andr.12338.
56. Majzoub A, Arafa M, Clemens H, et al. A systemic review and meta-analysis exploring the predictors of sperm retrieval in patients with non-obstructive azoospermia and chromosomal abnormalities. Andrologia. 2022;54(3):e14303. https://doi.org/10.1111/and.14303.
57. Pylyp LY, Zukin VD, Bilko NM. Chromosomal segregation in sperm of Robertsonian translocation carriers. J Assist Reprod Genet. 2013;30(9):1141–5. https://doi.org/10.1007/s10815-013-0067-1.
58. Collodel G, Moretti E, Capitani S, et al. TEM, FISH and molecular studies in infertile men with pericentric inversion of chromosome 9. Andrologia. 2006;38(4):122–7. https://doi.org/10.1111/j.1439-0272.2006.00725.x.
59. Ghorbel M, Baklouti-Gargouri S, ElGhazel H, et al. Pericentric inversion of chromosom 12 [Inv (12) (p12q12)] associated with idiopathic azoospermia in one infertile Tunisian

man. Biochem Biophys Res Commun. 2013;432(3):472–4. https://doi.org/10.1016/j.bbrc.2013.01.110.
60. Ichioka K, Yoshimura K, Honda T, Takahashi A, Terai A. Paracentric inversion of chromosome 7(q22-31) associated with nonobstructive azoospermia. Fertil Steril. 2005;83(2):455–6. https://doi.org/10.1016/j.fertnstert.2004.06.070.
61. Rhie A, Nurk S, Cechova M, et al. The complete sequence of a human Y chromosome. Nature. 2023;621(7978):344–54. https://doi.org/10.1038/s41586-023-06457-y.
62. Krausz C, Degl'Innocenti S. Y chromosome and male infertility: update, 2006. Front Biosci. 2006;11:3049–61. https://doi.org/10.2741/2032.
63. Tiepolo L, Zuffardi O. Localization of factors controlling spermatogenesis in the nonfluorescent portion of the human Y chromosome long arm. Hum Genet. 1976;34(2):119–24. https://doi.org/10.1007/bf00278879.
64. Vogt PH, Edelmann A, Kirsch S, et al. Human Y chromosome azoospermia factors (AZF) mapped to different subregions in Yq11. Hum Mol Genet. 1996;5(7):933–43. https://doi.org/10.1093/hmg/5.7.933.
65. Kuroda-Kawaguchi T, Skaletsky H, Brown LG, et al. The AZFc region of the Y chromosome features massive palindromes and uniform recurrent deletions in infertile men. Nat Genet. 2001;29(3):279–86. https://doi.org/10.1038/ng757.
66. Krausz C, Navarro-Costa P, Wilke M, Tüttelmann F. EAA/EMQN best practice guidelines for molecular diagnosis of Y-chromosomal microdeletions: State of the art 2023. Andrology. 2024;12(3):487–504. https://doi.org/10.1111/andr.13514.
67. Vogt PH, Zimmer J, Bender U, Strowitzki T. AZFa candidate gene UTY and its X homologue UTX are expressed in human germ cells. Reprod Fertil. 2021;2(2):151–60. https://doi.org/10.1530/raf-20-0049.
68. Ginalski K, Rychlewski L, Baker D, Grishin NV. Protein structure prediction for the male-specific region of the human Y chromosome. Proc Natl Acad Sci USA. 2004;101(8):2305–10. https://doi.org/10.1073/pnas.0306306101.
69. Tyler-Smith C, Krausz C. The will-o'-the-wisp of genetics–hunting for the azoospermia factor gene. N Engl J Med. 2009;360(9):925–7. https://doi.org/10.1056/NEJMe0900301.
70. Mohr S, Stryker JM, Lambowitz AM. A DEAD-box protein functions as an ATP-dependent RNA chaperone in group I intron splicing. Cell. 2002;109(6):769–79. https://doi.org/10.1016/s0092-8674(02)00771-7.
71. Dicke AK, Pilatz A, Wyrwoll MJ, et al. DDX3Y is likely the key spermatogenic factor in the AZFa region that contributes to human non-obstructive azoospermia. Commun Biol. 2023;6(1):350. https://doi.org/10.1038/s42003-023-04714-4.
72. Kamp C, Hirschmann P, Voss H, Huellen K, Vogt PH. Two long homologous retroviral sequence blocks in proximal Yq11 cause AZFa microdeletions as a result of intrachromosomal recombination events. Hum Mol Genet. 2000;9(17):2563–72. https://doi.org/10.1093/hmg/9.17.2563.
73. Repping S, Skaletsky H, Lange J, et al. Recombination between palindromes P5 and P1 on the human Y chromosome causes massive deletions and spermatogenic failure. Am J Hum Genet. 2002;71(4):906–22. https://doi.org/10.1086/342928.
74. Lo Giacco D, Chianese C, Sánchez-Curbelo J, et al. Clinical relevance of Y-linked CNV screening in male infertility: new insights based on the 8-year experience of a diagnostic genetic laboratory. Eur J Hum Genet. 2014;22(6):754–61. https://doi.org/10.1038/ejhg.2013.253.
75. Calogero AE, Garofalo MR, Barone N, et al. Spontaneous regression over time of the germinal epithelium in a Y chromosome-microdeleted patient: case report. Hum Reprod. 2001;16(9):1845–8. https://doi.org/10.1093/humrep/16.9.1845.
76. Oates RD, Silber S, Brown LG, Page DC. Clinical characterization of 42 oligospermic or azoospermic men with microdeletion of the AZFc region of the Y chromosome, and of 18 children conceived via ICSI. Hum Reprod. 2002;17(11):2813–24. https://doi.org/10.1093/humrep/17.11.2813.

77. Stouffs K, Vloeberghs V, Gheldof A, Tournaye H, Seneca S. Are AZFb deletions always incompatible with sperm production? Andrology. 2017;5(4):691–4. https://doi.org/10.1111/andr.12350.
78. Flannigan R, Schlegel PN. Genetic diagnostics of male infertility in clinical practice. Best Pract Res Clin Obstet Gynaecol. 2017;44:26–37. https://doi.org/10.1016/j.bpobgyn.2017.05.002.
79. Jaruzelska J, Korcz A, Wojda A, et al. Mosaicism for 45,X cell line may accentuate the severity of spermatogenic defects in men with AZFc deletion. J Med Genet. 2001;38(11):798–802. https://doi.org/10.1136/jmg.38.11.798.
80. Le Bourhis C, Siffroi JP, McElreavey K, Dadoune JP. Y chromosome microdeletions and germinal mosaicism in infertile males. Mol Hum Reprod. 2000;6(8):688–93. https://doi.org/10.1093/molehr/6.8.688.
81. Patsalis PC, Skordis N, Sismani C, et al. Identification of high frequency of Y chromosome deletions in patients with sex chromosome mosaicism and correlation with the clinical phenotype and Y-chromosome instability. Am J Med Genet A. 2005;135(2):145–9. https://doi.org/10.1002/ajmg.a.30712.
82. Siffroi JP, Le Bourhis C, Krausz C, et al. Sex chromosome mosaicism in males carrying Y chromosome long arm deletions. Hum Reprod. 2000;15(12):2559–62. https://doi.org/10.1093/humrep/15.12.2559.
83. Kasak L, Laan M. Monogenic causes of non-obstructive azoospermia: challenges, established knowledge, limitations and perspectives. Hum Genet. 2021;140(1):135–54. https://doi.org/10.1007/s00439-020-02112-y.
84. Boehm U, Bouloux PM, Dattani MT, et al. Expert consensus document: European Consensus Statement on congenital hypogonadotropic hypogonadism–pathogenesis, diagnosis and treatment. Nat Rev Endocrinol. 2015;11(9):547–64. https://doi.org/10.1038/nrendo.2015.112.
85. Young J, Xu C, Papadakis GE, et al. Clinical management of congenital hypogonadotropic hypogonadism. Endocr Rev. 2019;40(2):669–710. https://doi.org/10.1210/er.2018-00116.
86. Laitinen EM, Vaaralahti K, Tommiska J, et al. Incidence, phenotypic features and molecular genetics of Kallmann syndrome in Finland. Orphanet J Rare Dis. 2011;6:41. https://doi.org/10.1186/1750-1172-6-41.
87. Chan C, Wang CW, Chen CH, Chen CH. Live birth in male de novo Kallmann syndrome after cross-generational genetic sequencing. J Assist Reprod Genet. 2019;36(12):2481–4. https://doi.org/10.1007/s10815-019-01604-9.
88. Dodé C, Hardelin JP. Kallmann syndrome. Eur J Hum Genet. 2009;17(2):139–46. https://doi.org/10.1038/ejhg.2008.206.
89. Maione L, Dwyer AA, Francou B, et al. Genetics in endocrinology: genetic counseling for congenital hypogonadotropic hypogonadism and Kallmann syndrome: new challenges in the era of oligogenism and next-generation sequencing. Eur J Endocrinol. 2018;178(3):R55–r80. https://doi.org/10.1530/eje-17-0749.
90. Dodé C, Hardelin JP. Clinical genetics of Kallmann syndrome. Ann Endocrinol (Paris). 2010;71(3):149–57. https://doi.org/10.1016/j.ando.2010.02.005.
91. Thakker S, Persily J, Najari BB. Kallman syndrome and central non-obstructive azoospermia. Best Pract Res Clin Endocrinol Metab. 2020;34(6):101475. https://doi.org/10.1016/j.beem.2020.101475.
92. Liu Y, Zhi X. Advances in genetic diagnosis of Kallmann syndrome and genetic interruption. Reprod Sci. 2022;29(6):1697–709. https://doi.org/10.1007/s43032-021-00638-8.
93. Punab M, Poolamets O, Paju P, et al. Causes of male infertility: a 9-year prospective monocentre study on 1737 patients with reduced total sperm counts. Hum Reprod. 2017;32(1):18–31. https://doi.org/10.1093/humrep/dew284.
94. Tüttelmann F, Werny F, Cooper TG, Kliesch S, Simoni M, Nieschlag E. Clinical experience with azoospermia: aetiology and chances for spermatozoa detection upon biopsy. Int J Androl. 2011;34(4):291–8. https://doi.org/10.1111/j.1365-2605.2010.01087.x.
95. Yin H, Ma H, Hussain S, et al. A homozygous FANCM frameshift pathogenic variant causes male infertility. Genet Med. 2019;21(1):62–70. https://doi.org/10.1038/s41436-018-0015-7.

96. Krausz C, Riera-Escamilla A, Chianese C, et al. From exome analysis in idiopathic azoospermia to the identification of a high-risk subgroup for occult Fanconi anemia. Genet Med. 2019;21(1):189–94. https://doi.org/10.1038/s41436-018-0037-1.
97. Miyamoto T, Bando Y, Koh E, et al. A PLK4 mutation causing azoospermia in a man with Sertoli cell-only syndrome. Andrology. 2016;4(1):75–81. https://doi.org/10.1111/andr.12113.
98. Fakhro KA, Elbardisi H, Arafa M, et al. Point-of-care whole-exome sequencing of idiopathic male infertility. Genet Med. 2018;20(11):1365–73. https://doi.org/10.1038/gim.2018.10.
99. Llano E, Pendás AM. Synaptonemal complex in human biology and disease. Cells. 2023;12(13) https://doi.org/10.3390/cells12131718.
100. Ben Khelifa M, Ghieh F, Boudjenah R, et al. A MEI1 homozygous missense mutation associated with meiotic arrest in a consanguineous family. Hum Reprod. 2018;33(6):1034–7. https://doi.org/10.1093/humrep/dey073.
101. Bolcun-Filas E, Hall E, Speed R, et al. Mutation of the mouse Syce1 gene disrupts synapsis and suggests a link between synaptonemal complex structural components and DNA repair. PLoS Genet. 2009;5(2):e1000393. https://doi.org/10.1371/journal.pgen.1000393.
102. Maor-Sagie E, Cinnamon Y, Yaacov B, et al. Deleterious mutation in SYCE1 is associated with non-obstructive azoospermia. J Assist Reprod Genet. 2015;32(6):887–91. https://doi.org/10.1007/s10815-015-0445-y.
103. Yang F, Silber S, Leu NA, et al. TEX11 is mutated in infertile men with azoospermia and regulates genome-wide recombination rates in mouse. EMBO Mol Med. 2015;7(9):1198–210. https://doi.org/10.15252/emmm.201404967.
104. Yatsenko AN, Georgiadis AP, Röpke A, et al. X-linked TEX11 mutations, meiotic arrest, and azoospermia in infertile men. N Engl J Med. 2015;372(22):2097–107. https://doi.org/10.1056/NEJMoa1406192.
105. Nakamura S, Miyado M, Saito K, et al. Next-generation sequencing for patients with non-obstructive azoospermia: implications for significant roles of monogenic/oligogenic mutations. Andrology. 2017;5(4):824–31. https://doi.org/10.1111/andr.12378.
106. Sha Y, Zheng L, Ji Z, et al. A novel TEX11 mutation induces azoospermia: a case report of infertile brothers and literature review. BMC Med Genet. 2018;19(1):63. https://doi.org/10.1186/s12881-018-0570-4.
107. Okutman O, Muller J, Baert Y, et al. Exome sequencing reveals a nonsense mutation in TEX15 causing spermatogenic failure in a Turkish family. Hum Mol Genet. 2015;24(19):5581–8. https://doi.org/10.1093/hmg/ddv290.
108. Colombo R, Pontoglio A, Bini M. Two novel TEX15 mutations in a family with non-obstructive azoospermia. Gynecol Obstet Investig. 2017;82(3):283–6. https://doi.org/10.1159/000468934.
109. Luo M, Yang F, Leu NA, et al. MEIOB exhibits single-stranded DNA-binding and exonuclease activities and is essential for meiotic recombination. Nat Commun. 2013;4:2788. https://doi.org/10.1038/ncomms3788.
110. Souquet B, Abby E, Hervé R, et al. MEIOB targets single-strand DNA and is necessary for meiotic recombination. PLoS Genet. 2013;9(9):e1003784. https://doi.org/10.1371/journal.pgen.1003784.
111. Gershoni M, Hauser R, Barda S, et al. A new MEIOB mutation is a recurrent cause for azoospermia and testicular meiotic arrest. Hum Reprod. 2019;34(4):666–71. https://doi.org/10.1093/humrep/dez016.
112. Gershoni M, Hauser R, Yogev L, et al. A familial study of azoospermic men identifies three novel causative mutations in three new human azoospermia genes. Genet Med. 2017;19(9):998–1006. https://doi.org/10.1038/gim.2016.225.
113. He WB, Tu CF, Liu Q, et al. DMC1 mutation that causes human non-obstructive azoospermia and premature ovarian insufficiency identified by whole-exome sequencing. J Med Genet. 2018;55(3):198–204. https://doi.org/10.1136/jmedgenet-2017-104992.
114. Riera-Escamilla A, Enguita-Marruedo A, Moreno-Mendoza D, et al. Sequencing of a 'mouse azoospermia' gene panel in azoospermic men: identification of RNF212 and STAG3 muta-

tions as novel genetic causes of meiotic arrest. Hum Reprod. 2019;34(6):978–88. https://doi.org/10.1093/humrep/dez042.
115. van der Bijl N, Röpke A, Biswas U, et al. Mutations in the stromal antigen 3 (STAG3) gene cause male infertility due to meiotic arrest. Hum Reprod. 2019;34(11):2112–9. https://doi.org/10.1093/humrep/dez204.
116. Veitia RA, Nunes M, Quintana-Murci L, et al. Swyer syndrome and 46,XY partial gonadal dysgenesis associated with 9p deletions in the absence of monosomy 9p syndrome. Am J Hum Genet. 1998;63(3):901–5. https://doi.org/10.1086/302023.
117. Lopes AM, Aston KI, Thompson E, et al. Human spermatogenic failure purges deleterious mutation load from the autosomes and both sex chromosomes, including the gene DMRT1. PLoS Genet. 2013;9(3):e1003349. https://doi.org/10.1371/journal.pgen.1003349.
118. Krausz C, Riera-Escamilla A, Moreno-Mendoza D, et al. Genetic dissection of spermatogenic arrest through exome analysis: clinical implications for the management of azoospermic men. Genet Med. 2020;22(12):1956–66. https://doi.org/10.1038/s41436-020-0907-1.
119. Greenbaum MP, Iwamori T, Buchold GM, Matzuk MM. Germ cell intercellular bridges. Cold Spring Harb Perspect Biol. 2011;3(8):a005850. https://doi.org/10.1101/cshperspect.a005850.
120. Ruan J, He XJ, Du WD, et al. Genetic variants in TEX15 gene conferred susceptibility to spermatogenic failure in the Chinese Han population. Reprod Sci. 2012;19(11):1190–6. https://doi.org/10.1177/1933719112446076.
121. Saba R, Kato Y, Saga Y. NANOS2 promotes male germ cell development independent of meiosis suppression. Dev Biol. 2014;385(1):32–40. https://doi.org/10.1016/j.ydbio.2013.10.018.
122. Kusz-Zamelczyk K, Sajek M, Spik A, et al. Mutations of NANOS1, a human homologue of the Drosophila morphogen, are associated with a lack of germ cells in testes or severe oligo-astheno-teratozoospermia. J Med Genet. 2013;50(3):187–93. https://doi.org/10.1136/jmedgenet-2012-101230.
123. Nachtigal MW, Hirokawa Y, Enyeart-VanHouten DL, Flanagan JN, Hammer GD, Ingraham HA. Wilms' tumor 1 and Dax-1 modulate the orphan nuclear receptor SF-1 in sex-specific gene expression. Cell. 1998;93(3):445–54. https://doi.org/10.1016/s0092-8674(00)81172-1.
124. Cools M, Nordenström A, Robeva R, et al. Caring for individuals with a difference of sex development (DSD): a consensus statement. Nat Rev Endocrinol. 2018;14(7):415–29. https://doi.org/10.1038/s41574-018-0010-8.
125. Ferlin A, Rocca MS, Vinanzi C, Ghezzi M, Di Nisio A, Foresta C. Mutational screening of NR5A1 gene encoding steroidogenic factor 1 in cryptorchidism and male factor infertility and functional analysis of seven undescribed mutations. Fertil Steril. 2015;104(1):163–9.e1. https://doi.org/10.1016/j.fertnstert.2015.04.017.
126. Bashamboo A, Ferraz-de-Souza B, Lourenço D, et al. Human male infertility associated with mutations in NR5A1 encoding steroidogenic factor 1. Am J Hum Genet. 2010;87(4):505–12. https://doi.org/10.1016/j.ajhg.2010.09.009.
127. Eggers S, Sadedin S, van den Bergen JA, et al. Disorders of sex development: insights from targeted gene sequencing of a large international patient cohort. Genome Biol. 2016;17(1):243. https://doi.org/10.1186/s13059-016-1105-y.
128. Ferraz-de-Souza B, Lin L, Achermann JC. Steroidogenic factor-1 (SF-1, NR5A1) and human disease. Mol Cell Endocrinol. 2011;336(1–2):198–205. https://doi.org/10.1016/j.mce.2010.11.006.
129. Zare-Abdollahi D, Safari S, Mirfakhraie R, et al. Mutational screening of the NR5A1 in azoospermia. Andrologia. 2015;47(4):395–401. https://doi.org/10.1111/and.12274.
130. Köhler B, Biebermann H, Friedsam V, et al. Analysis of the Wilms' tumor suppressor gene (WT1) in patients 46,XY disorders of sex development. J Clin Endocrinol Metab. 2011;96(7):E1131–6. https://doi.org/10.1210/jc.2010-2804.
131. Arafat M, Har-Vardi I, Harlev A, et al. Mutation in TDRD9 causes non-obstructive azoospermia in infertile men. J Med Genet. 2017;54(9):633–9. https://doi.org/10.1136/jmedgenet-2017-104514.

132. Shoji M, Tanaka T, Hosokawa M, et al. The TDRD9-MIWI2 complex is essential for piRNA-mediated retrotransposon silencing in the mouse male germline. Dev Cell. 2009;17(6):775–87. https://doi.org/10.1016/j.devcel.2009.10.012.
133. Ayhan Ö, Balkan M, Guven A, et al. Truncating mutations in TAF4B and ZMYND15 causing recessive azoospermia. J Med Genet. 2014;51(4):239–44. https://doi.org/10.1136/jmedgenet-2013-102102.
134. Wyrwoll MJ, Temel ŞG, Nagirnaja L, et al. Bi-allelic mutations in M1AP are a frequent cause of meiotic arrest and severely impaired spermatogenesis leading to male infertility. Am J Hum Genet. 2020;107(2):342–51. https://doi.org/10.1016/j.ajhg.2020.06.010.
135. Zhao W, Sung P. Significance of ligand interactions involving Hop2-Mnd1 and the RAD51 and DMC1 recombinases in homologous DNA repair and XX ovarian dysgenesis. Nucleic Acids Res. 2015;43(8):4055–66. https://doi.org/10.1093/nar/gkv259.
136. Sansam CL, Pezza RJ. Connecting by breaking and repairing: mechanisms of DNA strand exchange in meiotic recombination. FEBS J. 2015;282(13):2444–57. https://doi.org/10.1111/febs.13317.
137. Al-Agha AE, Ahmed IA, Nuebel E, et al. Primary ovarian insufficiency and azoospermia in carriers of a homozygous PSMC3IP stop gain mutation. J Clin Endocrinol Metab. 2018;103(2):555–63. https://doi.org/10.1210/jc.2017-01966.
138. Griffin WC, Trakselis MA. The MCM8/9 complex: a recent recruit to the roster of helicases involved in genome maintenance. DNA Repair (Amst). 2019;76:1–10. https://doi.org/10.1016/j.dnarep.2019.02.003.
139. Tenenbaum-Rakover Y, Weinberg-Shukron A, Renbaum P, et al. Minichromosome maintenance complex component 8 (MCM8) gene mutations result in primary gonadal failure. J Med Genet. 2015;52(6):391–9. https://doi.org/10.1136/jmedgenet-2014-102921.
140. Klami R, Mankonen H, Perheentupa A. Successful microdissection testicular sperm extraction for men with non-obstructive azoospermia. Reprod Biol. 2018;18(2):137–42. https://doi.org/10.1016/j.repbio.2018.03.003.
141. Shin DH, Turek PJ. Sperm retrieval techniques. Nat Rev Urol. 2013;10(12):723–30. https://doi.org/10.1038/nrurol.2013.262.
142. Bernie AM, Mata DA, Ramasamy R, Schlegel PN. Comparison of microdissection testicular sperm extraction, conventional testicular sperm extraction, and testicular sperm aspiration for nonobstructive azoospermia: a systematic review and meta-analysis. Fertil Steril. 2015;104(5):1099–103.e1–3. https://doi.org/10.1016/j.fertnstert.2015.07.1136.
143. Saccà A, Pastore AL, Roscigno M, et al. Conventional testicular sperm extraction (TESE) and non-obstructive azoospermia: is there still a chance in the era of microdissection TESE? Results from a single non-academic community hospital. Andrology. 2016;4(3):425–9. https://doi.org/10.1111/andr.12159.
144. Ghalayini IF, Al-Ghazo MA, Hani OB, et al. Clinical comparison of conventional testicular sperm extraction and microdissection techniques for non-obstructive azoospermia. J Clin Med Res. 2011;3(3):124–31. https://doi.org/10.4021/jocmr542w.
145. Corona G, Minhas S, Giwercman A, et al. Sperm recovery and ICSI outcomes in men with non-obstructive azoospermia: a systematic review and meta-analysis. Hum Reprod Update. 2019;25(6):733–57. https://doi.org/10.1093/humupd/dmz028.
146. Bernie AM, Ramasamy R, Schlegel PN. Predictive factors of successful microdissection testicular sperm extraction. Basic Clin Androl. 2013;23:5. https://doi.org/10.1186/2051-4190-23-5.
147. Ramasamy R, Trivedi NN, Reifsnyder JE, Palermo GD, Rosenwaks Z, Schlegel PN. Age does not adversely affect sperm retrieval in men undergoing microdissection testicular sperm extraction. Fertil Steril. 2014;101(3):653–5. https://doi.org/10.1016/j.fertnstert.2013.11.123.
148. Gies I, Oates R, De Schepper J, Tournaye H. Testicular biopsy and cryopreservation for fertility preservation of prepubertal boys with Klinefelter syndrome: a pro/con debate. Fertil Steril. 2016;105(2):249–55. https://doi.org/10.1016/j.fertnstert.2015.12.011.
149. Aksglaede L, Juul A. Testicular function and fertility in men with Klinefelter syndrome: a review. Eur J Endocrinol. 2013;168(4):R67–76. https://doi.org/10.1530/eje-12-0934.

150. Hopps CV, Mielnik A, Goldstein M, Palermo GD, Rosenwaks Z, Schlegel PN. Detection of sperm in men with Y chromosome microdeletions of the AZFa, AZFb and AZFc regions. Hum Reprod. 2003;18(8):1660–5. https://doi.org/10.1093/humrep/deg348.
151. Stahl PJ, Masson P, Mielnik A, Marean MB, Schlegel PN, Paduch DA. A decade of experience emphasizes that testing for Y microdeletions is essential in American men with azoospermia and severe oligozoospermia. Fertil Steril. 2010;94(5):1753–6. https://doi.org/10.1016/j.fertnstert.2009.09.006.
152. Lu Y, Liu L, Zhang P, Sun Y, Ma C, Li Y. Risk of birth defects in children conceived with assisted reproductive technology: a meta-analysis. Medicine (Baltimore). 2022;101(52):e32405. https://doi.org/10.1097/md.0000000000032405.
153. Wilkes S, Chinn DJ, Murdoch A, Rubin G. Epidemiology and management of infertility: a population-based study in UK primary care. Fam Pract. 2009;26(4):269–74. https://doi.org/10.1093/fampra/cmp029.
154. Yu XW, Wei ZT, Jiang YT, Zhang SL. Y chromosome azoospermia factor region microdeletions and transmission characteristics in azoospermic and severe oligozoospermic patients. Int J Clin Exp Med. 2015;8(9):14634–46.
155. Sueoka K. Preimplantation genetic diagnosis: an update on current technologies and ethical considerations. Reprod Med Biol. 2016;15(2):69–75. https://doi.org/10.1007/s12522-015-0224-6.
156. Batzer FR, Ravitsky V. Preimplantation genetic diagnosis. In: The Penn Center guide to bioethics, vol. 339; 2009.
157. Liebaers I, Desmyttere S, Verpoest W, et al. Report on a consecutive series of 581 children born after blastomere biopsy for preimplantation genetic diagnosis. Hum Reprod. 2010;25(1):275–82. https://doi.org/10.1093/humrep/dep298.
158. De Wert G, Dondorp W, Shenfield F, et al. ESHRE task force on ethics and Law22: preimplantation genetic diagnosis. Hum Reprod. 2014;29(8):1610–7. https://doi.org/10.1093/humrep/deu132.

Chapter 4
Differentiation Between OA and NOA

Taymour Mostafa, Germar-Michael Pinggera, and Giovanni M. Colpi

Introduction

The prevalence of male infertility, which affects up to 6% of men in North America and at least 30 million men worldwide, is increasing within the global population, with azoospermia accounting for 10–15% of cases among infertile males [1, 2]. Furthermore, recent studies have elucidated a conspicuous downward trajectory in various semen parameters, a trend that has become increasingly evident over the past two decades and appears to impact even young males [3, 4]. Applying a meta-regression model adjusted for several confounding factors, the annual decreases in the sperm concentration (SC) and total sperm count (TSC) were −1.2% and −1.4%, respectively, before 1972, increasing to corresponding annual decreases of −2.6% and −2.5%, respectively, for the investigated period after 2000 [4]. Regardless of the cause of such sperm deterioration over time and the fact that sperm parameters such as SC or TSC are considered imperfect indicators of male fertility, these findings are nevertheless strongly negatively linked to fertility and/or pregnancy worldwide.

Azoospermia is an extreme case in male fertility diagnostics related to the inability to conceive spontaneously by natural means. The World Health Organization defines azoospermia as the absence of spermatozoa in the ejaculate following centrifugation and subsequent microscopy of the specimen on two separate semen analyses [5]. Yet, this definition in spermiogram evaluation is descriptive in nature

T. Mostafa (✉)
Faculty of Medicine, Department of Andrology, Sexology & STIs, Cairo University, Cairo, Egypt

G.-M. Pinggera
Department of Urology, Medical University Innsbruck, Innsbruck, Austria

G. M. Colpi
Andrology and IVF Center, Next Fertility Procrea, Lugano, Switzerland

W. Zohdy et al. (eds.), *Non-Obstructive Azoospermia*,
https://doi.org/10.1007/978-3-031-99431-9_4

and does not foretell about its etiology, nor does this examination allow any differential diagnosis in the evaluation of azoospermia. Thus, upon encountering a patient with azoospermia who wishes for paternity, a critical initial step for a reproductive specialist is to ascertain whether the condition is attributable to obstructive azoospermia (OA) or nonobstructive azoospermia (NOA).

Although NOA is generally more prevalent, OA is nonetheless significant, impacting an estimated 20–40% of men diagnosed with azoospermia [6]. The etiological factors contributing to both OA and NOA are diverse and include congenital, genetic, physiological, surgical, inflammatory, and environmental factors. This variability in origins necessitates a tailored approach to clinical management and treatment strategies, underlining the importance of a thorough diagnostic process. Identifying the specific type of azoospermia not only informs the choice of intervention but also has implications for the prognosis and potential for fertility restoration.

In general, for the diagnosis of NOA, confirmatory results from at least two sperm investigations are requested. Currently, surgical interventions such as microsurgical testicular sperm extraction (micro-TESE) and high-power optical field instruments for sperm retrieval, in combination with advancements in assisted reproductive technology (ART), are the central focus of NOA therapy [7]. On the other hand, reconstructive interventions such as vasovasostomy, epididymovasostomy, percutaneous epididymal sperm aspiration (PESA), microsurgical epididymal sperm aspiration (MESA), and TESE are offered for selected OA patients [8, 9].

This chapter aims to present the key points with a clinical focus, offering a guide to essential diagnostic algorithms and options while pointing to additional pertinent literature for further exploration.

Clinical Differentiation

The differentiation between OA and NOA has clinical value because it affects patient management. Severe spermatogenic dysfunction observed in NOA patients is usually a consequence of either primary testicular failure or hypothalamus–pituitary–gonadal axis dysfunction [10]. OA originates from a mechanical obstruction in the reproductive tract, and unlike NOA, spermatogenesis is preserved, and both reconstructive measures and sperm retrieval (SR) are efficacious in these patients [11]. NOA can be distinguished from OA in most cases based on a detailed history, clinical examination, semen analysis, hormonal assessment, imaging, and genetic testing.

A. **Detailed Medical History**

A detailed history is essential in these cases regarding the history of offsprings from previous marriage, delayed puberty, trauma to the genital organs, undescended or migrant testicles, drug allergies, medication history (gonadotropins, anabolic steroids, testosterone supplementation, toxins), chemotherapy, pesticide, hernia repair, and radiation exposure that must be obtained. Additionally, the history of genitourinary infections, sexually transmitted diseases, and endocrine surgery such as removal of adenomas must be evaluated in detail [10, 12].

B. **Clinical Examination**

1. Secondary sexual characteristics: Abnormal body hair distribution and gynecomastia may indicate hypogonadism or hormonal disturbances [13].
2. Inguinal region: Scars of previous surgeries that might injure the testicular blood supply or the vas deferens.
3. Penile anomalies (hypospadias, epispadias, fibrotic nodules).
4. The testis: Testicular size, texture, and consistency should be assessed. Testicular volume is estimated using Prader's orchidometer, with a mean testicular volume of 20.0 ± 5.0 mL. The testes of men with OA have a firm texture, while those of men with NOA usually are small (<15 mL) [14]. However, testicular size is not a reliable parameter for distinguishing OA from NOA, as both OA patients and those with NOA exhibiting maturation arrest (MA) may present with normal testicular volumes. Furthermore, no definitive threshold for testicular size has been established that can reliably predict the absence of successful SR in men with NOA patients [15].
5. The vas deferens and the epididymis: Patients with NOA typically have palpable vasa deferentia and flat epididymides. Congenital bilateral absence of the vas deferens (CBAVD) is associated with OA: in the majority of these cases, the head of the epididymis is only felt, and hypoplasia of the seminal vesicles is detected by trans-rectal ultrasound [16, 17].
6. Spermatic cord: Although varicocele is not uncommon in azoospermic men, it is debatable whether it is linked to spermatogenesis disruption in those patients. It has been shown that varicocele repair might ameliorate spermatogenesis and androgen production in some NOA patients [18].

C. **Semen Analysis**

An azoospermic ejaculate with a normal volume (>1.5 mL) should be followed by examination of the pelleted semen after centrifugation (3000 × g for >15 min) to exclude rare sperm in at least two consecutive semen analyses with an interval between them to avoid temporary azoospermia [19]. Ejaculates of men with NOA usually display normal semen volume and pH (>7.2), indicating functional seminal vesicles and patent ejaculatory ducts. A combination of a low volume (<1.5 mL), acidic ejaculate (pH <7.2), and low fructose (<13 μmol/ejaculate) indicates seminal vesicle hypoplasia or obstruction, which are usually associated with OA cases of CBAVD and ejaculatory duct obstruction [10, 20].

D. **Hormonal Assessment**

Serum follicle-stimulating hormone (FSH) and testosterone (T) are the essential hormones driving spermatogenesis. Adequate levels of intratesticular T are critical for sperm maturation, whereas FSH cooperates with intratesticular T to promote cell proliferation [21]. Usually, there is an inverse relationship between FSH levels and spermatogonial quantity and between the proportion of seminiferous tubules exhibiting Sertoli cell-only characteristics in testicular biopsies [22]. Often, patients with NOA present with elevated FSH (>7.6 mIU/mL) and frequently low T (<300 ng/dL) levels, whereas those with OA have normal FSH and T levels. Low FSH levels (<1.5 mIU/mL), combined with low luteinizing hormone (LH) (<1.5 mIU/mL), and low T levels (<300 ng/dL) indicate secondary hypogonadotropic hypogonadism. Serum estradiol (E2) should be measured in NOA men when there is an alteration in T concentration, obesity, a polluted workplace occupation, or before hormonal therapy [23]. In addition, elevated levels of serum prolactin (PRL) could have a detrimental effect on spermatogenesis by inhibiting the pulsatile release of gonadotropins from the anterior pituitary gland [24].

E. **Imaging**

The typical first question posed to scrotal ultrasound (US) concerns testicular size, symmetry in volumetry, the testicular parenchymal pattern, [25] blood flow patterns, intratesticular lesions, and the morphological appearance of the adjacent epididymis and the structures within the pampiniform plexus. (Figs. 4.1, 4.2, 4.3, and 4.8) In the case of NOA, there are often testicular dysgenesis (e.g., microlithiasis, heterogeneous testis architecture) or some characteristic signs related to a genetic specific condition, such as the pathological absence in approximately 45–95% of the vas deferens in cystic fibrosis transmembrane conductance regulator (CFTR) mutation carriers, a genetic disease found in approximately 10% of all OA patients, helping the clinician ascertain the correct first diagnosis [17, 26]. This condition often presents as part of the spectrum of CBAVD or, less commonly, with approximately 15% of all vasal abnormalities, such as unilateral absence (CUAVD), when only one vas deferens is missing [27] (Figs. 4.4, 4.5, 4.6, 4.7, 4.8, 4.9, and 4.10).

Imaging vascular networks using color and power Doppler plays a crucial role generally in evaluating a wide array of disease conditions, including testicular hyperemia, ischemia, infarction, and flow patterns in organs, tumors, and blood

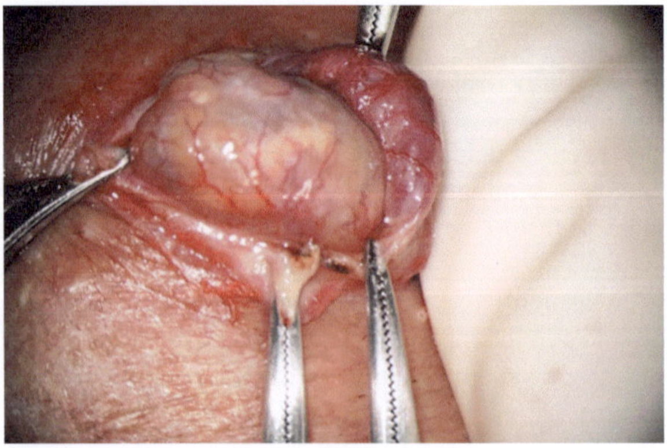

Fig. 4.1 Intraoperative exploration with signs of epididymal obstruction

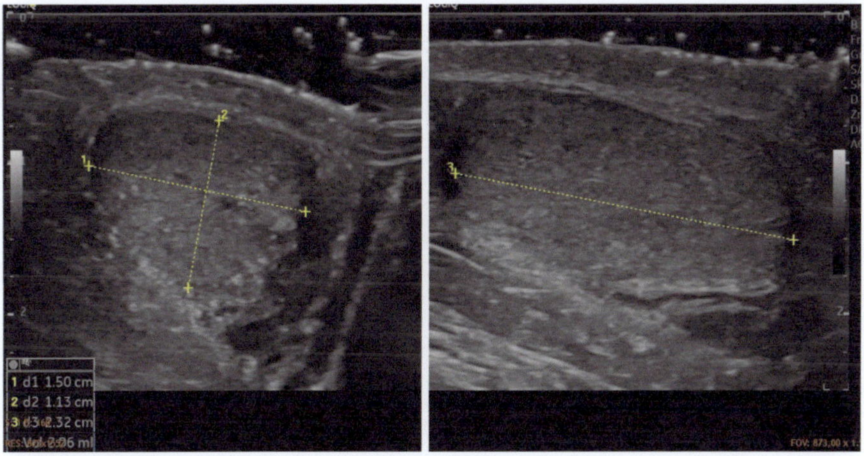

Fig. 4.2 Testicular volumetric measurements in the NOA
High-frequency ultrasound shows the testicle in two axes for volume determination, with a typically reduced testicular volume in idiopathic NOA (measured at 3 ml). On B-mode sonography, a somewhat more inhomogeneous parenchymal pattern is found with multiple punctiform brightening of an overall more inhomogeneous image and no dilatation of the epididymis

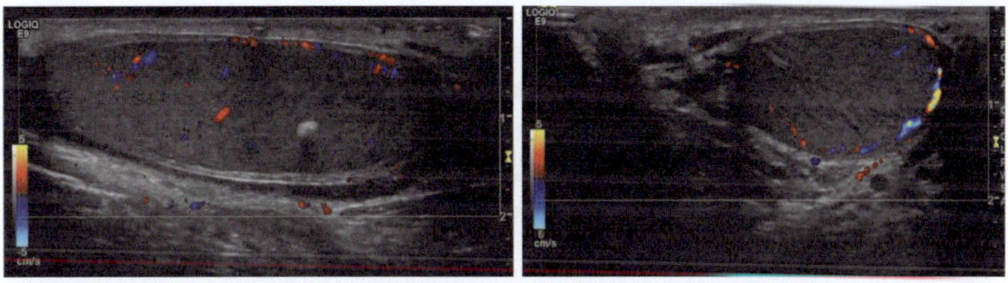

Fig. 4.3 Representative B-mode sonography in NOA testicle. (Courtesy of Dr. Aigner F)
Histologically confirmed SCO NOA testicles by B-mode ultrasound centrally showed solitary hyperechogenic calcification with corresponding dorsal shadowing. With the use of a high-frequency US probe, the retained lobular testicular structure is still recognizable; on Doppler sonography, there is reduced and primarily peripheral and subtunical blood flow with generally asymmetric reduced perfusion in the testicular parenchyma itself

vessels. Varicocele diagnosis is carried out by physical examination in a warm room and confirmed with scrotal Doppler ultrasound.

Moreover, high-resolution US, including microvascular color flow imaging and power Doppler US (PDUS) due to its improved flow sensitivity (with or without the use of specific contrast media or microbubble contrast agents, for example, by applying contrast-enhanced US (CEUS) or spectral Doppler analysis), has improved the assessment of testicular structure and blood flow, potentially indicating areas of

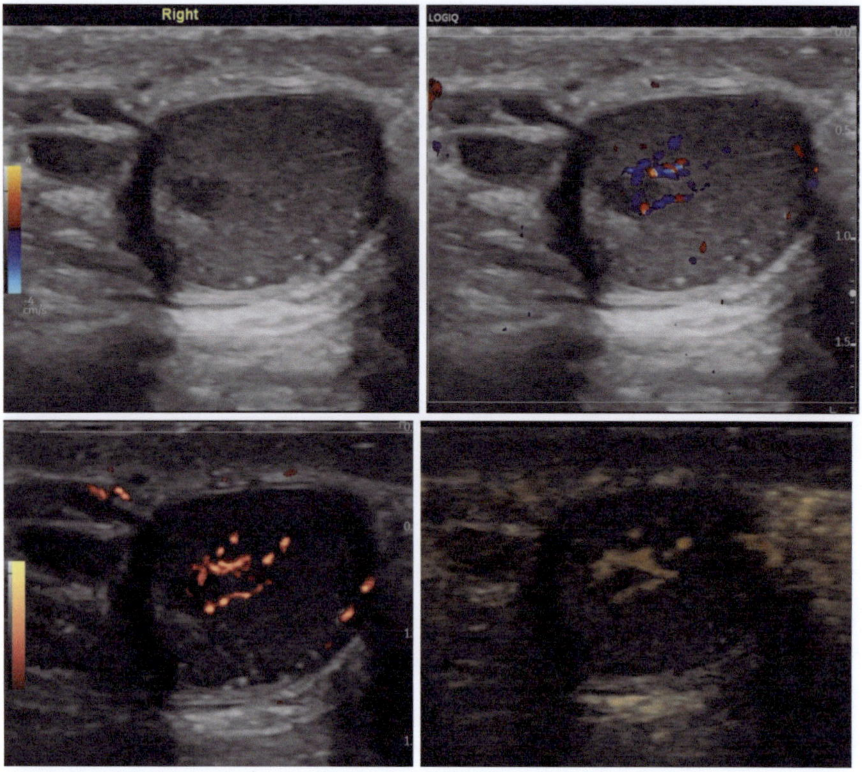

Fig. 4.4 Hypoplastic testicle in the genetically confirmed non-mosaic 47,XXY NOA investigated with different US modalities. (Courtesy of Dr. Aigner F)
In 47,XXY patients, solitary hypoechoic lesions are often found (left image), which histologically correspond to benign Leydig cell hyperplasia. Note the perilesional hypervascularization with central vessels in the simultaneous Doppler ultrasound examination (right image). Direct comparison of ultrasound examinations of the identical testis, using both Doppler (b) and Power Doppler US with central vessels in the simultaneous Doppler ultrasound examination (right image). Direct comparison of ultrasound examinations of the identical testis, using both Doppler (b) and Power Doppler US examination (left below) and differently color-coded measurements with microvascular imaging techniques (right below) in the detection of the smallest low flow capillaries intratesticular showing the higher sensitivity for Microvascular Flow Imaging (MVI) techniques in difficult cases, see Fig below in the actual version = 3,6 XXX

active spermatogenesis or identifying varicoceles that could impact testicular function [27].

Spectral Doppler waveforms are helpful for fast differentiation between arterial and venous blood flows within scrotal structures. Nevertheless, the limiting factor for all these previously mentioned techniques is their ability to detect blood flow in vessels larger than 0.2 mm in diameter [28]. Regarding the extra-testicular arterial supply for the testicle, Raman et al measured the diameter of the testicular artery in the range of 0.2 to 1.9 mm (mean 1.0), that of the vasal artery in the range of 0.2 to

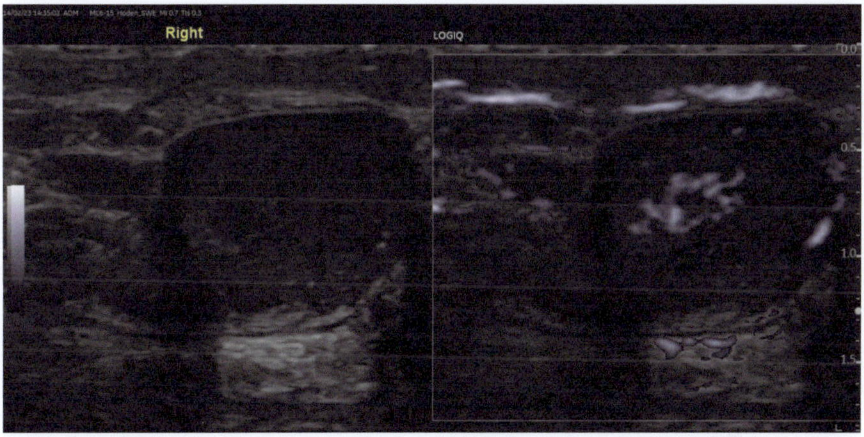

Fig. 4.5 Non-mosaic 47,XXY, B-mode ultrasound showing hypoechogenic lesions in the upper pole (left) and MVI measurements to detect low flow vascularization

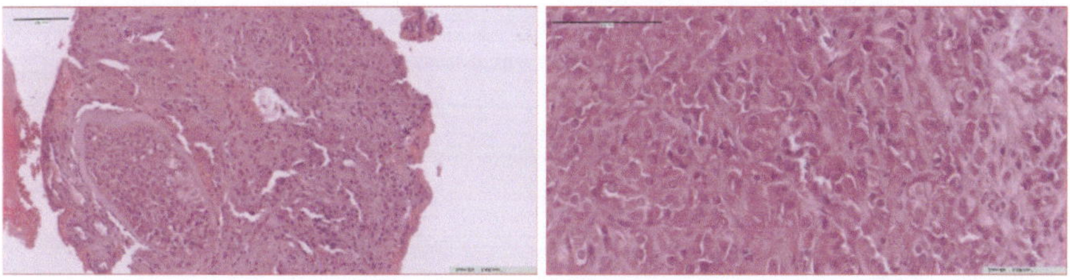

Fig. 4.6 H&E-stained histologic testicular specimen at 20× magnification at 47,XXY with azoospermia in (a) and at 400× magnification without any spermatocyte, corresponding to US investigation in Fig. 4.6. (Courtesy of Dr. Pipp)

1.8 mm (mean 0.6) and that of the cremasteric arteries between 0.1 and 1.5 mm (mean 0.5) [29]. Since intratesticular arteries and capillaries running in a radial fashion between single lobuli are smaller in diameter and exhibit greater variability, particularly in small testes, in NOA patients, there is a need for better microimaging techniques. Thus, to avoid the use of CEUS and to enhance perfusion detection, as defined as a measurement of blood flow over time, novel technical adaptations allowing the filtering of random motion effects in vessels and preserving the imaging of directional blood flow have recently been introduced. Compared with traditional ultrasound techniques, this advanced noncontrast media-based technique has improved microvascular flow imaging, particularly for slow flow vessels, as observed intratesticular. Different manufacturers have introduced such application tools in their high-end US machines under different names, such as Microvascular Imaging (MVI) by GE Healthcare; MicroFlow Imaging by Philips; Superb

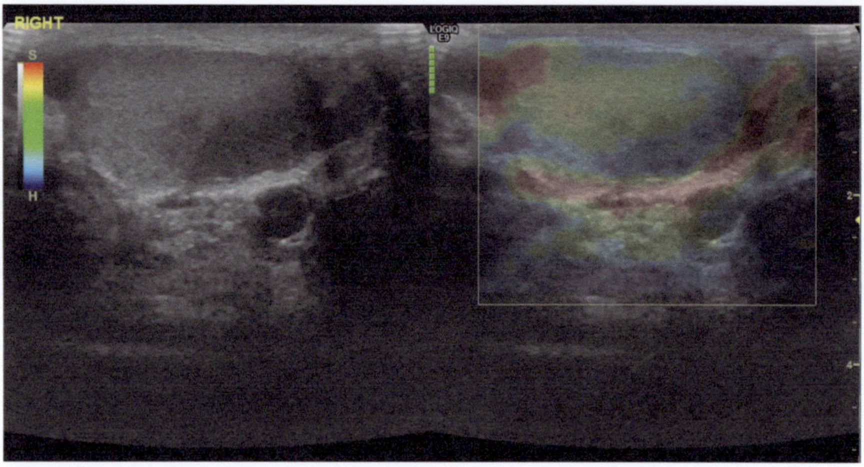

Fig. 4.7 Focal sclerosis after inflammation in 46,XY NOA with hypoplastic testicles, shown by elastography
High-resolution B-mode ultrasound revealed a focal hypoechoic circumscriptive area, which appeared hardened in the simulated elastography, coded in blue. By courtesy Dr. Aigner

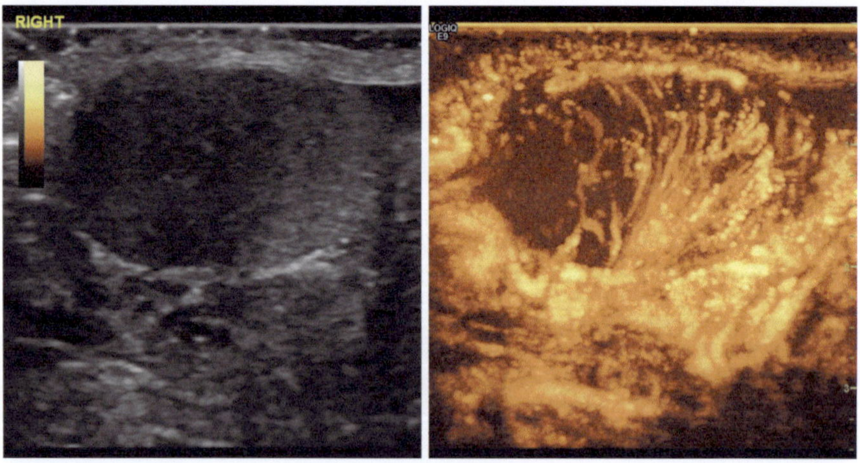

Fig. 4.8 Focal sclerosis with low perfusion lesion in NOA
In the same case as in Fig. 4.7, where no perfusion could be detected in the hypoechoic lesion by color Doppler ultrasound, this was confirmed by ultrasound examination after intravenous contrast agent administration (left image)

Microvascular Imaging (SMI) by Canon Medical; and MVflow by Samsung. In NOA testicles, an inhomogeneous vascular pattern can often be found after the application of Microvascular Imaging (MVI), showing a haphazard distribution in different sections. MVI can better visualize small vessel vascularity than can color Doppler imaging, which increases its diagnostic value in difficult cases [30]. In NOA patients, testicular fibrosis with sonographic features such as a striated

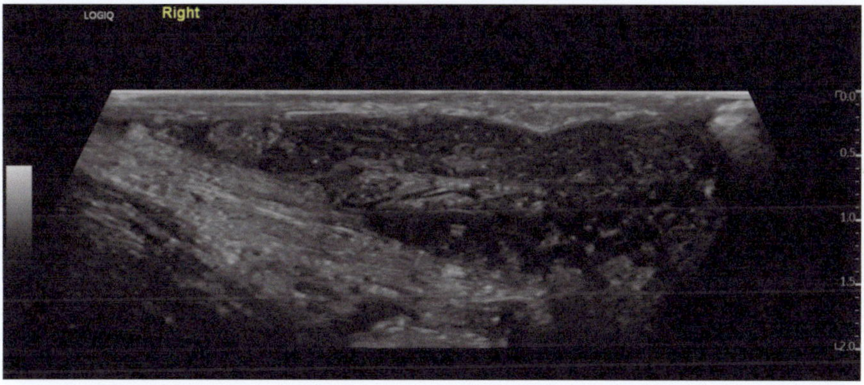

Fig. 4.9 Tubular ectasia in hypoplastic testicle, 46,XY, NOA
Both the epididymis and the partially imaged vas deferens show dilated, hypoechoic zones in a severely hypoplastic NOA testicle in panoramic view

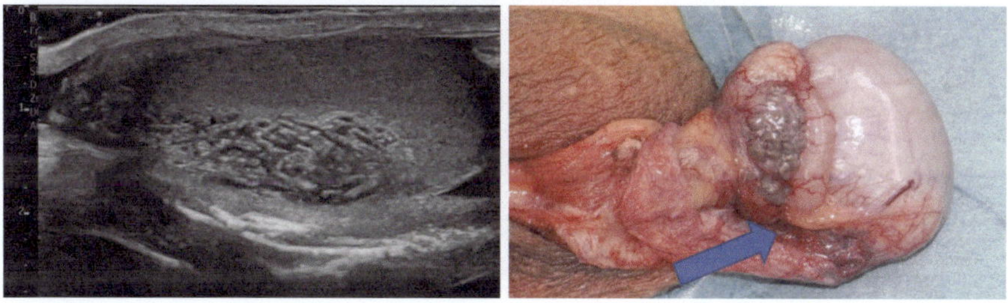

Fig. 4.10 CFTR-positive cystic fibrosis patient testicles, US image in (a) B-mode US image in the left picture and corresponding intraoperative situation in CF-related azoospermia and absent vas deferens by CBAVD and "blind-ending epididymis," marked by an arrow
In direct comparison to the case of a hypoplastic testis with NOA, as shown in Figure XYXY, a two (biallelic) CF mutation carrier presented a testis of normal volume with a regular, preserved isoechogenic parenchymal pattern, but, simultaneous dilatation of the rete testis tubular structures in terms of obstructive tubular ectasia in CBAVD/CFTR carriers

pattern, diffuse heterogeneity together with unilateral or bilateral focal hyperechoic masses or avascular hypoechoic masses can sometimes be detected. The SRR is such localized areas is in most of the cases negative [31].

Clinical investigations of the presence of intratesticular varicosities, defined as a condition characterized by the dilation of veins within the testicle, are lacking, underscoring the impact of such conditions. Fewer than 2% of symptomatic men who undergo testicular ultrasound, compared with those with extratesticular varicoceles, which are present in 15–35% of men, have such findings. According to some studies, it was assumed that intratesticular varicosities have a negative impact on spermatogenesis; therefore, more precise, high-end machine sonography for striking testicles, such as in NOA cases, might be required [31]. Numerous investigations are being conducted to better understand the consequences of intratesticular testosterone levels and the impact of varicoceles on spermatogenesis, as well as the association between intratesticular varicosity and male fertility. For example, despite lower serum testosterone levels, research on males with Klinefelter syndrome revealed normal or even higher intratesticular testosterone concentrations, indicating complicated connections between male fertility, hormone levels, and intratesticular varicosities [32, 33].

Shear wave elastography (SWE) and strain wave elastography, both relatively new ultrasound techniques, measure the stiffness of testicular tissue with established use for testicular tumor differentiation, but recent studies have shown their potential even in distinguishing between normal and abnormal testicular tissue, which may have implications for identifying regions within the testes that might yield sperm upon biopsy [34, 35]. One study investigated the predictive value of a positive SSR by measuring the rete testis thickness (RTT) and performing testicular SWE to differentiate OA from NOA patients [36]. By applying an RTT cutoff of 1.6 mm, they reported a sensitivity and specificity of 94.1% and 79.2%, respectively, for differentiating OA from NOA. In addition, US findings of tubular ectasia, which is considered a cystic dilatation in the rete testis, can help visualize kinds of obstruction and is a helpful indicator for differentiating the NOA from the OA. Typically, there are multiple anechoic, avascular dilated structures within the rete testis accompanied by ipsilateral spermatoceles or epididymal cysts, which resemble a partial or complete obliteration of the 12–20 efferent ductules merging in the head of the epididymis. Post-inflammatory conditions in the epididymis or previous vasectomy are typical causes of OA and not of NOA [37].

Ultrasound findings revealed a thickened epididymis in 32% of 309 infertile men [38]. An experienced clinician should also immediately request an ultrasound examination of the ductus deferens, as in the presence of an obstruction, the vas deferens also shows typical bead-like changes with caliber irregularities and dilatated lumina, which have been described as deferentitis nodosa. Essentially, enlargement of the epididymis detected on scrotal ultrasound may indicate specific clinical conditions and may be associated with male genital tract obstruction or inflammation in infertile men [39]. These findings underscore the importance of sonographic evaluation of the epididymis in the assessment of male infertility, helping to identify potential causes and guide treatment decisions.

Lately, laser Doppler has been introduced for visualizing intraoperatively regions of better testicular perfusion, where it is supposed to reveal a more distinctive and healthier environment for spermatogenesis [40], there are still some conflicting results about the role of the vascular pattern in increasing the sperm retrieval rate [41, 42].

Transrectal ultrasound (TRUS) is indicated for azoospermic patients with low semen volume and a seminal acidic pH if an obstruction is suspected. Using TRUS, seminal vesicle abnormalities and prostatic cysts can be detected for associated genitourinary anomalies (renal agenesis, dysgenesis, or autosomal dominant polycystic kidney disease). In addition, TRUS can confirm CBAVD as the seminal vesicles of these patients are absent or hypoplastic [43].

Magnetic resonance imaging (MRI) helps assess the distal parts of the seminal tract, the presence of prolactinomas, or the intra-abdominal location of an undescended testis. Renal imaging studies should be performed in men with anatomical vas deferens abnormalities and no evidence of CFTR mutations as unilateral absence of the vas deferens is usually associated with an ipsilateral absence of the kidney. Moreover, renal abnormalities (e.g., in the pelvic kidney) may be found in patients with CBAVD without CFTR mutations [44, 45].

In recent decades, novel sophisticated advanced protocols for testicular MRI, including functional MRI techniques such as diffusion-weighted imaging (DWI) and magnetic resonance spectroscopy (MRS), have been developed, providing additional detailed information about testicular physiology. Such MRI investigations may help identify spermatogenic active areas within the testes, although their role and utility in NOA are still being explored and are not yet routine [46]. As a next-generation technique, micro-MRI offers ultra-high-resolution imaging of the testicular structure and is currently under investigation. It potentially identifies spermatogenesis at the microscopic level, although its clinical application and accessibility are limited at this stage. New molecular imaging techniques target specific cellular or molecular markers of spermatogenesis. This approach could eventually enable noninvasive identification of spermatogenic active areas within the testes.

Genetic Counseling of the Couple and Family Planning

Male Infertility due to NOA Can Stem from Various Genetic and Nongenetic Factors

For couples experiencing male infertility, the path to parenthood is often laden and fraught with uncertainty and emotional challenges, particularly concerning potential genetic disease transmission to their offspring. Recent quantitative studies have shown that men diagnosed with male factor infertility experience significantly greater psychological distress than men in infertile couples where the infertility is attributed to female factors or remains unexplained. This suggests that the emotional impact on men is intensified when they are identified as the primary cause of infertility [47]. A cross-sectional study and a cohort study revealed that infertile men have a low quality of life and that a greater psychological burden affects their mental well-being [48, 49]. There is, undoubtedly, a pressing need to comprehend, just before any medical intervention, the realistic prospects for both successful testicular sperm retrieval and successful pregnancy, ultimately aiming to increase the likelihood of bringing a baby home, which is the primary request for couples. The identification of a genetic cause for infertility carries significant clinical importance as it may impact not only the reproductive health of infertile men but also the overall general health of the patient and potentially their children. The question in a genetic counseling session for a couple must be analyzed on at least three distinctive levels [50].

At the forefront, genetic clarification aids in the precise diagnosis and differentiation between NOA and OA. In both cases, infertility with azoospermia is present, yet the clinical and laboratory picture, despite certain probabilities, is not always clear-cut.

Second, it is important to provide the couple with information directly related to the potential risk of transmission of a genetic disorder.

Third, it is important to consider that infertile men with NOA, due to specific genetic traits and carrier status, have a lifelong disease risk compared to the general male population.

Genetic counseling should therefore keep all three aspects in mind and take them into consideration, and, depending on the patient's wishes or the couple's expectations, the relevant information should be presented during the consultation and infertility guidance. Confronting the challenge of infertility diagnosis represents significant distress for affected couples [51]. Although infertility is common, it remains a socially taboo subject, leading these couples to refrain from discussing their struggles, thereby intensifying their emotional burden. Furthermore, the female partner's age plays a pivotal role in the ability to conceive even in terms of assisted reproductive medicine; this must be considered an additional factor influencing psychological strain when family planning extends for several years. The delivery of unfavorable news encompasses not only life-threatening conditions but also scenarios that diminish hope and elicit anxieties regarding the future. Navigating the communication of such adverse news is undeniably complex. Various protocols for delivering difficult news, such as ABCDE, BREAKS, and SPIKES, can be adapted from oncologic psychotherapist settings and employed in these situations [52–54]. Notably, in many countries, the legal situation is well-defined and standardized and requires such counseling to be conducted by a specially trained human geneticist or genetic counsellor; therefore, these specific aspects will not be detailed here [55]. However, there is indeed a broader context concerning infertility in NOA. While cases of male infertility secondary to clear conditions such as post-vasectomy cases generally do not require detailed genetic testing, the underlying causes of NOA cases are more nuanced and require a different approach to clinical decision-making. Notably, men with a diagnosis of azoospermia are at the highest risk—approximately 20–25%—of carrying genetic abnormalities, a risk that gradually decreases as sperm production increases [56]. In instances of severe oligoasthenoteratozoospermia (OAT), characterized by a sperm concentration of < 5 million/mL, there is typically an increase in the risk of structural chromosomal abnormalities. This increase ranges from approximately four- to tenfold compared to the corresponding risk in men without reproductive abnormalities [57, 58]. These findings of variable genetic etiological predispositions to abnormal spermiogenesis have been incorporated into the various guidelines of professional societies and scientific organizations, which require a stepwise approach to genetic analysis depending on the quantitative disorders of spermatogenesis.

Occasionally, men with unfulfilled desires for children present with certain clinical abnormalities, and therefore, in these suspected cases, the presence of a genetic mutation should be promptly considered, as this can have implications for their health status, quality of life, expectations in couples counseling, diagnostic and therapeutic algorithms, and life expectancy. In NOA, the most common underlying conditions are Klinefelter syndrome (KS) and Kallmann syndrome (KAL). It is recommended that patients exhibiting a combination of infertility, bilateral atrophic testes, underdeveloped secondary sexual characteristics, and notably, anosmia or hyposmia be evaluated for KAL (see below). The European clinical guidelines advocate a threshold of <5 million spermatozoa/mL for initiating a genetic analysis [59].

The most common chromosomal anomaly leading to azoospermia or severe oligozoospermia is Klinefelter syndrome (karyotype 47,XXY or mosaic forms in 6.3% of cases with 47,XXY/46,XY), which occurs in approximately 1–2 out of 1000 male newborns, while it is found at a higher frequency in approximately 15% of men with azoospermia. (Figs. 4.5 and 4.7) Aside from other clinical symptoms and findings with small testes (1–8 mL), gynecomastia (~40% of cases), and hypogonadism in approximately 80% of patients, azoospermia remains a leading symptom. The results of semen analysis might be confirmed since in less than 10% of men with Klinefelter syndrome, a few sperm may intermittently be found in the ejaculate, suggesting a new therapeutic option. Nevertheless, over time, most of these men will require treatment for testosterone deficiency secondary to functional loss of Leydig cells [60]. To mitigate increased morbidity linked to a higher incidence of diabetes mellitus, obesity, or metabolic syndrome in hypogonadal KS men and thereby reduce the inherently elevated mortality rate of 7 years to a general life expectancy, it is imperative to provide patients with appropriate counseling and management following diagnostic genetic evaluation. On the other hand, the correct cytogenetic diagnosis and proper genetic counseling have immediate therapeutic consequences for the patient as testosterone replacement therapy should not be started before a testicular biopsy for TESE, and again, proper counseling for this genetic disorder is mandatory to avoid impeding future fertility treatment. It cannot be emphasized enough how crucial genetic testing and counseling are for this medical condition, as they set the decisive course for further treatment. Although men with Klinefelter syndrome have long been considered infertile, the success rate of surgical sperm retrieval, mainly by mTESE, in these men is approximately 50% as long as long-acting steroids are not prescribed for a prolonged period. Interestingly, once sperm can be harvested by TESE, the offspring will not exhibit the same genetic disposition, and this unique situation must be reassuringly explained to the couple [61].

For patients who exhibit a combination of infertility, bilateral atrophic testes, and underdeveloped secondary sexual characteristics, notably, anosmia or hyposmia, a diagnosis of Kallmann syndrome (KAL), with an estimated prevalence of 1 in 30,000 males, must be considered. The hormonal disorder is due to the underdevelopment of specific neurons, or nerves, in the brain that signal the hypothalamus [62], whereas the genetic diagnosis of KS is based on karyotyping. In KAL, there is sometimes a need for a more extensive investigation since aberrations in more than 20 genes have been linked to KAL. Mutations occurring within the ANOS1, CHD7, FGF8, FGFR1, PROK2, or PROKR2 genes are predominantly implicated in the etiology of this condition. Occasionally, individuals affected by this syndrome may exhibit mutations in multiple genes from this set.

Furthermore, a shortened Y chromosome, which often appears as a ring chromosome or isochromosome, can be examined for the presence or absence of azoospermia factor (AZF) loci. Knowledge of Yq microdeletions (YCMs) in AZF regions is important because YCMs are estimated to be the cause of severe spermatogenesis failure in 1:12 infertile patients worldwide and because there is an estimated incidence of approximately 1:4000 men in the general population [63]. Since the AZF loci are essential for spermatogenesis and their absence or damage can lead to azoospermia, AZF deletions are considered responsible for 2 to 10% of cases, whereas AZF deletions have never been found in normospermic men [6]. Microdeletion polymorphic variants in the long arm of the Y chromosome are the second most common genetic cause of azoospermia as they aggregate 26 genes involved in spermatogenesis regulation. The AZF interval has three subregions, AZFa, AZFb, and AZFc, with frequencies of 0.5–9%, 15–7%, and 70–80%, respectively, each of which includes vital genes for spermatogenesis control [64]. SR success is determined by the type of Y microdeletion detected, as in men with AZFc deletions, sperm may occasionally be found either in the ejaculate or through testicular sperm extraction in at least 50% of individuals, while complete AZFa and/or complete AZFb microdeletions are considered contraindications for performing surgical SR because deletions in these subregions are incompatible with residual spermatogenesis [10, 65]. Therefore, further genetic counseling regarding the risk of transmission to offspring is recommended in most guidelines since hereditary transmission from the affected father to his son is obligatory [66–68]. For the partial AZFc mutation gr/gr, there was a threefold increased risk for testicular germ cell tumors, with an OR = 3.1, 95% CI = 1.4–7.0 [69]. The EAU recommendation was strongly rated for Y-chromosome microdeletion testing when the sperm concentration was <5 million sperm/mL but was strongly rated with a mandatory recommendation when the sperm concentration was < 1 million sperm/mL. Indeed, in the case of azoospermia, the incidence of Y microdeletions is the highest, at 8–12%, and decreases to 3–7% in oligospermic patients, whereas the detection rate is poor for infertile men with sperm concentrations greater than 5 million/ml, with an approximate detection rate of only approximately 0.7% [70]. However, in contrast to this proposed cutoff for a sperm concentration of < 5 million sperm/mL, a recent meta-analysis, which reviewed 37 studies from Europe and North America involving 12,492 oligozoospermic men, revealed that microdeletions on the Y chromosome predominantly occur in men with sperm concentrations below 1 million sperm/mL; in contrast, <1% of these deletions were found in men with more than 1 million sperm/mL [71]. Adopting these findings as a precise criterion could lead to more efficient diagnostics by accelerating the time needed to obtain genetic results and enabling a cost-effective strategy. This approach assumes that omitting numerous genetic tests will not result in a substantial loss of diagnostic accuracy due to the absence of evidence.

CFTR mutations, such as those found in mucoviscidosis, usually result in CBAVD and idiopathic ejaculatory duct obstruction (EDO), and affected patients have OA. Approximately 8/10 patients with CBAVD harbor 2 CFTR mutations, usually in compound heterozygosity. CFTR gene mutation testing should be recommended for infertile men with congenital bilateral absence of the vas deferens (CBAVD), and also considered in men with unilateral vas agenesis (CUAVD). If the male partner is found to carry a CFTR mutation, the female partner should also be tested [16, 17, 72]. In men with NOA or severe asthenozoospermia and a history of recurrent sinusitis, bronchitis, pneumonia, pancreatitis, or otitis media, primary ciliary dyskinesia (PCD) should be suspected — particularly if CFTR testing is negative. A subtype of PCD is Kartagener syndrome, where, in addition to the aforementioned symptoms, a situs inversus is found, in 50% [73]. The phenotypic and genetic spectrum of PCD is diverse and is caused by biallelic (autosomal recessive) mutations in a large number of genes [74]. Therefore, sequencing of the associated genes (Exome or Multigene Panel Analysis) should be offered in cases of appropriate clinical suspicion.

Genome-wide association studies have revealed that several variants are associated with an increased risk of impaired spermiogenesis, among which the following gene mutation targets are of interest: MEIOB, TEX14, DNAH6, MTHFR, FSHR, USP8, and TGFβ, as well as putative mutations in TAF4B, ZMYND15, NPAS2, and TEX15. When utilizing sperm analysis techniques such as fluorescent in situ hybridization (FISH) or array-based analysis to identify chromosomal abnormalities or genetic defects in patients with NOA, which can encompass numerical anomalies such as trisomies or structural variations such as inversions or Robertsonian translocations, a general increase in chromosomal aneuploidy may be observed. The most frequently analyzed genes were 13, 15, 18, 21, X, and Y. In the case of extended research extending to additional chromosomes (4, 6–12, and 17), heightened aneuploidy levels might be observed, although with a lower diagnostic value than that of stringent genes, including 13, 18, 21, X, and Y [7]. In this context, the EAU guidelines released in 2023 were strongly favorable for standard karyotype analysis and genetic counseling for all men with azoospermia and oligozoospermia, starting with a cutoff spermatozoa concentration <10 million/mL for preoperative genetic diagnostic purposes [67].

Genetically Counseling for NOA Regarding the Risk for Malignancy

In the context of counseling, is it correct to limit the discussion to the aspects of fecundity potential and possible risks to offspring, or is the essential task of the treating physician to guide the infertile man in a comprehensive overview of those disease patterns that may be genetically determined in this context?

Indeed, several studies investigating the correlation between male infertility and cancer incidence have shown that the diagnosis of infertility itself is considered to be a harbinger of future health issues [75]. Eisenberg et al. mined claims data for 76,083 infertile US men and reported a 49% increased risk across a broad range of cancers (n = 18) compared to a control cohort [76]. Furthermore, an elevated risk of all cancers (SIR 2.9, 95% CI 1.4–5.4) was highlighted in cases of azoospermia [76]. A recent study investigating semen analysis of 10,511 men and 63,891 siblings revealed a twofold greater risk of any-site cancer and a threefold greater risk of acute lymphoblastic leukemia in the siblings of oligozoospermic men than in the siblings of fertile controls [77]. For instance, the risk for testicular cancer diagnosis increases by up to 20 times in men who exhibit abnormal semen parameters. Among various cancers, testicular cancer has the most significant impact on semen quality. Oligospermia, a condition marked by a low sperm count, was identified in 52% of semen samples collected from men with testicular cancer prior to treatment. This contrasts with the occurrence of oligospermia in approximately 12–30% of men diagnosed with other types of cancer, underscoring the unique reproductive challenges associated with testicular cancer [78, 79]. Furthermore, this risk is 52% greater among first-degree relatives, highlighting a significant genetic or familial predisposition to this condition. Lately, Ramsay and coworkers performed a retrospective data analysis of cancer incidence in a cohort of infertile men (n = 786, including 426 azoospermic men) and a matched cohort of healthy and fertile men as controls (n = 5674). In both groups, all family members who were third-degree relatives were identified, including a total cohort of 337,754 persons. Surprisingly, in the familial cohort of azoospermic men comprising 21,361 individuals, there was a greater incidence of five cancer types than in the control families: bone and joint cancer hazard ratio (HR) = 2.56 (95% CI = 1.48–4.42), soft tissue cancer HR = 1.56 (95% CI = 1.01–2.39), uterine cancer HR = 1.27 (95% CI = 1.03–1.56), Hodgkin lymphoma HR = 1.60 (95% CI = 1.07–2.39), and thyroid cancer HR = 1.54 (95% CI = 1.21–1.97). Similarly, among families with severe oligozoospermia, increased risk was observed for three cancer types: colon cancer, HR = 1.16 (95% CI = 1.01–1.32); bone and joint cancers, HR = 2.43 (95% CI = 1.30–4.54); and testis cancer, HR = 2.34 (95% CI = 1.60–3.42), along with a significant decrease in esophageal cancer risk, HR = 0.39 (95% CI = 0.16–0.97) [80].

In direct comparisons between men with azoospermia and men without azoospermia, several studies have revealed a 2.2-fold greater risk for cancer in the infertility group [76, 81]. Specifically, in patients with azoospermia, there is a 25% greater risk of testicular cancers than other malignancies [82]. This underscores the essential role of appropriate genetic counseling as a pivotal resource to guide couples through this journey, offering scientifically based information and guidance for optimal clinical decision-making. Indeed, with scientific progress in the field of genetic analysis, over 2000 genes involved in spermatogenesis have been discovered, as observed for primary testicular failure patients with quantitative impairment of spermatogenesis, which is responsible for approximately 75% of male factor infertility cases, thus making NOA the most prevalent cause followed etiologically by the obstructive conditions in OA. Therefore, currently, testing for these genetic factors can yield a genetic diagnosis for more than 20% of male infertility cases. Aside from the detection of numerical chromosomal aberrations by classical karyotyping, current novel techniques, such as single-nucleotide polymorphism (SNP), whole-exome and whole-genome analyses, are needed to develop further helpful diagnostic approaches for better characterizing male NOA infertility. The guideline recommendation strength rating was weak for the associated health risk in infertile men with abnormal semen parameters but was strong for providing genetic counseling in the case of either a genetic abnormality or an inheritable disease [67].

Genetic Testing in Men with Specific Sperm Defects

Studies have shown that the expression patterns of microRNA (miRNA) genes as small noncoding RNAs, among others, such as piRNAs or tsRNAs, play a crucial role in the regulation of several highly orchestrated developmental gene expression processes in the testicle; these include cell cycle regulation, apoptosis, and differentiation and are somewhat distinct among men facing infertility compared to those with normal fertility. These molecules are considered responsible for controlling spermatogenesis at different phases and across various cells within the male reproductive system [83]. Indeed, it was reported that miRNAs, such as miR-122, miR-449a, and miR-34b/c, are pivotal in the regulation and posttranscriptional processes of spermatogenesis and may be involved in the pathogenesis of azoospermia in NOA [8–87]. Consequently, microRNAs hold promise as valuable biomarkers for diagnosing and understanding male infertility, and further ongoing studies are evaluating their applicability and usefulness in measuring specific miRNAs for other health conditions or cancer diagnoses in addition to testicular tissue [88].

Biochemical Predictive Markers for OA vs. NOA Differentiation

Seminal fluid can serve as a medium to assess the status of spermatogenesis and presence or absence of certain markers that can help diagnose and differentiate azoospermia.

- Seminal Transferrin, Carnitine, and Fructose.

  Saeed et al. pointed out that these parameters when used in conjunction with each other could localize the site of obstruction in azoospermia [89]. Patients with an obstruction at the testis–epididymal junction had low levels of transferrin but normal levels of carnitine and fructose. Patients who had lower levels of transferrin and carnitine but normal levels of fructose had obstruction at the epididymal level, probably in the tail. Obstruction of the ejaculatory ducts was signified by lower levels of all parameters in the semen.

- Anti-Müllerian Hormone (AMH).

  AMH is a Sertoli cell-secreted glycoprotein responsible for Müllerian duct regression in male embryos. AMH is present in seminal plasma of most fertile men higher than the serum level (mean concentrations 153 pmol/l vs. 10.7 pmol/l). Seminal AMH concentrations are undetectable in all OA patients, confirming its testicular origin. In NOA, seminal AMH concentration is lower (mean 17 pmol/l) than in fertile men without correlation with plasma FSH levels [90]. It was shown that seminal plasma AMH is an absolute testicular marker that is absent in all OA cases but has a poor predictability for successful testicular SR in NOA cases [91].
- Seminal Lipocalin-Type Prostaglandin D Synthase (L-PGDS).

  Heshmat et al. suggested that seminal L-PGDS level can potentially be a biomarker for assessing patency in the seminal tract in azoospermia cases. In azoospermic men with high seminal L-PGDS (>100 ug/l), the diagnosis of NOA can be potentially made without biopsy [92].
- Cell-Free Seminal mRNA (cfs-mRNA).cfs-mRNA exists in human ejaculate at high concentrations and stability containing many tissue-specific transcripts secreted from the male reproductive system as germ cell-specific (DDX4), seminal vesicle-specific (SEMG1), and prostate-specific (TGM4). Li et al. detected DDX4 in all patients with MA and incomplete SCO but was absent in most cases of complete SCO (75.0%) or non-CBAVD (85.7%), and in all men with vasectomy or CBAVD [93]. The presence of DDX4 in some men with complete SCO or non-CBAVD suggests the presence of germ cells in the testis and incomplete obstruction. SEMG1 was undetectable in patients with CBAVD with bilateral absence of the seminal vesicles. Goel et al. evaluated the role of cell-free seminal markers: DDX4, PRM1, and PRM2, in diagnosing and differentiating between OA and NOA. DDX4 was more sensitive for NOA compared with OA. Among various subtypes of NOA, DDX4 positivity was higher in patients with MA and HS compared with SCOS [94].
- Drabovich et al. pointed out that the combined detections of TEX101 and ECM1 proteins could bring a diagnostic output with a high sensitivity and specificity. Similar results were observed for combined detection of TEX101 and SPAG1 [95].

Role of Testicular Histopathology

To identify and assess the underlying causes of NOA, the histopathology of testicular specimens is essential and typically performed at least at the same time as for mTESE since these findings are crucial for understanding the underlying pathology of NOA and can guide therapeutic decision-making, including the potential for sperm retrieval during assisted reproductive procedures [96]. Histopathological examination of testicular specimens typically focuses in NOA cases on identifying the spermatogenic potency within the seminiferous tubules, the presence of Sertoli cell-only syndrome, the presence of tubules with focal inflammation or post-inflammatory stage or other pathological findings in NOA patients to assess any maturation arrest at various stages of spermatogenesis and to understand the type of hypospermatogenesis. The 250–1000 seminiferous tubules of the testis are tightly coiled, and each tubule measures approximately 30–70 cm in length when uncoiled. Given the significant variation among individuals, the total length of seminiferous tubules, if stretched out end-to-end, could be approximately 250–300 meters per testis, but a greater decrease in the number of tubules or structural architectural defects is often observed in NOA patients than in OA patients. In NOA, cellular mechanisms within the seminiferous tubules are significantly altered, leading to impaired spermatogenesis. Tubular diameter preserved by normal size, such encountered in fertile men, frequently, though via mechanisms not yet fully elucidated, supports ongoing spermatogenic activity, in contrast to adjacent nondilated regions, which typically demonstrate an absence of such activity; such atrophic and nondilated tubules constitute a major part of the seminiferous tubules in NOA patients. Clinically, spermatozoa are harvested from these dilated tubules utilizing mTESE, facilitating the acquisition of viable sperm for ICSI procedures. Indeed, it was shown that the maximal diameter of dilated seminiferous tubules correlates with the sperm retrieval rate in NOA patients, and this is basically the search strategy when performing mTESE [95, 97]. In one study, it was demonstrated that the differentiation stage of Sertoli cells, the germ cell count, and the seminiferous tubule wall caliber varied among the various categories of NOA, highlighting that intratubular microenvironments exhibit distinctive characteristics across diverse NOA patient subgroups [98].

Role of Diagnostic Testicular Biopsy

Diagnostic testicular biopsy is the gold-standard method for discriminating OA from NOA in men with normal FSH, normal testicular size, and no apparent obstruction signs. Practically, the majority of these cases could be differentiated on the basis of detailed medical history, clinical examination, semen analysis, hormonal assessment, imaging, and genetic studies. Nevertheless, there are cases of doubt in which the differential diagnosis between OA and NOA remains unclear unless a testis biopsy followed by histopathology is carried out. Congenital intratesticular obstruction and congenital epididymal obstruction, which are not related to anatomic vas deferens abnormalities and functional obstruction of the distal parts of the ejaculatory ducts, can cause OA, and these conditions are not easily identifiable [99].

Histopathology findings included (i) absence of germ cells (only Sertoli cells), (ii) spermatogenic MA, (iii) hypospermatogenesis (HS), (iv) tubular hyalinization, and (v) normal spermatogenesis. These patterns occur alone or in combination (mixed pattern). In contrast, normal spermatogenesis is indicative of OA [100]. In addition, intratubular germ cell neoplasia in situ (GCNIS) might be revealed in biopsy specimens taken from patients with NOA, mainly those with a history of cryptorchidism and/or multiple foci of testicular microlithiasis.

Notably, diagnostic biopsies might harm the testis; therefore, they should be limited to selected cases because their routine use as a diagnostic tool for azoospermia type is not recommended by relevant guidelines. Consistent with the EAU guidelines recommendations, a biopsy should be taken for histopathology to confirm the type of azoospermia combined with TESE for possible sperm cryopreservation using isolated sperm suspensions or tissue fragments [101, 102].

Conclusions

Understanding the nuances and underlying mechanisms of both OA and NOA is important to guide the development of more effective treatments and patient care protocols. For NOA patients, the impact of an accurate diagnosis for treatment strategies and outcomes is significant. Therefore, multifaceted, tailored diagnostic and therapeutic approaches are looked-for to improve their outcomes and success rates. This requires a precise diagnostic algorithm to determine the optimal therapeutic approaches and better-informed decision-making regarding different treatment options.

References

1. Jarow JP, Espeland MA, Lipshultz LI. Evaluation of the azoospermic patient. J Urol. 1989;142(1):62–5.
2. Agarwal A, Mulgund A, Hamada A, Chyatte MR. A unique view on male infertility around the globe. Reprod Biol Endocrinol. 2015;13:37.
3. Luo X, Yin C, Shi Y, Du C, Pan X. Global trends in semen quality of young men: a systematic review and regression analysis. J Assist Reprod Genet. 2023;40(8):1807–16.
4. Levine H, Jørgensen N, Martino-Andrade A, Mendiola J, Weksler-Derri D, Jolles M, et al. Temporal trends in sperm count: a systematic review and meta-regression analysis of samples collected globally in the 20th and 21st centuries. Hum Reprod Update. 2023;29(2):157–76.5.
5. World Health Organization (WHO). WHO laboratory manual for the examination and processing of human semen. 6th ed. WHO; 2021.
6. Practice Committee of the American Society for Reproductive Medicine in collaboration with the Society for Male R, Urology. Electronic address aao. The management of obstructive azoospermia: a committee opinion. Fertil Steril. 2019;111(5):873–80.
7. Rambhatla A, Shah R, Ziouziou I, Kothari P, Salvio G, Gul M, et al. Global practice patterns and variations in the medical and surgical management of non-obstructive azoospermia: results of a world-wide survey, guidelines and expert recommendations. World J Mens Health; 2024.
8. Almekaty KM, Zahran MH, Lotfy Amer M, Hagras AM, Salem KA, Rashed AS, et al. Factors predicting the outcome of percutaneous epididymal sperm aspiration in men with obstructive azoospermia. Arch Ital Urol Androl. 2022;94(3):323–7.

9. Schwarzer JU, Steinfatt H. Current status of vasectomy reversal. Nat Rev Urol. 2013;10(4):195–205.
10. Esteves SC. Clinical management of infertile men with nonobstructive azoospermia. Asian J Androl. 2015;17(3):459–70.
11. Miyaoka R, Orosz JE, Achermann AP, Esteves SC. Methods of surgical sperm extraction and implications for assisted reproductive technology success. Panminerva Med. 2019;61(2):164–77.
12. Burrows PJ, Schrepferman CG, Lipshultz LI. Comprehensive office evaluation in the new millennium. Urol Clin North Am. 2002;29(4):873–94.
13. Esteves SC, Miyaoka R, Agarwal A. An update on the clinical assessment of the infertile male [corrected]. Clinics (Sao Paulo). 2011;66(4):691–700.
14. Boeri L, Capogrosso P, Ventimiglia E, Cazzaniga W, Pozzi E, Belladelli F, et al. Testicular volume in infertile versus fertile white-European men: a case-control investigation in the real-life setting. Asian J Androl. 2021;23(5):501–9.
15. Majzoub A, Arafa M, Khalafalla K, AlSaid S, Burjaq H, Albader M, et al. Predictive model to estimate the chances of successful sperm retrieval by testicular sperm aspiration in patients with nonobstructive azoospermia. Fertil Steril. 2021;115(2):373–81.
16. Cai Z, Li H. Congenital bilateral absence of the vas deferens. Front Genet. 2022;13:775123.
17. Rudnik-Schoneborn S, Messner M, Vockel M, Wirleitner B, Pinggera GM, Witsch-Baumgartner M, et al. Andrological findings in infertile men with two (biallelic) CFTR mutations: results of a multicentre study in Germany and Austria comprising 71 patients. Hum Reprod. 2021;36(3):551–9.
18. Jensen S, Ko EY. Varicocele treatment in non-obstructive azoospermia: a systematic review. Arab J Urol. 2021;19(3):221–6.
19. Andrade DL, Viana MC, Esteves SC. Differential diagnosis of azoospermia in men with infertility. J Clin Med. 2021;10(14)
20. Achermann APP, Esteves SC. Diagnosis and management of infertility due to ejaculatory duct obstruction: summary evidence. Int Braz J Urol. 2021;47:868–81.
21. Oduwole OO, Peltoketo H, Huhtaniemi IT. Role of follicle-stimulating hormone in spermatogenesis. Front Endocrinol (Lausanne). 2018;9:763.
22. Chao HH, Zhang Y, Dong PY, Gurunathan S, Zhang XF. Comprehensive review on the positive and negative effects of various important regulators on male spermatogenesis and fertility. Front Nutr. 2022;9:1063510.
23. Salama N, Blgozah S. Serum estradiol levels in infertile men with non-obstructive azoospermia. Ther Adv Reprod Health. 2020;14:2633494120928342.
24. Tao Y. Endocrine aberrations of human nonobstructive azoospermia. Asian J Androl. 2022;24(3):274–86.
25. Li X, Tian RH, Li P, Li CX, Yao MH, Yao CC, et al. Ultrasonographic evaluation of the rete testis thickness: a promising approach to differentiate obstructive from nonobstructive azoospermia. Asian J Androl. 2023;25(6):725–30.
26. Fedder J, Jørgensen MW, Engvad B. Prevalence of CBAVD in azoospermic men carrying pathogenic CFTR mutations – evaluated in a cohort of 639 non-vasectomized azoospermic men. Andrology. 2021;9(2):588–98.
27. Lotti F, Frizza F, Balercia G, Barbonetti A, Behre HM, Calogero AE, et al. The European Academy of Andrology (EAA) ultrasound study on healthy, fertile men: scrotal ultrasound reference ranges and associations with clinical, seminal, and biochemical characteristics. Andrology. 2021;9(2):559–76.
28. Ma Y, Li G, Li J, Ren WD. The diagnostic value of superb microvascular Imaging (SMI) in detecting blood flow signals of breast lesions: a preliminary study comparing SMI to color Doppler flow imaging. Medicine (Baltimore). 2015;94(36):e1502.
29. Raman JD, Goldstein M. Intraoperative characterization of arterial vasculature in spermatic cord. Urology. 2004;64(3):561–4.

30. Ates F, Sivri M, Durmaz MS, Sekmenli T, Gunduz M, Ciftci I. Comparison of conventional Doppler imaging techniques and superb microvascular imaging in determination of vascularization in undescended testes. J Ultrason. 2023;23(93):e66–72.
31. Bhat S, Sachin J, Ramaprasad JS. Striated pattern on scrotal ultrasonography: a marker for Non-hodgkins lymphoma of testis. Indian J Urol. 2014;30(1):113–4.
32. Bucci S, Liguori G, Amodeo A, Salamè L, Trombetta C, Belgrano E. Intratesticular varicocele: evaluation using grey scale and color Doppler ultrasound. World J Urol. 2008;26(1):87–9.
33. Tuttelmann F, Damm OS, Luetjens CM, Baldi M, Zitzmann M, Kliesch S, et al. Intratesticular testosterone is increased in men with Klinefelter syndrome and may not be released into the bloodstream owing to altered testicular vascularization- a preliminary report. Andrology. 2014;2(2):275–81.
34. Rocher L, Criton A, Gennisson JL, Izard V, Ferlicot S, Tanter M, et al. Testicular shear wave elastography in normal and infertile men: a prospective study on 601 patients. Ultrasound Med Biol. 2017;43(4):782–9.
35. Yavuz A, Yokus A, Taken K, Batur A, Ozgokce M, Arslan H. Reliability of testicular stiffness quantification using shear wave elastography in predicting male fertility: a preliminary prospective study. Med Ultrason. 2018;20(2):141–7.
36. Li X, Tian R-H, Li P, Li C-X, Yao M-H, Yao C-C, et al. Ultrasonographic evaluation of the rete testis thickness: a promising approach to differentiate obstructive from nonobstructive azoospermia. Asian J Androl. 2023;25(6):725–30.
37. Rasul B. The scrotal colour doppler ultrasound findings in infertile men from 2014 to 2017 in Sulaymaniyah/Iraq. J Sulaimani Med Coll. 2023;13(4):9.
38. Jarvis LJ, Dubbins PA. Changes in the epididymis after vasectomy: sonographic findings. AJR Am J Roentgenol. 1989;152(3):531–4.
39. Lotti F, Maggi M. Ultrasound of the male genital tract in relation to male reproductive health. Hum Reprod Update. 2014;21(1):56–83.
40. Herwig R, Tosun K, Schuster A, Rehder P, Glodny B, Wildt L, et al. Tissue perfusion-controlled guided biopsies are essential for the outcome of testicular sperm extraction. Fertil Steril. 2007;87(5):1071–6.
41. Schwarzer JU, Steinfatt H, Schleyer M, Kohn FM, Fiedler K, von Hertwig I, et al. No relationship between biopsy sites near the main testicular vessels or rete testis and successful sperm retrieval using conventional or microdissection biopsies in 220 non-obstructive azoospermic men. Asian J Androl. 2013;15(6):795–8.
42. Mandourah H, Alghafees M, Alali H, Alsuhaibani S, Gutub E, Aldosari L, et al. Comparison of sperm retrieval rate between superficial and deep dissection during microscopic testicular sperm extraction. Urol Ann. 2024;16(1):108–12.
43. Sihag P, Tandon A, Pal R, Bhatt S, Sinha A, Sumbul M. Sonography in male infertility: a useful yet underutilized diagnostic tool. J Ultrasound. 2022;25(3):675–85.
44. Peng Y, Ouyang L, Lin Z, Zhang F, Wang H, Guan J. MRI findings of nonobstructive azoospermia: lesions in and out of pelvic cavity. Abdom Radiol (NY). 2020;45(7):2213–24.
45. Wang H, Peng Y, Fu W, Hu X, Li C, Guan J. MRI findings of obstructive azoospermia: lesions in and out of pelvic cavity. Abdom Radiol (NY). 2020;45(3):851–64.
46. Hesham Said A, Ragab A, Zohdy W, Ibrahim AS, Abd El Basset AS. Diffusion-weighted magnetic resonance imaging and magnetic resonance spectroscopy for non-invasive characterization of azoospermia: a prospective comparative single-center study. Andrology. 2023;11(6):1096–106.
47. Lee TY, Sun GH, Chao SC. The effect of an infertility diagnosis on the distress, marital and sexual satisfaction between husbands and wives in Taiwan. Hum Reprod. 2001;16(8):1762–7.
48. Saleh RA, Ranga GM, Raina R, Nelson DR, Agarwal A. Sexual dysfunction in men undergoing infertility evaluation: a cohort observational study. Fertil Steril. 2003;79(4):909–12.
49. Gabr AA, Omran EF, Abdallah AA, Kotb MM, Farid EZ, Dieb AS, et al. Prevalence of sexual dysfunction in infertile versus fertile couples. Eur J Obstet Gynecol Reprod Biol. 2017;217:38–43.

50. Pelzman DL, Hwang K. Genetic testing for men with infertility: techniques and indications. Transl Androl Urol. 2021;10(3):1354–64.
51. Cao D, Bai C, Zhang G. Psychological distress among infertility patients: a network analysis. Front Psychol. 2022;13:906226.
52. Soosaipillai G, Archer S, Ashrafian H, Darzi A. Breaking bad news training in the COVID-19 era and beyond. J Med Educat Curri Develop. 2020;7:2382120520938706.
53. Narayanan V, Bista B, Koshy C. 'BREAKS' protocol for breaking bad news. Indian J Palliat Care. 2010;16(2):61–5.
54. Baile WF, Buckman R, Lenzi R, Glober G, Beale EA, Kudelka AP. SPIKES-a six-step protocol for delivering bad news: application to the patient with cancer. Oncologist. 2000;5(4):302–11.
55. Schwaninger G, Benjamin C, Rudnik-Schoneborn S, Zschocke J. The genetic counseling profession in Austria: stakeholders' perspectives. J Genet Couns. 2021;30(3):861–71.
56. Krausz C. Male infertility: pathogenesis and clinical diagnosis. Best Pract Res Clin Endocrinol Metab. 2011;25(2):271–85.
57. Vincent MC, Daudin M, De MP, Massat G, Mieusset R, Pontonnier F, et al. Cytogenetic investigations of infertile men with low sperm counts: a 25-year experience. J Androl. 2002;23(1):18–22. discussion 44-5
58. Clementini E, Palka C, Iezzi I, Stuppia L, Guanciali-Franchi P, Tiboni GM. Prevalence of chromosomal abnormalities in 2078 infertile couples referred for assisted reproductive techniques. Hum Reprod. 2005;20(2):437–42.
59. Colpi GM, Francavilla S, Haidl G, Link K, Behre HM, Goulis DG, et al. European academy of andrology guideline management of oligo-astheno-teratozoospermia. Andrology. 2018;6(4):513–24.
60. Pena VN, Kohn TP, Herati AS. Genetic mutations contributing to non-obstructive azoospermia. Best Pract Res Clin Endocrinol Metab. 2020;34(6):101479.
61. Hockner M, Pinggera GM, Gunther B, Sergi C, Fauth C, Erdel M, et al. Unravelling the parental origin and mechanism of formation of the 47,XY,i(X)(q10) Klinefelter karyotype variant. Fertil Steril. 2008;90(5):2009 e13–7.
62. Stamou MI, Georgopoulos NA. Kallmann syndrome: phenotype and genotype of hypogonadotropic hypogonadism. Metabolism. 2018;86:124–34.
63. Fakhro KA, Robay A, Rodriguez-Flores JL, Crystal RG. Genetic evaluation of male infertility. In: Arafa M, Elbardisi H, Majzoub A, Agarwal A, editors. Genetics of male infertility: a case-based guide for clinicians. Cham. Springer; 2020. p. 95–118.
64. Krausz C, Navarro-Costa P, Wilke M, Tüttelmann F. EAA/EMQN best practice guidelines for molecular diagnosis of Y-chromosomal microdeletions: state of the art 2023. Andrology. 2024;12(3):487–504.
65. Yuen W, Golin AP, Flannigan R, Schlegel PN. Histology and sperm retrieval among men with Y chromosome microdeletions. Transl Androl Urol. 2021;10(3):1442–56.
66. Toth B, Baston-Bust DM, Behre HM, Bielfeld A, Bohlmann M, Buhling K, et al. Diagnosis and therapy before assisted reproductive treatments. Guideline of the DGGG, OEGGG and SGGG (S2k Level, AWMF Register Number 015-085, February 2019) – part 1, basic assessment of the woman. Geburtshilfe Frauenheilkd. 2019;79(12):1278–92.
67. EAU_Guidelines_Sexual_and_Reproductive_Health. EAU guidelines sexual and reproductive health 2023. Available from: http://uroweb.org/guidelines/compilations-of-all-guidelines/http://uroweb.org/guidelines/compilations-of-all-guidelines/.
68. Luddi A, Margollicci M, Gambera L, Serafini F, Cioni M, De Leo V, et al. Spermatogenesis in a man with complete deletion of USP9Y. N Engl J Med. 2009;360(9):881–5.
69. Moreno-Mendoza D, Casamonti E, Paoli D, Chianese C, Riera-Escamilla A, Giachini C, et al. gr/gr deletion predisposes to testicular germ cell tumour independently from altered spermatogenesis: results from the largest European study. Eur J Hum Genet. 2019;27(10):1578–88.

70. Kohn TP, Kohn JR, Owen RC, Coward RM. The prevalence of Y-chromosome microdeletions in oligozoospermic men: a systematic review and meta-analysis of European and North American studies. Eur Urol. 2019;76(5):626–36.
71. Li L, Qu X, Cui C, Feng K, Xia Y, Wan F, et al. Compound heterozygous mutations in CFTR causing congenital bilateral absence of the vas deferens in a Chinese pedigree. Mol Genet Genomic Med. 2024;12(1):e2364.
72. Sironen A, Shoemark A, Patel M, Loebinger MR, Mitchison HM. Sperm defects in primary ciliary dyskinesia and related causes of male infertility. Cell Mol Life Sci. 2020;77(11):2029–48.
73. Shapiro A J, Davis S D, Ferkol T, Dell S D, Rosenfeld M, Olivier K N, et al. Laterality defects other than situs inversus totalis in primary ciliary dyskinesia: insights into situs ambiguus and heterotaxy. Chest. 2014;146(5):1176-86.
74. Pang MG, Hoegerman SF, Cuticchia AJ, Moon SY, Doncel GF, Acosta AA, et al. Detection of aneuploidy for chromosomes 4, 6, 7, 8, 9, 10, 11, 12, 13, 17, 18, 21, X and Y by fluorescence in-situ hybridization in spermatozoa from nine patients with oligoasthenoteratozoospermia undergoing intracytoplasmic sperm injection. Hum Reprod. 1999;14(5):1266–73.
75. Nagirnaja L, Aston KI, Conrad DF. Genetic intersection of male infertility and cancer. Fertil Steril. 2018;109(1):20–6.
76. Eisenberg ML, Betts P, Herder D, Lamb DJ, Lipshultz LI. Increased risk of cancer among azoospermic men. Fertil Steril. 2013;100(3):681–5.
77. Anderson RE, Hanson HA, Lowrance WT, Redshaw J, Oottamasathien S, Schaeffer A, et al. Childhood cancer risk in the siblings and cousins of men with poor semen quality. J Urol. 2017;197(3 Pt 2):898–905.
78. Williams DHT, Karpman E, Sander JC, Spiess PE, Pisters LL, Lipshultz LI. Pretreatment semen parameters in men with cancer. J Urol. 2009;181(2):736–40.
79. Maiolino G, Fernandez-Pascual E, Ochoa Arvizo MA, Vishwakarma R, Martinez-Salamanca JI. Male infertility and the risk of developing testicular cancer: a critical contemporary literature review. Medicina (Kaunas). 2023;59(7).
80. Ramsay JM, Madsen MJ, Horns JJ, Hanson HA, Camp NJ, Emery BR, et al. Describing patterns of familial cancer risk in subfertile men using population pedigree data. Hum Reprod. 2024;
81. Pang KH, Osman NI, Muneer A, Alnajjar HM. The relationship between testicular tumour characteristics and azoospermia: a systematic review. Int J Impot Res. 2022;34(6):543–51.
82. Rives N, Perdrix A, Hennebicq S, Saias-Magnan J, Melin MC, Berthaut I, et al. The semen quality of 1158 men with testicular cancer at the time of cryopreservation: results of the French National CECOS Network. J Androl. 2012;33(6):1394–401.
83. Munoz X, Mata A, Bassas L, Larriba S. Altered miRNA signature of developing germ-cells in infertile patients relates to the severity of spermatogenic failure and persists in spermatozoa. Sci Rep. 2015;5:17991.
84. Tuttelmann F, Ruckert C, Ropke A. Disorders of spermatogenesis: perspectives for novel genetic diagnostics after 20 years of unchanged routine. Med Genet. 2018;30(1):12–20.
85. Bahmyari S. MicroRNAs in male fertility. DNA Cell Biol. 2024;
86. Barceló M, Mata A, Bassas L, Larriba S. Exosomal microRNAs in seminal plasma are markers of the origin of azoospermia and can predict the presence of sperm in testicular tissue. Hum Reprod. 2018;33(6):1087–98.
87. Li Z, Zheng Z, Ruan J, Li Z, Zhuang X, Tzeng CM. Integrated analysis miRNA and mRNA profiling in patients with severe oligozoospermia reveals miR-34c-3p downregulates PLCXD3 expression. Oncotarget. 2016;7(33):52781–96.
88. Larriba S, Vigues F, Bassas L. Using small non-coding RNAs in extracellular vesicles of semen as biomarkers of male reproductive system health: opportunities and challenges. Int J Mol Sci. 2023;24(6)
89. Saeed S, Khan FA, Khan DA, Naveed AK, Ahmad M. Demonstration of the site of obstruction in azoospermia by biochemical markers. J Pak Med Assoc. 1994;44(6):140–2.

90. Fenichel P, Rey R, Poggioli S, Donzeau M, Chevallier D, Pointis G. Anti-Mullerian hormone as a seminal marker for spermatogenesis in non-obstructive azoospermia. Hum Reprod. 1999;14(8):2020–4.
91. Mostafa T, Amer MK, Abdel-Malak G, Nsser TA, Zohdy W, Ashour S, et al. Seminal plasma anti-Mullerian hormone level correlates with semen parameters but does not predict success of testicular sperm extraction (TESE). Asian J Androl. 2007;9(2):265–70.
92. Heshmat SM, Mullen JB, Jarvi KA, Soosaipillai A, Diamandis EP, Hamilton RJ, et al. Seminal plasma lipocalin-type prostaglandin D synthase: a potential new marker for the diagnosis of obstructive azoospermia. J Urol. 2008;179(3):1077–80.
93. Li H, Wu C, Gu X, Xiong C. A novel application of cell-free seminal mRNA: non-invasive identification of the presence of germ cells or complete obstruction in men with azoospermia. Hum Reprod. 2012;27(4):991–7.
94. Goel R, Batra H, Kumar M, Dada R, Kumar R. Evaluation of cell-free seminal mRNA for the diagnosis of obstruction as the cause of azoospermia in infertile men: a prospective cohort study. Andrologia. 2022;54(9):e14364.
95. Drabovich AP, Dimitromanolakis A, Saraon P, Soosaipillai A, Batruch I, Mullen B, Jarvi K, Diamandis EP. Differential diagnosis of azoospermia with proteomic biomarkers ECM1 and TEX101 quantified in seminal plasma. Sci Transl Med. 2013;5(212):212ra160. https://doi.org/10.1126/scitranslmed.3006260. PMID: 24259048.
96. Mostafa T, Bocu K, Malhotra V. A review of testicular histopathology in nonobstructive azoospermia. Asian J Androl. 2025;27(3):370-374.
97. Amer M, GamalEl Din SF, Zeidan A, Adel A, Elsisi I, Fakhry E, et al. Intrasurgical seminiferous tubular diameter correlates with total motile sperm count in azoospermia: a prospective cohort study. Reprod Sci. 2022;29(6):1836–43.
98. Jensen CFS, Wang D, Mamsen LS, Giwercman A, Jørgensen N, Fode M, et al. Sertoli and germ cells within atrophic seminiferous tubules of men with non-obstructive azoospermia. Front Endocrinol. 2022;13
99. Font MD, Pastuszak AW, Case JR, Lipshultz LI. An infertile male with dilated seminal vesicles due to functional obstruction. Asian J Androl. 2017;19(2):256–7.
100. McLachlan RI, Rajpert-De Meyts E, Hoei-Hansen CE, de Kretser DM, Skakkebaek NE. Histological evaluation of the human testis–approaches to optimizing the clinical value of the assessment: mini review. Hum Reprod. 2007;22(1):2–16.
101. Schlegel PN, Sigman M, Collura B, De Jonge CJ, Eisenberg ML, Lamb DJ, et al. Diagnosis and treatment of infertility in men: AUA/ASRM guideline part II. J Urol. 2021;205(1):44–51.
102. Schlegel PN, Sigman M, Collura B, De Jonge CJ, Eisenberg ML, Lamb DJ, et al. Diagnosis and treatment of infertility in men: AUA/ASRM guideline part I. J Urol. 2021;205(1):36–43.

Chapter 5
Imaging Used in the Evaluation of NOA

Abheesh Varma Hegde, Tuncay Toprak, and Eric Chung

Diagnostic Imaging in Hypogonadotropic Hypogonadism, Indication, and Interpretations

Hypogonadotropic hypogonadism (HH) is a medical condition characterized by reduced or absent gonadal function due to a lack of appropriate gonadotropin-releasing hormone (GnRH) stimulation [1]. This results in low levels of luteinizing hormone (LH) and follicle-stimulating hormone (FSH), which are crucial for normal reproductive function. Although there has been a significant increase in the number of patients referred to endocrine outpatient clinics for evaluation of HH in recent years, most men have no identifiable lesions in the pituitary region [2]. Their clinical and biochemical manifestations are strongly linked to risk factors such as obesity [3], androgenic anabolic steroid use [4], type 2 diabetes [5], and advanced age [6]. Serum testosterone and gonadotropin levels vary significantly as a result of episodic secretion, circadian rhythms, and measurement variation [7, 8]. Acquired HH can be caused by trauma, systemic diseases such as sarcoidosis, histiocytosis, and hemochromatosis, drugs such as GnRH analogs and anabolic steroids, radiation, abusive use of alcohol and illicit drugs, and pituitary lesions [1, 9]. Therefore, it can be difficult to determine which patients will need pituitary imaging based on a single threshold of biochemical results. In one study, lesions were detected in only 18.8% of patients in pituitary magnetic resonance imaging (MRI) performed with

A. V. Hegde (✉)
Department of Urology, Father Muller Medical College Hospital, Mangalore, India

T. Toprak
Department of Urology, University of Health Sciences, Hamidiye Faculty of Medicine, FSM Health Practice & Research Center, Istanbul, Turkey

E. Chung
Department of Urology, Princess Alexandra Hospital, University of Queensland, Brisbane, QLD, Australia

W. Zohdy et al. (eds.), *Non-Obstructive Azoospermia*, https://doi.org/10.1007/978-3-031-99431-9_5

the diagnosis of hypogonadism [2], and this was supported by other studies in the literature [10, 11]. Most had micro−/macroadenomas or partially or completely empty sella [2], and these findings were consistent with those of other authors, who often recommended no significant surgical treatment [10–12].

Therefore, the decision to perform a pituitary MRI scan should be based on the patient's complete history and clinical evaluation. The Endocrine Society has recommended pituitary MRI to men with secondary hypogonadism if there are persistent hyperprolactinemia, panhypopituitarism, low total testosterone (TT) levels (< 5.2 nmol/L), or with symptoms of tumor mass effect (visual impairment, headache, or visual field defect) to improve the diagnostic yield [13]. There still remains significant uncertainty and debate among clinicians when evaluating patients with HH, particularly when deciding which patients need pituitary MRI, because routine imaging of all patients is not clinically justified or financially feasible. So, diagnostic imaging is not typically the primary method for diagnosing hypogonadotropic hypogonadism, but certain imaging studies may be useful in specific situations or to rule out other underlying causes [2]. Figure 5.1 shows MRI appearance of a pituitary adenoma.

Here are some imaging modalities that may be considered in the evaluation of hypogonadotropic hypogonadism.

1. **Brain Magnetic Resonance Imaging (MRI)**
   - **Indication:** Brain MRI is often performed to assess the structure of the hypothalamus and pituitary gland.
   - **Interpretation:** Hypogonadotropic hypogonadism can be caused by structural abnormalities in the hypothalamus or pituitary gland, such as tumors, cysts, or malformations. The MRI can help identify such abnormalities.
2. **Pituitary Dynamic Contrast-Enhanced Magnetic Resonance Imaging (DCE-MRI)**
   - **Indication:** DCE-MRI may be used to assess the blood flow in the pituitary gland and identify abnormalities.
   - **Interpretation:** Abnormal blood flow patterns in the pituitary gland may indicate vascular issues or abnormalities that could be contributing to hypogonadotropic hypogonadism.
3. **Computed Tomography (CT) Scan**
   Indication: CT scans may be used in cases where an MRI is contraindicated or not available.
   Interpretation: Similar to MRI, CT scans can help identify structural abnormalities in the hypothalamus and pituitary gland.

It is important to note that while imaging studies can provide valuable information, the diagnosis of hypogonadotropic hypogonadism is usually based on

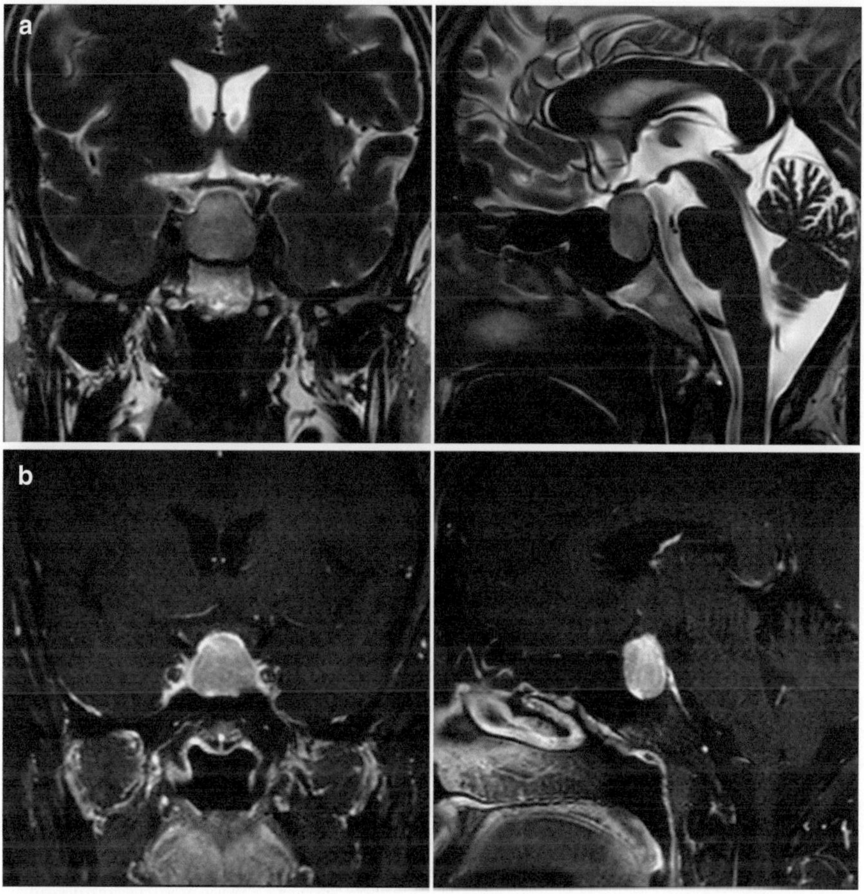

Fig. 5.1 MRI appearance of a pituitary adenoma. (**a**) T2-weighted, coronal, and sagittal views. (**b**) With contrast coronal and sagittal views

clinical and laboratory assessments [2]. Blood tests measuring hormone levels (LH, FSH, testosterone, etc.) and a thorough medical history are typically the primary tools for diagnosis [2]. If structural abnormalities are identified through imaging, further endocrinological and genetic testing may be necessary to determine the specific cause of hypogonadotropic hypogonadism [2].

It is crucial to consult with a healthcare professional, typically an endocrinologist or reproductive specialist, to determine the most appropriate diagnostic approach based on the individual's clinical presentation and medical history. Table 5.1 summarizes the purposes and indications of diagnostic imaging modalities in hypogonadotrophic hypogonadism.

Table 5.1 Diagnostic imaging in hypogonadotropic hypogonadism

Imaging	Purpose and indication
Pituitary MRI	Secondary hypogonadism if there are persistent hyperprolactinemia, panhypopituitarism, low TT levels (< 5.2 nmol/L), or with symptoms of tumor mass effect (visual impairment, headache, or visual field defect)
Brain MRI	To assess the structure of the hypothalamus and pituitary gland
DCE-MRI	To assess the blood flow in the pituitary gland and identify abnormalities
CT	It is used when an MRI is contraindicated or not available

MRI magnetic resonance imaging, *TT* total testosterone, *DCE* pituitary dynamic contrast-enhanced, *CT* computed tomography

Role of Imaging in Differentiating the Cause of NOA

Nonobstructive azoospermia (NOA) is a severe and common form of male infertility [14]. There is an absence of sperm in the ejaculate due to a failure in sperm production or maturation. Using noninvasive diagnostic methods before any intervention is very important to prevent unnecessary surgical interventions and increase the success of surgery [15].

Imaging studies may play a limited role in differentiating the various causes of NOA, but the primary diagnostic tools for evaluating NOA involve clinical assessments, hormone testing, and testicular biopsies. Here are some areas where the imaging method can be used:

Testicular ultrasound: Testicular ultrasound is often used to assess the size and structure of the testicles. It can help identify structural abnormalities such as testicular atrophy, tumors, or cysts. However, ultrasound alone may not provide a definitive diagnosis of the cause of NOA. Pezzella et al. [16] measured the epididymal head diameter by ultrasonography and found that it did not provide any clinical significance for patients with NOA. This measurement also did not predict success in sperm retrieval by TESE in patients with NOA. Signs of testicular dysgenesis, such as microlithiasis or heterogeneous testis architecture, could be detected in men with NOA [17, 18]. Figures 5.2 and 5.3 show ultrasound-detected lesions in the testis.

1. **Magnetic Resonance Imaging (MRI):** MRI may be considered in cases where ultrasound results are inconclusive or when more detailed imaging is needed. MRI can provide additional information about the testicular structure, blood flow, and the presence of any abnormalities within the testicles. Wang et al. [19] found that functional MRI, including magnetization transfer MRI and diffusion-weighted MRI, gives promising results for evaluating male infertility with a lower magnetization transfer ratio and with a higher apparent diffusion coefficient in testicular hypospermatogenesis. Another study suggested that testicular metabolite concentrations measured by 3 T proton spectroscopy could be used as noninvasive bio-

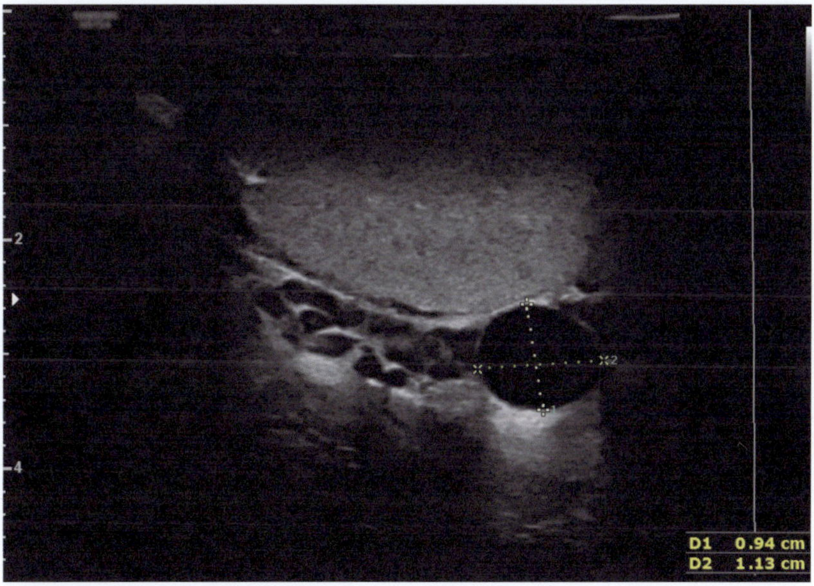

Fig. 5.2 Epididymal cyst on ultrasound

markers to predict spermatogenesis [20]. Another study found that phosphocholine concentrations were significantly higher in normal testicles compared to Sertoli cells only [21]. This finding demonstrated that the metabolic profile of spermatogenesis could be identified by proton magnetic resonance spectroscopy in men with NOA. In conclusion, MRI has certain clinical value in assessing spermatogenic status, but its use in differentiating NOA from OA is limited.

2. **High-Resolution Transrectal Ultrasonography (TRUS):** TRUS has become a first-line diagnostic tool for the diagnosis of ejaculatory duct obstruction (EDO) as a noninvasive testing method. The diagnostic criteria of Turek et al., such as a dilated ejaculatory duct (bigger than 2.3 mm), a dilated seminal vesicle (bigger than 1.5 cm in transverse diameter), presence of a cyst near the verumontanum, and a presense of calcification or stones in verumontanum or ejaculatory duct, are recognized as the criteria for TRUS evaluation [22].

Despite the role of imaging, the definitive diagnosis of the cause of NOA often requires a combination of measurement of hormone levels such as follicle-stimulating hormone (FSH), luteinizing hormone (LH), testosterone, and estradiol can provide insights into the functioning of the testicular axis, clinical examination, and genetic evaluations to identify any underlying genetic abnormalities that could contribute to impaired spermatogenesis, as well as a testicular biopsy that involves the extraction of tissue samples from the testicles for microscopic examination. This is a crucial step in determining the cause of NOA and may reveal information about the presence or absence of sperm, as well as the histological pattern of testicular tissue.

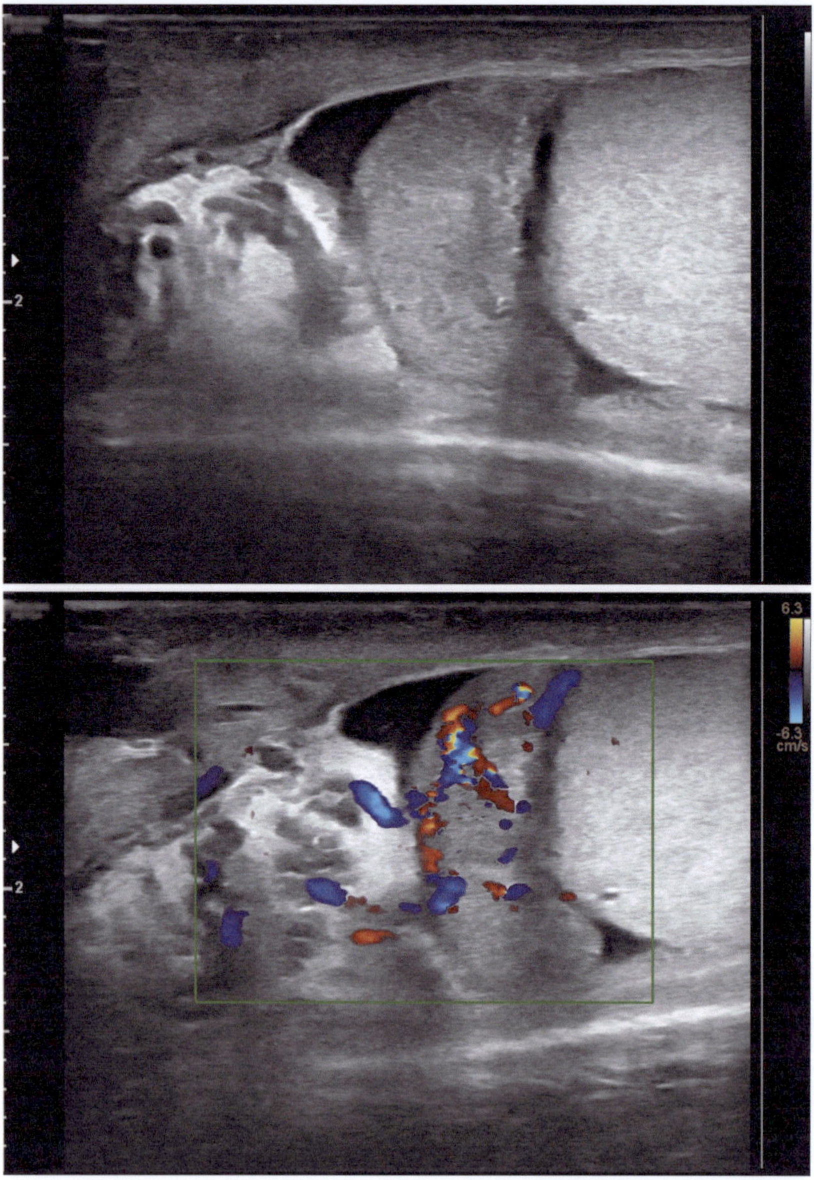

Fig. 5.3 Funiculitis with epididymitis (**a**) on grayscale ultrasound (**b**) on color Doppler

It is important to consult with a reproductive endocrinologist or urologist who specializes in male infertility to determine the most appropriate diagnostic approach based on individual clinical findings. Table 5.2 summarizes the role of imaging in distinguishing the cause of NOA (Table 5.3).

Table 5.2 Role of imaging in differentiating the cause of NOA

Imaging	Advantages	Disadvantages
Testicular USG	It assesses the size and structure of the testicles It can help identify structural abnormalities such as testicular atrophy, tumors, or cysts	Ultrasound alone may not provide a definitive diagnosis of the cause of NOA
Scrotal MRI	It provides more details and additional information about the testicular structure, blood flow, and the presence of any abnormalities within the testicles	Expensive, difficult to access, takes a long time, sometimes clear images cannot be obtained, its use in differentiating NOA from OA is limited
TRUS	It can detect ejaculatory duct obstruction. It is cheap, easily accessible, and radiation free	Process difficulty, possibility of personal interpretation

USG ultrasonography, *MRI* magnetic resonance imaging, *TRUS* high-resolution transrectal ultrasonography

Table 5.3 Newer methods of imaging in nonobstructive azoospermia (NOA)

Modality	Basis
Diffusion tensor imaging	A functional MRI technique
Shear wave elastography	Predicts stiffness of tissue utilizing acoustic radiofrequency signals
Multiphoton microscopy	Utilizes nonlinear excitation as a means of exciting fluorescence providing real-time images of tissues in vivo
Full-field optical coherence tomography	Uses white light interference microscopy to generate quick high-resolution tomographic images of fresh (unprocessed and unstained) tissue
Narrow-band imaging	Optical filter allows light to pass at a short wavelength of 400–430 nm

Role of Ultrasonography, CT, and MRI in Locating Undescended Testicles

Locating undescended testicles is essential for proper diagnosis and management. Various imaging modalities, such as ultrasonography, computed tomography (CT), and magnetic resonance imaging (MRI), may be employed for this purpose. Ultrasonography is a commonly used imaging modality for evaluating undescended testicles, especially in infants and children. It is often the initial imaging choice due to its noninvasive nature and lack of ionizing radiation. Ultrasonography can help visualize the position of the testicles within the inguinal canal and rarely within the abdomen. It provides real-time images and is particularly useful for assessing blood flow, ruling out associated abnormalities, and guiding the decision for surgical intervention. However, it cannot localize nonpalpable intra-abdominal testes. In children who are diagnosed with hypospadias or ambigiuous genitalia, an ultrasound also detects presence of Mullerian structures [23].

CT scans may be used in certain situations, especially when the testicle is located high in the abdomen and traditional imaging methods are inconclusive. CT is generally reserved for cases where more detailed anatomical information is needed. CT scans can provide cross-sectional images that help locate undescended testicles, detect pathologies such as testicular tumors in cryptorchid testes, and assess their relationship to surrounding structures. However, due to ionizing radiation exposure, especially in children, CT is typically used judiciously and when other modalities are insufficient [24].

MRI can be used to locate undescended testicles, especially when detailed soft tissue imaging is required. MRI may be considered when ultrasonography results are inconclusive or when additional anatomical details are needed. MRI provides high-resolution images without using ionizing radiation, which is important in the pediatric population. It can offer detailed information about the position of the testicles and surrounding structures, aiding in surgical planning. Addition of DWI and fat suppression T2WI improved the yield in nonpalpable undescended testis [25]. In general, the choice of imaging modality depends on the specific clinical scenario, age of the patient, and the suspected location of the undescended testicle. Ultrasonography is often the initial and preferred imaging method, while CT and MRI may be reserved for cases where further details are required or when ultrasonography is inconclusive. Ultrasound has 45% sensitivity and 78% specificity for detection of undescended testis. MRI has a sensitivity and specificity of 89.5% and 87.5%, but it is costlier, not easily available, and would need sedation to image children. Diagnostic laparoscopy has the highest yield in cryptorchidism, and all diagnostic modalities have been compared with it [23–25]. Figure 5.4 shows the images of undescended testis on ultrasound and MRI.

Varicocele Diagnosis and Prognosis After Varicocele Repair (VR)

Diagnosis of varicocele typically involves a physical examination, often performed while standing, as well as imaging studies such as scrotal ultrasound. US is the preferred imaging modality, but the need for US is debated because there is no clear consensus on which technique should be used, how the diagnosis should be made, and which of the many classification systems should be used [26–28]. Despite all this, there is also evidence that accurate imaging of varicoceles helps in treatment decisions [29, 30]. There are several different sonographic classifications for varicocele evaluation. However, the lack of standardization has led to variability in US technique and diagnostic criteria, which has prevented the adoption of a clear method. There is also a wide variation in the recommended threshold venous diameter for varicocele diagnosis, where the measurement is taken, the position in which the patient should be positioned, and the need for Valsalva [31–35]. A venous diameter of 3 mm is commonly considered to be the threshold for diagnosis of a

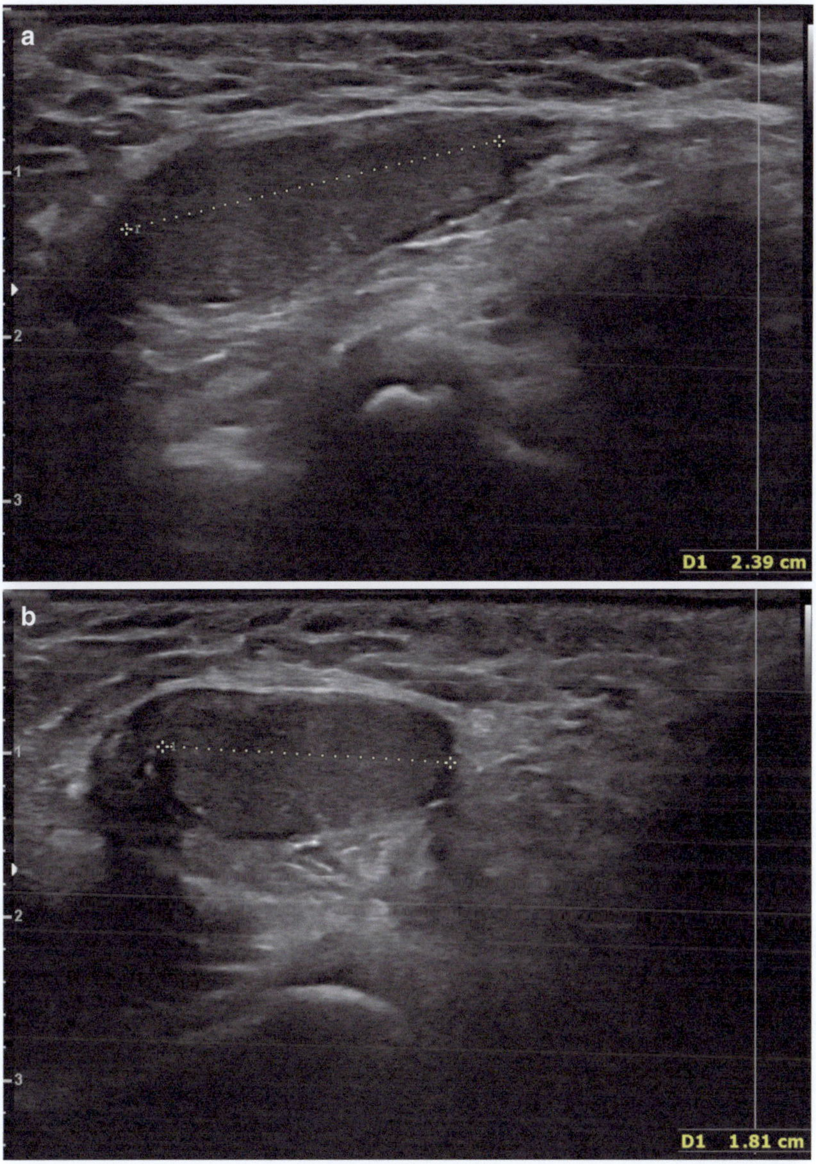

Fig. 5.4 Left inguinal testis, ultrasound appearance (**a**, **b**), on MRI (**c**)

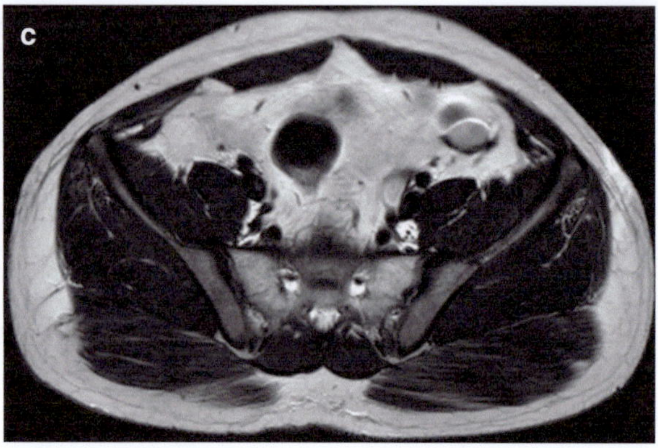

Fig. 5.4 (continued)

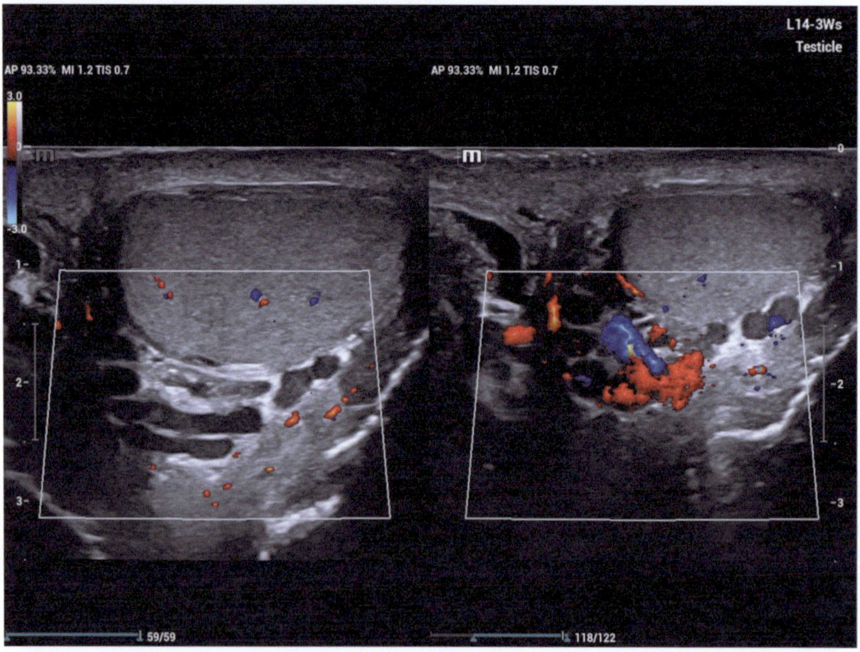

Fig. 5.5 Varicocele shown on ultrasound and color Doppler

varicocele, although higher and lower values have been advocated [34, 36, 37]. It is important to determine the patient's position and the area to be imaged. This is often done by examining the patient in both the supine and upright positions and both at rest and during Valsalva. It is generally recommended to measure the largest vein [38, 39]. Figure 5.5 shows the ultrasound appearance of a varicocele.

Evaluation of reflux is important for the diagnosis of varicocele and monitoring of treatment results. Assessment of flow direction and changes with Valsalva are done with color Doppler and confirmed with spectral Doppler, which also measures the duration of reflux [40]. The predicted venous reflux time for varicocele diagnosis and grading varies among studies [41–43]. Short-term reflux (< 1 s) during Valsalva is generally considered physiological [40, 43]. Moderate reflux is defined as reflux lasting less than 2 s and ending before the end of Valsalva. It is considered an indeterminate finding. Persistent reflux lasts longer than 2 s and plateaus during Valsalva and is always associated with abnormality on venography. Therefore, reflux lasting longer than 2 s is considered the most useful parameter for the diagnosis of varicocele [44, 45]. Color Doppler ultrasonography shows the normal pattern of venous flow at rest, with increased velocities with the Valsalva maneuver and the onset of retrograde filling [46, 47].

The AUA/ASRM guidelines recommend VR if there is infertility and palpable varicocele associated with abnormal semen parameters [48]. Diagnosis after VR involves a comprehensive approach, combining clinical evaluation, imaging studies, and patient feedback. The goal is to ensure that the varicocele has been successfully addressed, symptoms have resolved, and, if applicable, improvements in fertility parameters have been achieved. Regular follow-up with a healthcare provider is critical to monitor the postoperative course. AUA/ASRM guidelines (statement 21) do not recommend performing routine scrotal US to investigate varicocele recurrence [48].

EAU guidelines (10.4.3.2) recommend scrotal Doppler US to investigate residual/recurrent varicoceles if there is no improvement in semen parameters after VR.

According to the results of a survey conducted by the Global Andrology Forum with 521 participants worldwide who are experts in the field, there were significant disagreements about post-VR follow-up. While 14.8% (77/521) of the participants routinely recommended post-VR USG to all patients, 21.7% (113/521) never requested post-op USG. Others recommended it conditionally [49].

Routine Doppler US after VR may serve as a quality control method and help the clinician demonstrate that there is no residual varicocele and that the artery has been successfully preserved. However, this has many disadvantages other than time spent and additional cost. Performing Doppler US after VR may also detect a varicocele that is not clinically significant, leading to misdiagnosis of failed surgery. In a study conducted to control varicocele in adolescents after VR, significant differences were observed between ultrasound findings and clinical examination; ultrasound reported residual/recurrent varicocele in 12 of 15 patients [50]. If residual varicocele is detected by ultrasound after VR, this may lead to unjustified patient anxiety and management dilemma. According to a study, a 60% recurrence rate was reported if a Doppler US check was performed 5 years after VR; This suggests that Doppler US may overestimate recurrence after VR [51]. The recommendation made according to the results of the survey conducted by GAF; If there is no improvement in semen parameters or if the pain does not subside and there are findings suggestive of residual or recurrent varicocele on physical examination, repeat US may be considered [49].

Value of Ultrasound and Duplex in Differentiating Tubular Duct Ectasia from Intratesticular Varicocele

Both tubular duct ectasia and intratesticular varicocele may present with symptoms such as testicular pain or discomfort. Clinical correlation, including the patient's symptoms and history, is essential for accurate diagnosis.

Ultrasound and Duplex Doppler imaging are valuable diagnostic tools that can aid in differentiating between tubular duct ectasia and intratesticular varicocele, two conditions that may present with similar symptoms but have distinct underlying causes.

The key lies in assessing the morphology of the dilated structures and evaluating blood flow characteristics. These imaging modalities, along with clinical correlation, contribute to a comprehensive diagnostic approach, helping healthcare providers make informed decisions regarding further management or intervention.

On ultrasound, tubular duct ectasia may present as dilated tubular structures within the testicular parenchyma. These dilated tubules are often tortuous and can be seen as hypoechoic areas. Blood flow within these tubules is typically minimal or absent. Color Doppler imaging may show little to no vascularity within the dilated structures. Tubular duct ectasia is usually localized within the testicular parenchyma and may not involve the pampiniform plexus (the network of veins in the spermatic cord).

Varicoceles are characterized by dilated veins. In intratesticular varicocele, these dilated veins are within the testicular parenchyma, and they may appear as hypoechoic or anechoic tubular structures. In the case of intratesticular varicocele, Doppler imaging can show increased blood flow within the dilated veins, helping to differentiate it from other conditions.

Role of Ultrasound in Detecting Focal Lesions in Men with NOA

Ultrasound can play a role in assessing men with NOA by helping to detect focal lesions in the testicles. Ultrasound can provide detailed images of the testicles, allowing the assessment of size, shape, and overall morphology. Testicular size and shape abnormalities may indicate underlying issues contributing to NOA. Ultrasound can also detect focal lesions such as tumors, cysts, calcifications, or other masses within the testicles.

Diagnosis and Clinical Importance of Testicular Microlithiasis in Men with NOA

The scrotal imaging subcommittee of the European Society of Radiology (ESUR) classifies microlithiasis as limited (less than five per field of view) and classic (more than or equal to five per view). They appear as intratubular microcalcifications that are echogenic and measure 3 mm or less. The 15 MHz linear transducer is used for scrotal ultrasound. Large scrotums need lower frequencies. Incidence of microliths ismore with higher frequency ultrasound machines [52]. Testicular microlithiasis are seen in almost 9% of patients undergoing ultrasonography of the scrotum. Those with subfertility have microlithiasis in almost 20% cases [53]. It is often found in testicular dysgenesis and signifies spermatogenesis failure [54]. In a prospective study, it was found that testicular microlithiasis patients had poor sperm retrieval rates compared to those without (6.2% versus 39.4%) and smaller testicular diameters [55]. These patients should also be counseled about the risk for developing germ cell cancers and taught testicular self-examination. Risk factors such as personal/family history of germ cell tumors, ectopic testis, orchidopexy, and atrophic testis warrant further evaluation and follow up (routinely up to the age of 55 years). Patients with microlithiasis and no other risk factors need not undergo any additional investigations [52].

Klinefelter Syndrome

A large number of patients with Klinefelter syndrome also suffer from infertility and/or testicular atrophy. Patients with testicular atrophy will need surveillance, whereas patients with microlithiasis and only infertility need not undergo surveillance. Incidental testicular nodules that are mostly benign Leydig cell nodules/hyperplasia are more commonly found in Klinefelter syndrome patients [52].

Imaging Utility in Surgical Sperm Retrieval

Color Duplex Ultrasonography

Color duplex ultrasonography is a new addition to guide FNA or TESE by locating areas of better vascularity that could harbor zones of active spermatogenesis. When conducted before TESE, a high-resolution color duplex ultrasonography focusing on testicular perfusion correlated positively with the quality and quantity of harvested spermatozoa. This could help take targeted biopsies and reduce the biopsy passes into testicular tissue preventing damage. However, more studies are needed to establish the role of color Doppler in predicting areas of active spermatogenesis [56].

Value of Ultrasound in the Measurement of Seminiferous Tubule Diameters Before Micro-TESE

Seminiferous tubules are readily visible on grayscale US images of the testis. In micro-TESE, the aim is to obtain targeted biopsies of the tubules in which active spermatogenesis occurs. These are larger and more opaque than other tubules. It is based on the premise that the larger tubule has more chances of spermatogenesis. A grayscale and color Doppler ultrasonography using a high-frequency transducer (10–14 MHz) is obtained prior to surgery. Multiple grayscale images are obtained in the transverse and longitudinal planes and the grayscale images of the testicles in JPEG format are used for evaluation of the morphology of seminiferous tubules on a personal computer. In the water immersion method, normal seminiferous tubules appear hyperechogenic. Seminiferous tubules could be visualized by a simple two-step procedure of adjusting the contrast and brightness of images.

Thick, cell-rich tubules are displayed as hyperechoic bands, whereas narrow tubules and stromal tissue disappeared on processing the images. Once a seminiferous tubule is identified, the tubular diameter is measured on the first-visualized image and classified as 100 μm (very thin), 200 μm (thin), 250 μm (thick), or 300 μm (evidently thick). The maximum tubule size is used as the value for each patient. US image-derived tubule size by the immersion method roughly correlated with the width of the surgically retrieved tubules. 10–20 minutes of image analysis are needed for every patient. Such a US-generated image analysis protocol prior to surgery provided similar information as histology post micro-TESE [57].

Intraoperatively, the highest motile spermatozoa group was seen in those patients with dilated tubules (>300Um), and they had uneventful TESE. Occasionally, in patients with maturation arrest, the homogeneous appearance makes it difficult to differentiate dilated tubules from surroundings. Preop ST diameter is the strongest predictor for uneventful mTESE. Knowing the ST diameters and utilizing the information also reduce the chances of repeat mTESE in Sertoli-only syndrome patients [58].

Diffusion Tensor Imaging Parameters and Value in Testes with Nonobstructive Azoospermia

A functional magnetic resonance imaging technique, diffusion tensor imaging (DTI), shows the velocity and diffusion of a molecule of water in biological tissues. Mean diffusivity (MD) and functional anisotropy (FA) values are derived, which provide an idea about the structure and composition of organs and tissues. The quantitative readings of DTI help differentiate between NOA and controls. It can also predict sperm retrieval rates in nonobstructive azoospermia patients prior to mTESE [59].

Role of Ultrasonography in Follow-Up After TESE/TESA

Postprocedure ultrasound study is advised when patients have to be assessed for complications like testicular atrophy, hematoma, abscess, and scar tissue, which have to be ruled out before planning the next intervention. Viable testicular area can also be localized by serial USG follow-ups. Each testis should be measured in three dimensions and the volume calculated by use of the formula for an ellipsoid. Testicular texture should be evaluated in terms of echogenicity of the parenchyma, presence, and size of focal lesions, intratesticular hematoma, and color flow Doppler imaging. The presence of extratesticular hematoma or hydrocele should be also documented, as well as changes in size and texture of the head of the epididymis. In a study conducted to know the effects of sperm extraction on testicular tissue, sonographic and color Doppler imaging were obtained before the surgical procedures, and then at 1, 2 weeks, 2 and 6 months after the TESA/TESE procedures. The study included 14 patients in the nonobstructive azoospermia group and six obstructive azoospermia patients. At the end of 6 months, no sonological abnormalities remained in both groups [60]. Repeat TESE for those with no sperms found in the first attempt has been advocated with success rates of up to 18.4% with experienced surgeon and good technical infrastructure [61]. Figures 5.6, 5.7, and 5.8 show ultrasound images of orchitis, testicular hematoma, and atrophy.

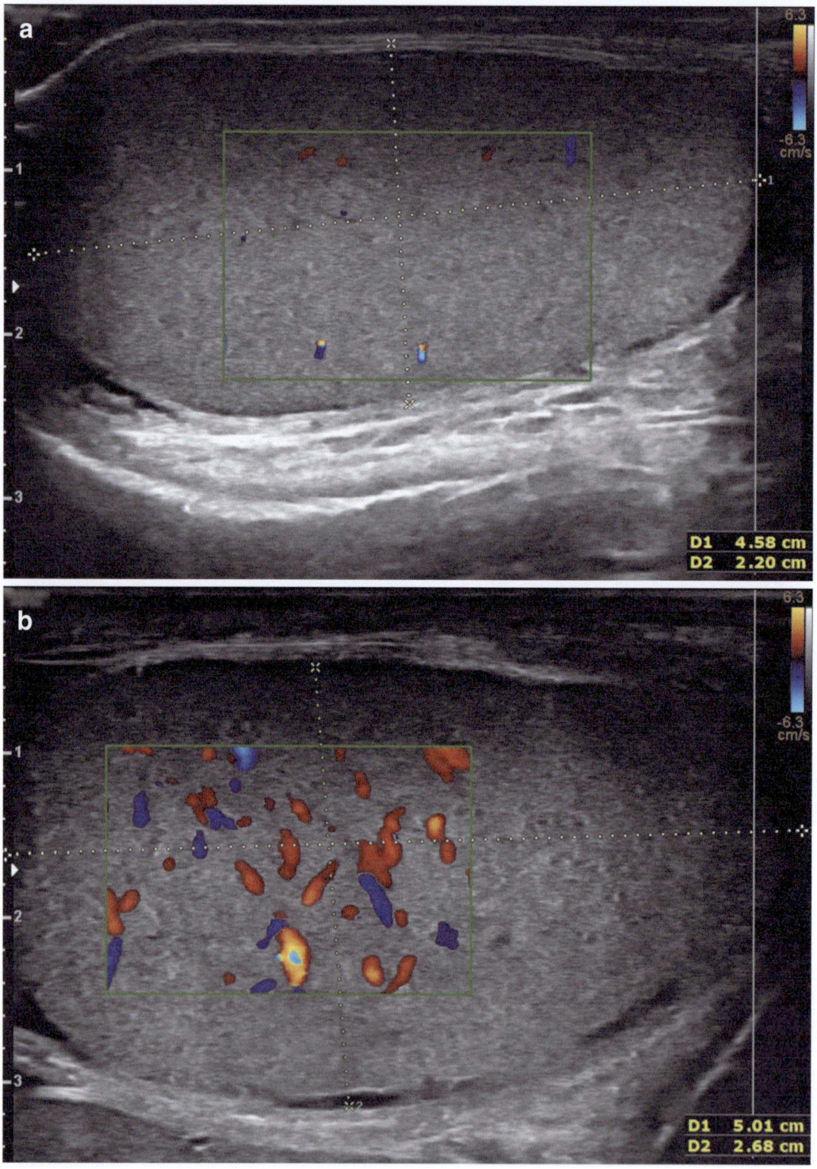

Fig. 5.6 Orchitis of the left testis as seen on ultrasound. (**a**) Grayscale; (**b**) color Doppler showing increased signals

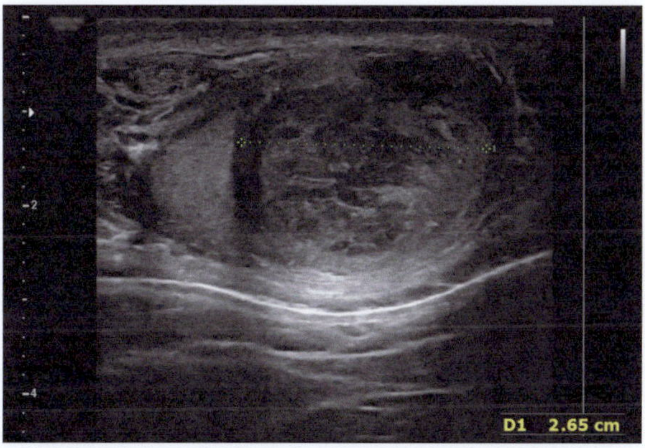

Fig. 5.7 Testicular hematoma, ultrasound appearance

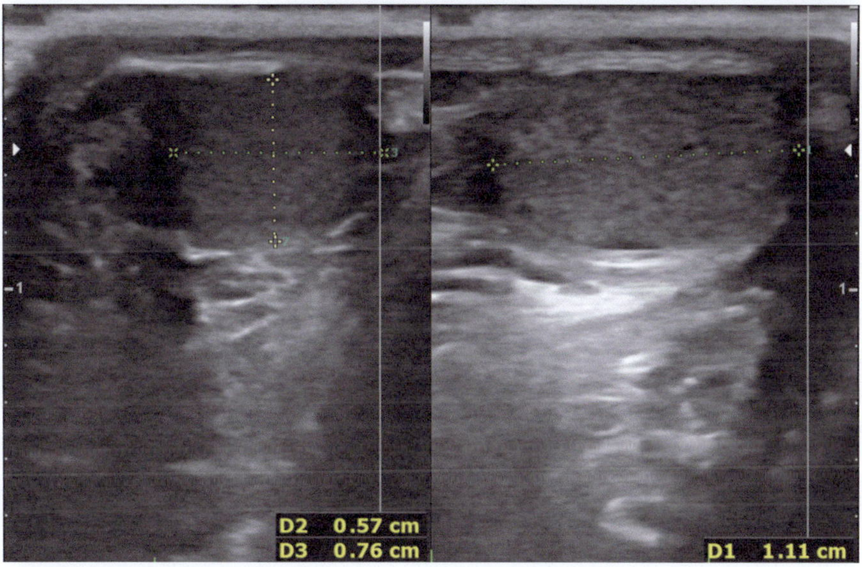

Fig. 5.8 Testicular atrophy on ultrasound

Shear Wave Elastography (SWE) in Predicting Testicular Pathology and TESE Outcome

Shear wave elastography (SWE) gives information regarding the inherent elasticity of tissues. An acoustic radiofrequency signal, sometimes termed "acoustic wind," produces shear waves that travel the surrounding tissue and provide information regarding tissue quality or stiffness. The pattern of the testicular elasticity is related to its function and volume. Testicular SWE serves as an adjunct to conventional US to identify non-neoplastic lesions when findings are discordant. SWE can distinguish testicles with spermatogenic changes from those without such changes.

Hence, it can noninvasively be used to evaluate the tissue alterations of the organ. SWE is used to investigate testicular pathologies, particularly neoplastic processes, varicocele, orchitis, infarction, and torsion. SWE is an inexpensive, noninvasive, and a well-tolerated diagnostic procedure. Measurements are expressed as kPa or cm/s since it is proportional to the speed of the waves. Acoustic pulses can be used to focus at different areas in the tissue at supersonic speed and are enhanced by forming a Mach cone that increases shear wave propagation. SWE values are calculated in the longest longitudinal plan. SWE images are viewed in dual mode, elasticity mode (kPa), and propagation (arrival time contour) mode. Tissue elasticity is presented in a range of colors between dark blue (lowest stiffness) and red (highest stiffness). Four SWE measurements are calculated for each testis (upper medial, upper lateral, lower medial, and lower lateral regions of the testis), and the average is considered the SWE value of the corresponding testis. In fact, SWE could be more accurate in evaluating testicular stiffness than the palpation method performed during the physical examination to assess parenchymal elasticity [62].

There is a negative correlation between testicular SWE parameters and testicular volumes and sperm counts. It could also be utilized in predicting parenchymal damage and hence abnormal sperm quantity by assessing stiffness in infertility patients. Lower testicular volumes and increased SWE may predict the degree of parenchymal damage. A consensus SWE cutoff value to differentiate oligospermia and azoospermia has not been arrived at yet [62, 63].

Role of TRUS in Men with NOA (Including Hypogonadism)

Transrectal ultrasound (TRUS) enables high-resolution imaging of the prostate, seminal vesicles, and vas deferens and is the modality of choice in diagnosing congenital and acquired abnormalities. A high-frequency endorectal transducer should be used with a condom cover. Systematic evaluation of the terminal vas deferens, seminal vesicles, ejaculatory duct, and prostate was carried out in axial and sagittal planes. TRUS is also used to guide prostatic cyst aspiration. Its role is limited only to eliminate obstructive azoospermia and rule out the pathologies of seminal vesicles and prostate [64].

Future Directions

- **Multiphoton Microscopy (MPM).**

  MPM is an optical imaging technology that utilizes nonlinear excitation as a means of exciting fluorescence. MPM, first demonstrated over 20 years ago, has proven to be extremely useful in biological imaging and has become the standard for fluorescence microscopy both ex vivo and in vivo imaging. MPM has been used in neuroscience, oncology, and immunology because it enables the visualization of various biological processes at the cellular level in vivo. Further, MPM is able to provide real-time images of unstained tissue in vivo. MPM could provide urologists with another novel technology that can aid in the diagnosis and evaluation. It provides distinctive optical signals that enables imaging of animal and human tissue with minimal phototoxicity to cells. The images can provide detailed information on cellular morphology and tissue architecture at submicron resolution in three dimensions to a depth over 1 mm below the sample surface depending on the tissue [65].

Microdissection testicular sperm extraction is the first-line procedure for sperm retrieval in men with nonobstructive azoospermia. This procedure, coupled with intracytoplasmic sperm injection into oocytes in vitro, has made it possible for men with impaired sperm production to father children. The efficacy of this procedure is limited by the ability of the operating surgeon to identify seminiferous tubules containing spermatozoa. In searching for areas of spermatogenesis within the testis, the seminiferous tubules are currently evaluated by subjective assessment of their size and opacity using the operating microscope. With the current technique, sperm has been retrieved in 40–60% of cases, depending on the underlying cause of low sperm production. MPM provides the operating surgeon with the opportunity for real-time visualization of seminiferous tubules in living tissue. The use of MPM in microdissection testicular sperm extraction has the potential to improve the success of this procedure. Safety of MPM laser must be addressed before MPM can be used in microdissection testicular sperm extraction. There are investigators currently working on several prototypes to make the laser imaging technique accessible. These prototypes will need to be small enough so they can be utilized within the confines of the operating room. MPM safety concerns include thermal damage to tissue and, more importantly, nonlinear damage to DNA. Although the rodent model showed minimal phototoxicity, this must be confirmed in a human model. Once these obstacles are overcome, MPM may take on a large role in the evaluation of men with nonobstructive azoospermia [65].

Full-Field Optical Coherence Tomography

Full-field optical coherence tomography (FFOCT) uses white light interference microscopy to generate quick high-resolution tomographic images of fresh (unprocessed and unstained) tissue. Furthermore, by using a nonlaser safe light source (150 W halogen lamp) for tissue illumination, it ensures that the sperm extracted for in vitro fertilization are not photo-damaged or mutagenized. FFOCT is a high-resolution "optical biopsy" technique that can render quick images of freshly excised (unprocessed and unstained) tissue. This technique makes use of a simple tungsten halogen lamp and is based on the principle of white light interference microscopy. FFOCT has recently been utilized in several areas of clinical research, including ophthalmology, cardiology, gastroenterology, and pulmonology [66].

FFOCT can directly visualize tubules that have the potential to improve success in micro-TESE procedures, while minimizing the removal of unnecessary biopsies and thus reducing operative time and associated potential complications. Additionally, FFOCT-guided testis biopsy could prevent loss of Leydig cells in interstitial testicular tissue, thereby potentially decreasing the risk of male hypogonadism. One specific advantage of FFOCT over other competing optical biopsy techniques, most of which use powerful lasers as the illumination source, is the fact that this technology uses very safe incident light, coming from a 150 W halogen lamp. Since the sperm isolated during this procedure will be used for ICSI, it is imperative that they not be photo-damaged—even at subclinical levels—by exposure to intense and potentially mutagenic light. The use of this safe illumination makes FFOCT especially suitable for the application in NOA [66].

Narrow-Band Imaging System (NBI)

In NBI mode, an optical filter allows a narrow-band light to pass at a short wavelength of 400–430 nm (centered at 415 nm), that only penetrates the mucosa superficially enhancing the mucosal vasculature. It evaluates the angiogenic potential in testicular specimens. An immunofluorescence study of blood vessels in the testes can be carried out. The number of blood vessels in the specimens of hypospermatogenesis will be significantly greater than that in the specimens of maturation arrest and Sertoli cell only. Significant differences in visual color between atrophic and normal lesions will be noted using NBI. The number of seminiferous tubules with spermatozoa in atrophic regions will be significantly lower than that in normal regions, and a significantly small number of blood vessels in atrophic regions will also be noted compared with that in normal regions. NBI can also identify patchy spermatogenesis in the busulfan-induced NOA patients. An NBI system can distinguish spermatogenically active regions through the visualization of blood vessels in the testes. This system may have the potential to provide useful information during micro-TESE for men with NOA but still in the experimental phase [67]. Table 5.3 summarizes the newer methods in imaging nonobstructive azoospermia.

References

1. Hayes FJ, Seminara SB, Crowley WF. Hypogonadotropic hypogonadism. Endocrinol Metab Clin. 1998;27:739–63.
2. Das G, Surya A, Okosieme O, Vali A, Tennant BP, Geen J, Abusahmin H. Pituitary imaging by MRI and its correlation with biochemical parameters in the evaluation of men with hypogonadotropic hypogonadism. Endocr Pract. 2019;25:926–34.
3. Corona G, Rastrelli G, Monami M, Saad F, Luconi M, Lucchese M, et al. Body weight loss reverts obesity-associated hypogonadotropic hypogonadism: a systematic review and meta-analysis. Eur J Endocrinol. 2013;168:829–43.

4. Rahnema CD, Lipshultz LI, Crosnoe LE, Kovac JR, Kim ED. Anabolic steroid–induced hypogonadism: diagnosis and treatment. Fertil Steril. 2014;101:1271–9.
5. Kapoor D, Aldred H, Clark S, Channer KS, Jones TH. Clinical and biochemical assessment of hypogonadism in men with type 2 diabetes: correlations with bioavailable testosterone and visceral adiposity. Diabetes Care. 2007;30:911–7.
6. Huhtaniemi I. Late-onset hypogonadism: current concepts and controversies of pathogenesis, diagnosis and treatment. Asian J Androl. 2014;16:192.
7. Bremner WJ, Vitiello MV, Prinz PN. Loss of circadian rhythmicity in blood testosterone levels with aging in normal men. J Clin Endocrinol Metabol. 1983;56:1278–81.
8. Brambilla DJ, O'Donnell AB, Matsumoto AM, McKinlay JB. Intraindividual variation in levels of serum testosterone and other reproductive and adrenal hormones in men. Clin Endocrinol. 2007;67:853–62.
9. Darby E, Anawalt BD. Male hypogonadism: an update on diagnosis and treatment. Treat Endocrinol. 2005;4:293–309.
10. Hirsch D, Benbassat C, Toledano Y, S'chigol I, Tsvetov G, Shraga-Slutzky I, et al. Pituitary imaging findings in male patients with hypogonadotrophic hypogonadism. Pituitary. 2015;18:494–9.
11. Citron JT, Ettinger B, Rubinoff H, Ettinger VM, Minkoff J, Hom F, et al. Prevalence of hypothalamic-pituitary imaging abnormalities in impotent men with secondary hypogonadism. J Urol. 1996;155:529–33.
12. Rhoden EL, Estrada C, Levine L, Morgentaler A. The value of pituitary magnetic resonance imaging in men with hypogonadism. J Urol. 2003;170:795–8.
13. Bhasin S, Brito JP, Cunningham GR, Hayes FJ, Hodis HN, Matsumoto AM, et al. Testosterone therapy in men with hypogonadism: an endocrine society clinical practice guideline. J Clin Endocrinol Metabol. 2018;103:1715–44.
14. Gao S, Yang X, Xiao X, Yin S, Guan Y, Chen J, Chen Y. Outcomes and affecting factors for ICSI and microTESE treatments in nonobstructive azoospermia patients with different etiologies: a retrospective analysis. Front Endocrinol (Lausanne). 2022;13:1006208.
15. Qi L, Liu YP, Zhang NN, Su YC. Predictors of testicular sperm retrieval in patients with non-obstructive azoospermia: a review. J Int Med Res. 2021;49:03000605211002703.
16. Pezzella A, Barbonetti A, D'Andrea S, Necozione S, Micillo A, Di Gregorio A, et al. Ultrasonographic caput epididymis diameter is reduced in non-obstructive azoospermia compared with normozoospermia but is not predictive for successful sperm retrieval after TESE. Hum Reprod. 2014,29.1368–74.
17. Fedder J, Jørgensen MW, Engvad B. Prevalence of CBAVD in azoospermic men carrying pathogenic CFTR mutations – evaluated in a cohort of 639 non-vasectomized azoospermic men. Andrology. 2021;9(2):588–98.
18. Rudnik-Schoneborn S, Messner M, Vockel M, Wirleitner B, Pinggera GM, Witsch-Baumgartner M, et al. Andrological findings in infertile men with two (biallelic) CFTR mutations: results of a multicentre study in Germany and Austria comprising 71 patients. Hum Reprod. 2021;36(3):551–9.
19. Wang H, Guan J, Lin J, Zhang Z, Li S, Guo Y, Cai H. Diffusion-weighted and magnetization transfer imaging in testicular spermatogenic function evaluation: preliminary results. J Magn Reson Imaging. 2018;47:186–90.
20. Storey P, Gonen O, Rosenkrantz AB, Khurana KK, Zhao T, Bhatta R, Alukal JP. Quantitative proton spectroscopy of the testes at 3 tesla: towards a noninvasive biomarker of spermatogenesis. Investig Radiol. 2018;53:87.
21. Aaronson DS, Iman R, Walsh TJ, Kurhanewicz J, Turek PJ. A novel application of 1H magnetic resonance spectroscopy: non-invasive identification of spermatogenesis in men with non-obstructive azoospermia. Hum Reprod. 2010;25:847–52.
22. Turek PJ, Magana JO, Lipshultz LI. Semen parameters before and after transurethral surgery for ejaculatory duct obstruction. J Urol. 1996;155:1291–3.

23. Hartigan S, Tasian GE. Unnecessary diagnostic imaging: a review of the literature on preoperative imaging for boys with undescended testes. Transl Androl Urol. 2014;3(4):359–64. https://doi.org/10.3978/j.issn.2223-4683.2014.11.05.
24. Tasian GE, Copp HL, Baskin LS. Diagnostic imaging in cryptorchidism: utility, indications, and effectiveness. J Pediatr Surg. 2011;46(12):2406–13. https://doi.org/10.1016/j.jpedsurg.2011.08.008. PMID: 22152893; PMCID: PMC3712862
25. Mohammed NEA, Badwey ME, Nagla SA, et al. Diffusion-weighted imaging and conventional magnetic resonance imaging for detection of non-palpable undescended testis. Egypt J Radiol Nucl Med. 2022;53:169. https://doi.org/10.1186/s43055-022-00854-5.
26. Practice Committee of the American Society for Reproductive Medicine; Society for Male Reproduction and Urology. Report on varicocele and infertility: a committee opinion. Fertil Steril. 2014;102(6):1556–60.
27. Khera M, Lipshultz LI. Evolving approach to the varicocele. Urol Clin North Am. 2008;35(2):183–9.
28. Dubin L, Amelar RD. Varicocele size and results of varicocelectomy in selected subfertile men with varicocele. Fertil Steril. 1970;21(8):606–9.
29. Jungwirth A, Giwercman A, Tournaye H, et al. European Association of Urology guidelines on male infertility: the 2012 update. Eur Urol. 2012;62(2):324–32.
30. Agarwal A, Deepinder F, Cocuzza M, et al. Efficacy of varicocelectomy in improving semen parameters: new metaanalytical approach. Urology. 2007;70(3):532–8.
31. Hoekstra T, Witt MA. The correlation of internal spermatic vein palpability with ultrasonographic diameter and reversal of venous flow. J Urol. 1995;153(1):82–4.
32. Wolverson MK, Houttuin E, Heiberg E, Sundaram M, Gregory J. High-resolution real-time sonography of scrotal varicocele. AJR Am J Roentgenol. 1983;141(4):775–9.
33. Orda R, Sayfan J, Manor H, Witz E, Sofer Y. Diagnosis of varicocele and postoperative evaluation using inguinal ultrasonography. Ann Surg. 1987;206(1):99–101.
34. Pilatz A, Altinkilic B, Kohler E, Marconi M, Weidner W. Color Doppler ultrasound imaging in varicoceles: is the venous diameter sufficient for predicting clinical and subclinical varicocele? World J Urol. 2011;29(5):645–50.
35. Kim YS, Kim SK, Cho IC, Min SK. Efficacy of scrotal Doppler ultrasonography with the Valsalva maneuver, standing position, and resting-Valsalva ratio for varicocele diagnosis. Korean J Urol. 2015;56(2):144–9.
36. Chiou RK, Anderson JC, Wobig RK, et al. Color Doppler ultrasound criteria to diagnose varicoceles: correlation of a new scoring system with physical examination. Urology. 1997;50(6):953–6.
37. Eskew LA, Watson NE, Wolfman N, Bechtold R, Scharling E, Jarow JP. Ultrasonographic diagnosis of varicoceles. Fertil Steril. 1993;60(4):693–7.
38. Ultrasound evaluation of varicoceles: guidelines and recommendations of the European Society of Urogenital Radiology Scrotal and Penile Imaging Working Group (ESUR-SPIWG) for detection, classification, and grading.
39. European Radiology. https://doi.org/10.1007/s00330-019-06280-y.
40. Patil V, Shetty SC, Das SK. Redefining the criteria for grading varicoceles based on reflux times: a clinicoradiological correlation. Ultrasound Q. 2016;32(1):82–5.
41. Dhabuwala CB, Kumar AB, Kerkar PD, Bhutawala A, Pierce J. Patterns of Doppler recordings and its relationship to varicocele in infertile men. Int J Androl. 1989;12(6):430–8.
42. Oyen RH. Scrotal ultrasound. Eur Radiol. 2002;12(1):19–34.
43. Iosa G, Lazzarini D. Hemodynamic classification of varicoceles in men: our experience. J Ultrasound. 2013;16(2):57–63.

44. Cornud F, Belin X, Amar E, Delafontaine D, Helenon O, Moreau JF. Varicocele: strategies in diagnosis and treatment. Eur Radiol. 1999;9(3):536–45.
45. Cornud F, Amar E, Hamida K, Thiounn N, Helenon O, Moreau JF. Imaging in male hypofertility and impotence. BJU Int. 2000;86:153–63.
46. Dogra V, Gottlieb H, Oka M, Rubens D. Sonography of the scrotum. Radiology. 2003;227:18–36.
47. Rubenstein RA, Dogra VS, Seftel AD, Resnick MI. Benign intrascrotal lesions. J Urol. 2004;171:1765–72.
48. Esteves SC, Chan P. A systematic review of recent clinical practice guidelines and best practice statements for the evaluation of the infertile male. Int Urol Nephrol. 2015;47:1441–56.
49. Shah R, Agarwal A, Kavoussi P, Rambhatla A, Saleh R, Cannarella R, et al. Consensus and diversity in the management of varicocele for male infertility: results of a global practice survey and comparison with guidelines and recommendations. World J Men's Health. 2023;41:164.
50. Lund L, Roebuck D, Lee K, Sørensen H, Yeung C. Clinical assessment after varicocelectomy. Scand J Urol Nephrol. 2000;34:119–22.
51. Turgut M, Ozkan R. Recurrence rate after varicocelectomy in infertile men. Tanisal ve Girisimsel Radyoloji: Tibbi Goruntuleme ve Girisimsel Radyoloji Dernegi Yayin Organi. 2004;10:144–6.
52. Richenberg J, Belfield J, Ramchandani P, et al. Testicular microlithiasis imaging and follow-up: guidelines of the ESUR scrotal imaging subcommittee. Eur Radiol. 2015;25:323–30.
53. Yao M, Satchi M. Testicular microlithiasis: a cause for concern? Trends Urol Men Health. 2023;14:19–23.
54. Chiba K, Enatsu N, Fujisawa M. Management of non-obstructive azoospermia. Reprod Med Biol. 2016;15(3):165–73.
55. Barda S, Hauser R, Mano R, Savin Z, Molad-Hayo Y, Lehavi O, Kleiman SE, Azem F, Yossepowitch O, Dekalo S. Testicular microlithiasis defines a subgroup of azoospermic men with low rates of sperm retrieval. Int J Urol. 2022;29:65–8.
56. Ishikawa T. Surgical recovery of sperm in non-obstructive azoospermia. Asian J Androl. 2012 Jan;14(1):109–15.
57. Nariyoshia S, Nakano K, Sukegawa G, Sho T, Tsuji Y. Ultrasonographically determined size of seminiferous tubules predicts sperm retrieval by microdissection testicular sperm extraction in men with nonobstructive azoospermia. Fertil Steril. 2020;113(1):97–104.
58. Amer M, GamalEl Din SF, Zeidan A, et al. Intrasurgical seminiferous tubular diameter correlates with total motile sperm count in azoospermia: a prospective cohort study. Reprod Sci. 2022;29:1836–43.
59. Gao S, Yang J, Chen D, Min X, Fan C, Zhang P, Wang Q, Li Z, Cai W. Noninvasive prediction of sperm retrieval using diffusion tensor imaging in patients with nonobstructive azoospermia. J Imaging. 2023;9:182.
60. Ron-El R, Strauss S, Friedler S, Strassburger D, Komarovsky D, Raziel A. Serial sonography and colour flow Doppler imaging following testicular and epididymal sperm extraction. Hum Reprod. 1998;13(12):3390–3. https://doi.org/10.1093/humrep/13.12.3390.
61. Özman O, Tosun S, Bayazıt N, Cengiz S, Bakırcıoğlu ME. Efficacy of the second micro–testicular sperm extraction after failed first micro–testicular sperm extraction in men with nonobstructive azoospermia. Fertil Steril. 2021;115(4):915–21. https://doi.org/10.1016/j.fertnstert.2020.10.005.
62. Abdelaal AMA, El-Azizi HM, GamalEl Din SF, Abdulsalam Mohammad Azzazi O, Shokr MM. Evaluation of the potential role of shear wave elastography as a promising predictor of sperm retrieval in non-obstructive azoospermic patients: a prospective study. Andrology. 2021;9(5):1481–9.

63. Cantisani V, Di Leo N, Bertolotto M, et al. Role of multiparametric ultrasound in testicular focal lesions and diffuse pathology evaluation, with particular regard to elastography: review of literature. Andrology. 2021;9:1356–68. https://doi.org/10.1111/andr.13067.
64. Ammar T, Sidhu PS, Wilkins CJ. Male infertility: the role of imaging in diagnosis and management. Br J Radiol. 2012;85(1):S59–68. https://doi.org/10.1259/bjr/31818161. Epub 2012 Jul 4. PMID: 22763036; PMCID: PMC3746399
65. Katz MJ, Huland DM, Ramasamy R. Multiphoton microscopy: applications in Urology and Andrology. Transl Androl Urol. 2014;3(1):77–83.
66. Ramasamy R, Sterling J, Manzoor M, Salamoon B, Jain M, Fisher E, Li PS, Schlegel PN, Mukherjee S. Full field optical coherence tomography can identify spermatogenesis in a rodent sertoli-cell only model. J Pathol Inform. 2012;3:4. https://doi.org/10.4103/2153-3539.93401. Epub 2012 Feb 29
67. Enatsu N, Miyake H, Chiba K, Fujisawa M. Identification of spermatogenically active regions in rat testes by using narrow-band imaging system. Urology. 2015;86(5):929.

Chapter 6
Management of Primary Hypogonadism in Men with NOA

Kadir Böcü and Murat Gül

Understanding Male Hypogonadism: Definitions, Prevalence, and Classification

Definition

Male hypogonadism constitutes a clinical syndrome characterized by a spectrum of symptoms, which may be present with or without observable clinical signs, in conjunction with laboratory evidence of decreased testosterone levels. This disorder is associated with impaired testicular function, resulting in reduced androgen production and potentially impacting sperm production [1]. This could be the result of malfunctioning testicles (hypergonadotropic hypogonadism or primary hypogonadism) or due to insufficient activation of the testes by the hypothalamic–pituitary axis (hypogonadotropic hypogonadism or secondary hypogonadism). In rarer instances, it might be due to testosterone's reduced ability to activate the androgen receptor inside cells. Hypogonadism can adversely affect the operation of different organs and decrease the quality of life [2].

This section covers all the potential causes of male hypogonadism, with a particular focus on primary hypogonadism. It outlines how to differentiate primary from secondary hypogonadism and describes their clinical characteristics. Additionally, it provides detailed information on how to manage male infertility resulting from primary hypogonadism.

K. Böcü (✉)
Department of Urology, Niğde Ömer Halisdemir University Faculty of Medicine, Niğde, Turkey

M. Gül
Department of Urology, Selçuk University School of Medicine, Konya, Türkiye

Department of Andrology, Selçuk University School of Medicine, Konya, Türkiye

W. Zohdy et al. (eds.), *Non-Obstructive Azoospermia*,
https://doi.org/10.1007/978-3-031-99431-9_6

Prevalence of Male Hypogonadism

The occurrence and frequency of organic hypogonadism in males stemming from identifiable diseases affecting the testes, pituitary gland, and hypothalamus are still not determined. A minimal percentage of males undergoing testosterone treatment in the United States are diagnosed with conditions related to the testes, pituitary gland, and hypothalamus [3]. Numerous studies in epidemiology have gauged the frequency of testosterone reduction due to aging. The variation in these frequency estimates can be attributed to differences in the populations studied, the criteria for defining low testosterone, and the methodologies employed to assess testosterone levels in the bloodstream [4, 5]. A reduction in testosterone levels with advancing age can be attributed to dysfunctions throughout the hypothalamic–pituitary–testicular axis. Variables, including body mass index, weight gain, pre-existing health conditions, prescribed medications, and genetic factors, influence the rate of this decrease [6]. The term late-onset hypogonadism (LOH) emerged from this situation. It highlights the fact that in certain middle-aged and older men, a decrease in testosterone levels due to aging can lead to a group of symptoms and signs similar to those seen in men with traditional androgen deficiency [7].

Recent investigations have demonstrated that approximately 10–14% of men residing in community settings aged 65 years and older exhibit diminished testosterone levels [4, 5, 7, 8]. The European Male Aging Study has disclosed that the frequency of late-onset hypogonadism, distinguished by specific symptoms and a total testosterone concentration less than 220 ng/dL (8 nmol/L), is reported to be 3.2% among men aged 60–69 years. This percentage increases to 5.1% for individuals within the 70- to 79-year age bracket [9].

Distinction and Classification of Male Hypogonadism

Hypogonadism in males is characterized by a diminished function in one or both testes' principal functions: the production of sperm and the synthesis of testosterone. Generally, this ailment originates from either a malfunction of the testes, referred to as primary hypogonadism, or complications impacting the pituitary gland or hypothalamus, termed secondary hypogonadism [10]. The differentiation between primary and secondary hypogonadism is established by assessing serum levels of luteinizing hormone (LH) and follicle-stimulating hormone (FSH) [11]. Primary hypogonadism is diagnosed when the levels of serum testosterone and sperm count are lower than normal while the levels of serum LH and FSH are above normal. Secondary hypogonadism is considered where there is a subnormal level in both testosterone concentration in the bloodstream and sperm count in semen analysis but without a corresponding rise in LH and FSH concentrations (Fig. 6.1) [12]. Primary hypogonadism predominantly impacts sperm production rather than testosterone production. Various testicular conditions harm both the seminiferous tubules

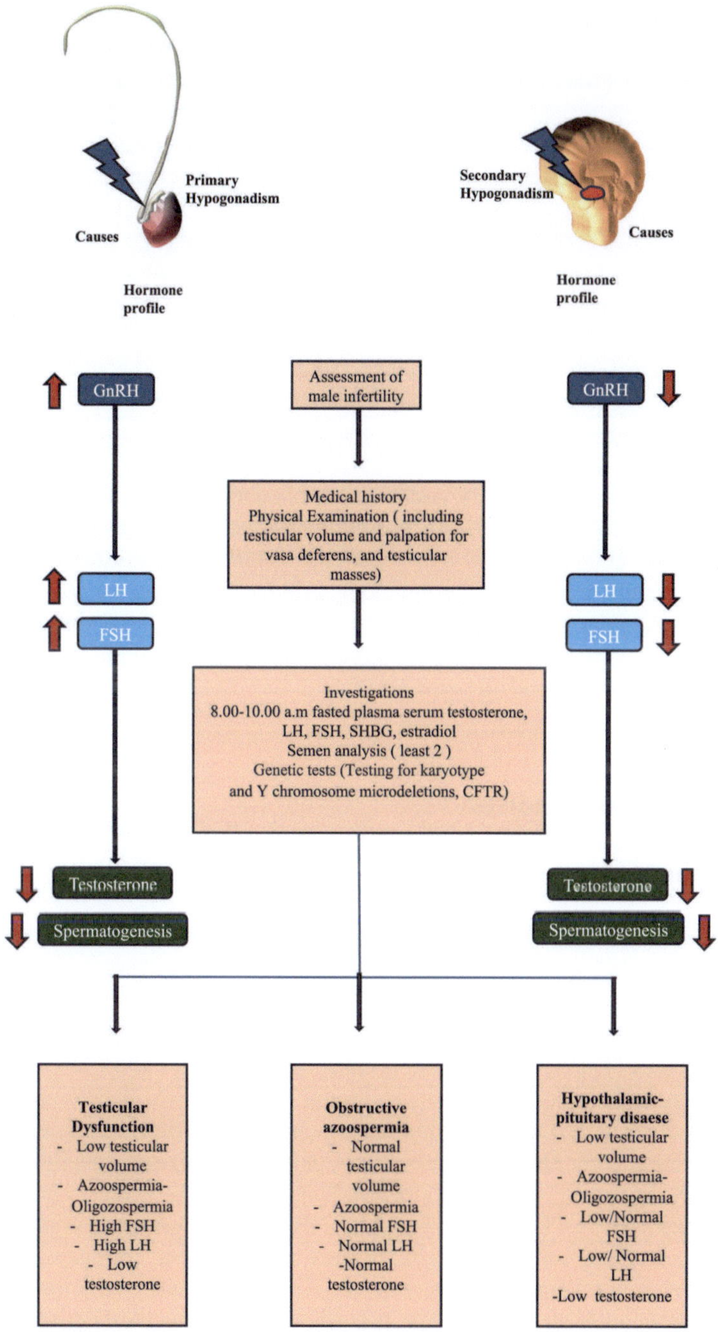

Fig. 6.1 A graphical representation displaying the process of evaluating a man experiencing infertility and differentiating male hypogonadism. *CBAVD* congenital bilateral absence of vasa deferens, *FSH* follicle-stimulating hormone, *LH* luteinizing hormone, *NOA* nonobstructive azoospermia, *SHBG* sex hormone binding globulin

and Leydig cells, but the damage is often more severe in the seminiferous tubules. As a result, individuals might exhibit a reduced sperm count with normal or elevated levels of serum FSH while their serum testosterone levels stay within the normal range.

On the other hand, in cases of secondary hypogonadism, there is a corresponding decrease in both testosterone and sperm production. Gynecomastia is frequently associated with primary hypogonadism, a condition thought to arise due to the significantly elevated serum levels of FSH and LH, which enhance aromatase activity within the testes. Consequently, this augmentation in aromatase activity catalyzes an increased conversion of testosterone into estradiol, amplifying estradiol production relative to testosterone by the testicles [13].

Various forms of hypogonadism necessitate specific therapeutic approaches, underscoring the importance of accurate patient classification. Both primary and secondary hypogonadism can result from an extensive array of congenital and acquired conditions [14] (Table 6.1). A rare manifestation of this disorder involves mutations in androgen receptors, resulting in a phenotype exhibiting partial or complete resistance to androgens [15]. Furthermore, late-onset hypogonadism represents a more comprehensive classification, including types that manifest in adulthood due to either organic or functional origins and may be identified as either primary or secondary. This variant of hypogonadism is often diagnosed without a clear etiological cause and becomes increasingly prevalent with advancing age, especially in males beyond 40 years [16].

Primary Hypogonadism

Congenital Causes

Klinefelter Syndrome

Klinefelter syndrome (KS) is identified as the predominant genetic manifestation of primary hypogonadism, with an incidence rate between 1:500 and 1:700 among newborn males [17]. This syndrome is categorized within a spectrum of chromosomal anomalies characterized by an additional X chromosome in the standard male karyotype of 46, XY. The most common genetic configuration found in KS is the 47, XXY karyotype. However, most cases exhibit mosaicism, specifically a 46, XY/47, XXY pattern [18]. Furthermore, although infrequently, other chromosomal irregularities such as 48, XXXXY and 49, XXXXY, are observed in approximately 1:50,000 and 1:100,000 male births, respectively. A direct correlation typically exists between the number of supplementary sex chromosomes and the degree of clinical presentation observed in KS. It is uncommon for individuals exhibiting a 47, XXY karyotype to display a mosaic genotype within testicular tissue. Conversely, individuals with a phenotypically normal karyotype may present with a KS genotype exclusively at the sperm level [19].

Table 6.1 Classification of hypogonadism

Primary hypogonadism	
Congenital or developmental disorders	
Common causes	**Uncommon causes**
Klinefelter syndrome Uncorrected cryptorchidism (including INSL3 and LGR8 mutations) Y chromosome microdeletions	Rare chromosomal abnormalities XX male syndrome 47 XYY syndrome 48 XXYY syndrome Defects of testosterone biosynthesis: STAR/20–22 desmolase 3β-HSD 17α-HSD/17–20 lyase 17β-HSD CAH (testicular adrenal rest tumors) Disorders of sex development (gonadal dysgenesis) LHCGR gene mutations Myotonic dystrophy (including type I and II) Uncorrected cryptorchidism (including INSL3 and LGR8 mutations) Bilateral congenital anorchia Sickle cell disease Noonan syndrome Down syndrome Autosomal translocations Adrenoleukodystrophy Myotonic dystrophy (including type I and II) Sertoli-cell only syndrome Primary ciliary dyskinesia Down syndrome FSH receptor gene mutations/ polymorphism Autosomal translocations
Acquired disorders	
Localized problems	
Bilateral surgical castration or trauma Drug-induced Chemotherapy agents Alkylating agents Methotrexate Inhibitors of testosterone Synthesis Ketoconazole Aminoglutethimide Mitotane Metyrapone Testicular radiation	Orchitis (including mumps) Autoimmune testicular failure

(continued)

Table 6.1 (continued)

Systemic diseases with testis localization	
Chronic systemic diseases Chronic organ failures Glucocorticoid excess (Cushing syndrome) Aging Orchitis Testicular irradiation Chemotherapy agents Malignancy Lymphoma Testicular cancer Idiopathic	Malignancy Lymphoma Testicular cancer Spinal cord injury Vasculitis Infiltrative diseases (amyloidosis leukemia) Environmental toxins Spinal cord injury
Androgen resistance /decreased testosterone bioactivity	
Congenital or developmental disorders	
Common causes	**Uncommon causes**
	Aromatase deficiency Kennedy diseases (spinal and bulbar muscular atrophy) and other extensions of CAG repeats Partial or complete androgen insensitivity 5α reductase type II deficiency
Acquired disorders	
Drug-induced AR blockage *Steroidal antiandrogen Cyproterone acetate Spironolactone *Non-steroidal antiandrogen Flutamide Bicalutamide Nilutamide Drug-induced 5α reductase activity blockade Finasteride Dutasteride Drug-induced ER blockade Clomiphene Tamoxifen Raloxifene Drug-induced aromatase activity blockade Letrozole Anastrazole Exemestane Increased Sex Hormone Binding Protein Drug-induced (antiepileptic, estrogen, thyroid hormones) Hyperthyroidism Liver diseases Aging	Celiac disease

(continued)

Table 6.1 (continued)

Secondary hypogonadism	
Congenital or developmental disorders	
Common causes	**Uncommon causes**
Constitutional delay of puberty Hemochromatosis	Combined hormone pituitary deficiency Idiopathic hypogonadotropic hypogonadism (IHH) with variants Normosmic IHH Kallmann syndrome Isolated LH β gene mutations Non-Kallmann syndromic form Congenital adrenal hyperplasia 21-hydroxylase deficiency 11β-hydroxylase deficiency Isolated FSHβ gene mutations
Acquired disorders	
Systemic diseases	
Chronic systemic diseases Metabolic diseases (Metabolic syndrome, Obesity, Type 2 diabetes mellitus) HIV infection Chronic organ failure Chronic kidney diseases(CKD) Chronic obstructive pulmonary disease (COPD) Chronic liver diseases Chronic heart failure Malignancy Glucocorticoid excess (Cushing syndrome) Eating disorders Starvation, malnutrition Morbid obesity Endurance exercise Acute a critical illness Aging Drug-induced Testosterone or androgenic anabolic steroids Malignancy Hodking diseases Testicular cancer	Spinal cord injury Transfusion-related iron overload (β-thalassemia) Androgen or hCG-secreting tumors

The extra X chromosome in 47, XXY may come from errors during egg or sperm formation or early zygote development. The chance of such mistakes rises with the mother's age. Roughly 66% of KS cases come from the mother and about 33% from the father [20]. Research links the source of the extra X chromosome in KS men to variations in health problems because the X chromosome has genes essential for cell death, sugar processing, and inflammation [21]. This could explain the health issues seen in these men. This genetic change leads to a swift loss of germ cells from birth and overgrowth of Leydig cells, affecting testosterone levels based on the Leydig cells' number and function [22].

Pre-puberty indicators of KS include undescended testicles, small testicle size, taller height for age, and cognitive and speech impairments. Post-puberty, KS is characterized by small testicles (1–3 mL), symptoms of low testosterone, increased height, breast tissue development, sparse body hair, osteopenia/osteoporosis, varicose veins, type 2 diabetes, and metabolic syndrome [23]. KS individuals often have a disproportionate body structure with longer legs than the torso, contributing to a unique physical appearance. Infertility is common in KS due to affected reproductive ducts, with a rare occurrence of temporary sperm production, primarily in milder cases. Although testosterone levels might initially be normal at puberty's onset, a premature decline typically leads to worsened low testosterone symptoms over time [24].

Other Uncommon Chromosome Abnormalities

46, XX Male Syndrome

XX male syndrome is a rare condition, affecting about 1 in 20,000–25,000 male births. It leads to a range of symptoms, including unclear or developing male genitalia and different levels of masculinization. This is usually because genetic material from the Y chromosome ends up on one of the X chromosomes, often during prenatal development, affecting the SRY gene, which is crucial for developing male gonads. About 90% of XX males have this scenario, causing infertility due to missing the Y chromosome's azoospermic factor [25].

About 10% of XX males lack the SRY gene. In these cases, it is thought that another gene, named "Z," or other genes might interfere with testis development and allow ovaries to form instead [26].

47, XYY Syndrome

47, XYY syndrome is a condition where males have an extra Y chromosome, resulting in a 47, XYY karyotype. Physically, these individuals appear normal except for being taller and having bigger teeth compared to the average person. Unlike men with KS, those with this syndrome maintain normal fertility and cognitive abilities [26].

48, XXYY Syndrome

The 48, XXYY syndrome is a type of KS recognized and affects one in every 17,000 male births, showing traits like taller height, breast development, less body hair, high gonadotropins but low gonadal function, small testicles, and infertility [27]. However, it also often leads to unique facial features, birth defects, lower IQ, and more intense behavior and psychiatric problems such as attention-deficit hyperactivity disorder, autism, and mood and tic disorders [19].

Y-Chromosome Microdeletions

Microdeletions in the Y chromosome's long arm are the top genetic cause of infertility in men, aside from KS. These deletions disrupt spermatogenesis, which is crucial for producing sperm, and are mainly found in three areas: AZFa, AZFb, and AZFc [28]. Recent advances show that AZFb and AZFc deletions overlap due to three deletion patterns [29]. Men without sperm have more microdeletions than those with low sperm counts. The larger the deletion, the worse the infertility, as extensive deletions can lead to a condition where only Sertoli cells are seen in testicular biopsies, indicating a complete absence of germ cells. This condition, leading to infertility, is mainly caused by Y-chromosome microdeletions [30]. The impact of these deletions varies; complete deletion of AZFa always results in this condition and infertility. Deletions in the AZFb and AZFbc regions could also stop sperm production. Identifying a complete deletion in these regions means there is almost no chance to extract sperm. However, partial deletions in AZFc may allow for a 50% chance of sperm retrieval. Testosterone and LH levels are typically normal, but FSH might increase due to less inhibin B production and missing feedback regulation [31, 32].

Disorders of Androgen Synthesis

Alterations in the genes responsible for producing the enzymes necessary for testosterone synthesis can reduce testosterone levels in the bloodstream. Such uncommon genetic changes disrupt functions, including the dismantling of cholesterol's side chain and the performance of specific enzymes like 3β-hydroxysteroid dehydrogenase and 17α-hydroxylase, present in both the adrenal glands and testicles, as well as 17β-hydroxysteroid dehydrogenase, which is exclusive to the testicles. The degree of these genetic alterations influences the varying degrees of masculinization before birth [33].

Alterations in Gonadotropin Receptors

LH and FSH influence the cells within the testes by attaching to distinct receptors, which are part of the family of G-protein-coupled transmembrane receptors. These gonadotropin receptors can undergo mutations that might either activate or inactivate them. Such mutations have the potential to either change or maintain the gene function and the structure of the resulting protein [34].

Alterations in LH and FSH receptors constitute infrequent etiologies of primary hypogonadism. The genetic variation within the FSH receptor engenders a fluctuating sperm count, which predominantly assumes a lower range, alongside altered inhibin B and FSH concentrations. Conversely, mutations in the LH receptor incite hypoplasia and a deficiency in Leydig cell testosterone production during the first trimester of intrauterine development. This leads to varying extents of disorders of sexual development [35].

Congenital Anorchia

Anorchia is characterized by the absence of one or both testicles. It is less frequently observed to affect both testicles, with an incidence rate of 1 in 20,000 males, whereas unilateral absence is four times more prevalent [36]. This condition may be congenital due to genetic mutations, such as those found in the SRY gene, or it may develop later in life because of infections, injuries, tumors, surgical interventions, or testicular torsion. Congenital anorchia is often associated with mutations in the SF1 gene, which leads to the condition known as vanishing testis syndrome, wherein affected individuals also exhibit significantly reduced penile size [37]. The principal cause of anorchia acquired postnatally is torsion, which occurs before birth. The physical manifestations of individuals with bilateral anorchia vary depending on the onset timing of the condition. If the onset was prenatal and testosterone was produced, the individual will exhibit male characteristics; conversely, without prenatal testosterone production, they will display female characteristics and lack both Müllerian and Wolffian ducts. In the absence of testosterone replacement therapy, a distinctive eunuchoid body shape emerges. In cases of bilateral anorchia, certain hormone levels are markedly elevated, and there is an absence of testosterone response to stimulatory tests. In men with solitary testis, the remaining one typically compensates by producing sufficient hormones to avoid issues with sexual development and hypogonadism less likely [13].

Cryptorchidism

Cryptorchidism is when one or both testicles are absent from the scrotum at birth. This issue is encountered in about 1% of newborn boys, making it the most frequent congenital anomaly of the male reproductive organs [38]. The exact causes of this condition remain a mystery, highlighting the complex processes that govern the formation and lowering of the testes [39]. Theories suggest both hormonal influences and environmental factors might play a role. In this context, abnormalities in the gene responsible for insulin-like factor (INSL)-3 and its receptor and in the AR, gene have been identified as potential explanations for a small number of cryptorchidism cases [40]. Nonetheless, the significance of additional genetic variants, for instance, mutations in the leucine-rich repeat-containing G-protein-coupled receptor (LGR)-8 gene, is still under investigation [41].

Leaving cryptorchidism untreated can result in the loss of testicular function and lead to permanent hypogonadism (PHG) and sterility. Despite the possibility of resolving the condition early with successful intervention, the effects of cryptorchidism can persist, possibly resulting in decreased fertility and an increased risk of developing testicular cancer later in life [42].

Noonan Syndrome

Noonan syndrome (NS) is a genetic disorder that affects approximately 1 in every 1000–2000 infants and is characterized by a spectrum of congenital abnormalities [43]. These abnormalities comprise cardiac defects, stature notably below average, a distinctive broad and webbed neck, chest deformities, variable developmental delays, cryptorchidism, an increased propensity for bleeding, and facial features that are unique and change over time. The genesis of NS is attributed to mutations in the RAS/mitogen-activated protein kinase (MAPK) pathway, which plays a pivotal role in cell cycle regulation, growth, and senescence. In males, Noonan syndrome often leads to cryptorchidism, delayed onset of puberty, and potential fertility issues [44].

Down Syndrome or Trisomy 21

Down syndrome, referred to as Trisomy 21, represents the most prevalent genetic disorder, impacting approximately 1 in every 700–800 live births. In over 90% of instances, it is attributed to the presence of an additional chromosome 21. A relatively rare variant, seen in fewer than 2% of occurrences, is known as mosaic Down syndrome. Males affected by Down syndrome commonly face challenges in sperm production, primarily owing to insufficient sperm production and occasionally reduced testosterone levels [45].

Sertoli Cell-Only Syndrome

Sertoli cell-only syndrome (SCOS) , also known as Del Castillo syndrome, is a significant pathological condition linked with primary hypogonadism. It is characterized by the exclusive presence of Sertoli cells within the seminiferous tubules of the testis. The absence of germ cells in these tubules leads to infertility, making SCOS one of the primary causes of azoospermia and male infertility [46].

Acquired Disorders

Testicular Trauma

The testicles are at an increased risk of injury due to their external positioning relative to the body. Despite this vulnerability, there is a notable lack of research concerning the impact of scrotal injuries on the functionality and dimensions of the testicles. A prospective study involving ten men who sustained blunt trauma to the scrotum revealed that a mere 50% exhibited symptoms of testicular atrophy after the incident. Scrotal ultrasonography has proven to be exceedingly effective in the detection of testicular ruptures resulting from such injuries, thereby facilitating optimal decision-making concerning the requisite surgical intervention [47].

Testicular Torsion

Testicular torsion represents a predominant cause for the prepubertal loss of a testicle. This condition entails a rotation of the spermatic cord, precipitating significant blood flow disruption to the testicle [48]. Absent spontaneous resolution or timely surgical intervention to correct this torsion, the testicle may be lost due to insufficient blood supply. The extent of harm is contingent upon the duration of the torsion; instances extending beyond eight hours can induce damage sufficient to reduce sperm production. Notably, even if the torsion affects only one testicle, both may suffer impairment, though the mechanisms of such bilateral damage remain uncertain [49].

Varicocele

A varicocele is characterized by the enlargement of veins within the pampiniform plexus, a condition found in approximately 15% of the male demographic [50]. This ailment can adversely affect testicular functionality, leading to potential complications such as discomfort, testicular atrophy, and a spectrum of fertility issues, extending from diminished sperm count to complete sperm absence [51]. Furthermore, it can precipitate a decline in testosterone secretion by the testicles, which may result in hypogonadism in specific individuals [52]. The adverse effects associated with a varicocele relate to an elevated testicular temperature, which can impair sperm production, compromise the efficiency of Sertoli cells, detrimentally modify the metabolism of testicular proteins, and reduce testosterone output by Leydig cells within the testicles, according to research conducted by Rajfer and his team in 1987 [53]. However, it is essential to acknowledge that the majority of men afflicted with a varicocele exhibit no symptoms and retain normal fertility levels.

Mumps Orchitis

Numerous infections can potentially damage the testicles, among which mumps is a significant cause. Orchitis, a frequently observed condition, mainly occurs in adults. The proliferation of immunization programs has notably decreased incidences of such afflictions. Testicular mumps result in the enlargement and severe discomfort of the testicles and may further develop into atrophy. Damage is predominantly sustained by the seminiferous tubules, potentially leading to infertility, significantly when both testicles are affected. Additionally, harm to the Leydig cells can transpire, culminating in diminished testosterone production [54].

Chronic Disorders

Numerous chronic disorders, including metabolic syndromes, HIV, chronic renal failure, and pulmonary diseases, frequently correlate with male hypogonadism. The underlying etiologies are intricate and remain incompletely elucidated. Such conditions may influence testosterone synthesis via disruptions in both the central and peripheral systems, resulting in secondary, primary, or, more prevalently, mixed forms of hypogonadism [55–57].

Medications

Chemotherapy

Alkylating chemotherapy agents, such as cyclophosphamide, significantly impair male fertility, with the extent of damage contingent upon the cumulative dosage. These pharmaceuticals frequently result in a prolonged absence of sperm in approximately 90% of men, whereas platinum-based medications have a similar effect in 50% of cases [58]. The seminiferous tubules within the testes are predominantly affected, although Leydig cells exhibit a higher resilience. The onset of detriment to sperm production can commence as early as 2 weeks following the initiation of treatment and is notably more severe in individuals who have completed puberty. Additionally, chemotherapy treatments can precipitate a decrease in testosterone levels [59]. The potential for recovery is contingent upon the viability of certain stem cells, with the possibility of sperm production resuming within a period of 12 weeks after the conclusion of treatment. While chemotherapy reduces sperm count in cancer survivors, it appears that the integrity of sperm DNA may improve over time. However, the precise timeline for recovery remains uncertain. To safeguard fertility, the cryopreservation of sperm is advised [60].

Inhibitors of Testosterone Synthesis

Ketoconazole effectively impedes testosterone synthesis, resulting in diminished production of the hormone [61]. Prolonged administration of glucocorticoids is noted to decrease testosterone levels in roughly one-third of individuals. The precise mechanism remains unclear; nonetheless, it is suggested that this reduction may occur in both the testes and the pituitary gland [62].

Radiation

Cancer radiotherapy can cause varying degrees of testicular damage, contingent on the targeted area, the cumulative radiation dose, and the distribution of this dosage over time. It has been observed that different testicular cell types exhibit varied responses to radiation. Specifically, Leydig cells demonstrate more resistance to radiation effects than germ cells [63]. Adolescent males undergoing cancer radiotherapy often proceed through normal puberty and retain typical hormone levels, albeit their spermatogenic capability may be impaired. Should the radiation dosage not surpass 30 Gray (Gy), Leydig cell functionality is largely unaffected. Nevertheless, exposure to doses over 30 Gy may precipitate dysfunction in these cells. The repercussions on germinal cells are directly proportional to the dosage and fractionation, with single-dose radiation exerting a milder effect than its multiple-dose counterpart. Azoospermia, defined as the complete absence of sperm, is foreseeable with doses exceeding 1.5 Gy. The recuperation to baseline sperm levels post-treatment is generally expected to span 10–24 months, though recovery durations might extend with higher doses [64].

Androgen Insensitivity/Decreased Testosterone Bioactivity

Androgen resistance is characterized by the body's tissues' failure to respond to androgens adequately. The primary cause of 46 XY sex development disorders identified is androgen insensitivity syndrome (AIS). This syndrome occurs due to the inability of androgens to engage with the androgen receptor effectively. The clinical presentation of AIS is notably diverse, ranging from a fully female phenotype in cases of complete AIS to a male phenotype with potential breast development or infertility in instances of partial AIS, contingent upon the residual functionality of the androgen receptor [65].

Over 400 mutations have been identified in the androgen receptor, impacting all eight exons of its gene [66]. The management strategy for this condition comprises a multifaceted approach, including counseling, support for mental and social well-being, hormonal therapies, and, as deemed necessary, surgical interventions. Nevertheless, the application of hormone replacement therapy and the determination of optimal timings for surgical interventions continue to be subjects of ongoing discussion.

Diminished androgen activity or resistance may arise from complications associated with key enzymes involved in the conversion of testosterone (T) into dihydrotestosterone (DHT)—this includes a deficiency in 5α-reductase type 2—or its transformation into estrogens, indicative of an aromatase deficiency [67]. Similarly, a variety of pharmaceuticals, including cyproterone acetate, spironolactone, flutamide, bicalutamide, finasteride, and letrozole, have been identified as altering androgen metabolism and function, subsequently reducing their biological efficacy [68, 69]. Moreover, men diagnosed with celiac disease may exhibit signs of diminished androgen levels attributed to the malnutrition associated with this condition. A noted reduction in DHT levels among these individuals further corroborates this observation. The presence of 5α-reductase in the intestinal tract and its reduced activity in individuals with active celiac disease may partially explain the decreased DHT levels [70].

Late-Onset Hypogonadism

The delineation and clinical significance of LOH, alongside the benefits derived from its treatment, continue to be subjects of debate. The symptomatic manifestations associated with diminished testosterone (T) levels are not distinct and resemble the physiological alterations occurring with normal aging. Recent findings from the European Male Ageing Study (EMAS) have elucidated that within the general European demographic, reduced T levels in conjunction with three specific sexual symptoms constitute a symptomatic androgen deficiency correlated with an elevated risk of reduced muscular strength, decreased bone density and hemoglobin levels, compromised well-being and quality of life, and altered metabolic markers [9]. The EMAS results indicate that the severity of LOH is contingent upon the testosterone concentrations, which may be moderately (8–11 nmol/L) or significantly (<8 nmol/L) reduced [9]. Notably, LOH with markedly low T levels exhibits a stronger association with symptoms of androgen deficiency and impacted glucometabolic conditions, implying that severe LOH more accurately represents a genuine state of androgen deficiency. Furthermore, the EMAS study has linked LOH with an increase in overall and cardiovascular (CV) mortality, a connection that is particularly evident in severe instances of LOH [71]. The observation that sexual symptoms and total T levels below 8 nmol/L, independently, are associated with elevated mortality rates complicates the interpretation of LOH's clinical importance. It remains unclear whether LOH constitutes a pathological condition that directly affects general well-being and health or is merely a biomarker of preexisting health conditions, serving more as an indicator of vulnerability than a causative factor. In the absence of results from long-term, rigorously conducted RCTs, the efficacy and safety of testosterone replacement therapy (TRT) in individuals with LOH are still under scrutiny. The decision to proceed with TRT necessitates carefully evaluating each patient's potential benefits and risks, with vigilant monitoring for any adverse responses, in adherence to prevailing medical guidelines [72, 73].

Evaluation of Male Infertility Attributable to Testicular Dysfunction

Testicular failure often becomes apparent during fertility investigations. Undertaking a comprehensive history and physical examination, particularly concerning the testicles, is paramount in the assessment and management of male infertility. A thorough clinical evaluation can identify the underlying causes of testicular failure and highlight reversible factors, thereby providing therapeutic advantages to both individuals involved (Fig. 6.1).

Medical and Sexual History

Identifying the frequency of sexual activity and how long the infertility has persisted is crucial. Signs of low testosterone, like a reduced sex drive and fewer morning erections, might be present. It is essential to initially gather information on the onset of puberty, previous fatherhood, and any instances of testes not descending or recent infections in the urinary or genital areas. A review of any medications that could harm the gonads and any previous scrotal or pelvic exposure to radiation, surgery, or injury is also necessary [74]. Furthermore, this moment provides an ideal chance to check for accompanying systemic health issues such as obesity and to identify reversible risk factors, including excessive alcohol consumption, smoking, and the use of recreational drugs [75].

Physical Examination

During the physical examination, it is imperative to meticulously assess for the manifestation of secondary sexual characteristics and indicators suggestive of Klinefelter syndrome (KS). This entails evaluating traits such as an above-average stature, the formation of breast tissue in males, and challenges associated with behavior or cognitive development. Examining the urethral opening's placement is equally critical, which may signify insufficient androgen exposure during prenatal growth. Furthermore, the dimensions of the testes ought to be precisely measured utilizing a Prader orchidometer. Testicular volumes less than 15 ml, as determined by the orchidometer, indicate potential hypogonadism or testicular dysfunction [76, 77].

Certain individuals may not have undergone treatment for cryptorchidism or they may have received an orchidopexy procedure during their childhood or adulthood. Should a man possess a diminutive testicle that previously failed to descend, this may signify a malfunction of the testicle. Furthermore, individuals afflicted with undescended testicles (UDT) are at an elevated risk of developing germ cell tumors. An augmentation or congestion in the epididymis may indicate the presence of an obstruction. The most efficacious method for detecting varicoceles involves instructing the patient to stand and execute the Valsalva maneuver. A lack of vasa deferentia could suggest the existence of a condition referred to as Congenital Bilateral Absence of the Vas Deferens (CBAVD) [78].

Diagnostic Tests

The assessment comprises evaluations for hormone levels, including testosterone, LH, FSH, estradiol, and SHBG, which are conducted in the morning following a fasting period, in addition to semen analyses, ultrasound examinations of the testicles, and essential genetic tests [79]. The testosterone concentration in the bloodstream shows variation throughout the day, reaching its zenith in the early morning [80]. This peak can be further elevated by fasting overnight, whereas consuming food can result in a slight decrease. Moreover, acute or mild illnesses and certain medications can also affect these levels [81, 82]. A typical hormone profile, including testicular size, is usually present in obstructive azoospermia. In contrast, indications of testicular failure are characterized by elevated FSH levels, while LH and testosterone levels may not exhibit substantial alterations [83]. However, relying solely on FSH levels to differentiate between conditions proves unreliable towards the higher end of the normal spectrum due to potential overlaps between obstructive azoospermia and nonobstructive azoospermia [84]. It is recommended to perform a semen analysis on two separate occasions, adhering to a sexual abstinence period of 2–7 days, in alignment with the rigorous protocols established by the WHO [85]. Men encountering infertility issues, especially those suspected of having nonobstructive azoospermia or severe oligozoospermia, are advised to undergo comprehensive testing, including analyses for chromosomal structure and Y chromosome microdeletions. Moreover, testing for CFTR gene mutations is advocated for individuals presumed to have obstructive azoospermia [74].

Testicular Histologic Findings

A testicular biopsy is typically conducted concurrently with the surgical extraction of sperm. The process of spermatogenesis is categorized histologically into four principal patterns: complete spermatogenesis, observable in healthy testes and cases of obstructive azoospermia; hypospermatogenesis, where all cellular components are present in the correct proportion yet in diminished quantities; maturation arrest, denoting the cessation of spermatogenesis beyond a particular developmental stage; and Sertoli cell-only (SCO) syndrome, characterized by the complete absence of germ cells. Among these histological patterns, SCO syndrome represents the most extreme, with an outright lack of germ cells [86].

Management of Primary Testicular Failure

At present, there are no officially approved pharmacological interventions for enhancing sperm production in instances of primary testicular failure. Consequently, severe forms of male infertility, characterized by conditions such as azoospermia (no sperm count) or oligozoospermia (low sperm count), necessitate the utilization of assisted reproductive technologies (ART), such as in vitro fertilization (IVF) or intracytoplasmic sperm injection (ICSI) [87]. While these techniques have proven effective, their accessibility may be limited for some couples, and they may not receive support from specific healthcare frameworks. Additionally, these methods carry potential risks for women, including the possibility of ovarian hyperstimulation syndrome [88]. The deployment of ART is contingent upon several factors, including the availability of reproductive technology infrastructure, national healthcare policies, and financial support from either government entities or insurance plans. Current proven treatment modalities and empirical treatments for managing primary testicular failure are presented under subheadings.

Lifestyle Changes

In the absence of effective pharmacological interventions, offering recommendations for lifestyle modifications emerges as a critical approach to support pairs grappling with male infertility. The beneficial effects of lifestyle enhancements on general health and well-being are universally recognized. Contemporary studies, utilizing both animal models and human subjects, suggest that alleviating adverse lifestyle habits, notably the diminution of alcohol consumption and cessation of tobacco use, may significantly improve male fertility and quality of life indicators [89, 90]. Although improvements in semen quality have been observed, their effect on pregnancy rates and live births continues to be limited. An elevated body mass index (BMI) frequently results in diminished male fertility outcomes. However, evidence from research concentrating on intervention strategies fails to definitively establish whether weight loss directly ameliorates issues related to male infertility [91, 92]. Among the various techniques to address obesity, bariatric surgery is the most efficacious weight reduction method. Yet, a longitudinal study by Legro et al. disclosed an unexpected decline in sperm count during the initial 6 months following bariatric surgery [93].

Recent research indicates that minimal weight reduction can enhance sperm quality among overweight men facing fertility challenges [94]. A study conducted by Hakonsen et al., involving 43 obese individuals, uncovered that participants who achieved a substantial weight loss—ranging from 17.2% to 25.4% of their total body weight—exhibited improved sperm count, semen volume, and testosterone levels compared to baseline measurements [95]. Similarly, investigations led by Mir and his associates have demonstrated that weight reduction significantly decreases the DNA fragmentation index, consequently improving sperm morphology [96]. However, there is a notable lack of data concerning the impact of assisted reproductive technologies (ARTs) in such scenarios. Recent comprehensive reviews have elucidated that adopting moderate-intensity physical exercises can increase sperm density and enhance motility [97].

In conclusion, providing advice on health before becoming a father can enhance lifestyle choices, which positively affects the quality of sperm.

Potential Hormone Treatments for Testicular Dysfunction

Individuals diagnosed with azoospermia frequently undergo treatment regimens that incorporate gonadotropin replacement therapy and antiestrogens, encompassing selective estrogen receptor modulators (SERMs) and aromatase inhibitors, as an initial phase before undertaking surgical sperm extraction procedures. Nevertheless, it is significant to note the pronounced lack of compelling evidence corroborating the efficacy of these therapeutic interventions [98].

Gonadotropins

Administration of gonadotropin has demonstrated considerable effectiveness in mitigating gonadotropin deficiency, a conclusion supported by many research studies [99, 100]. Nevertheless, its success rate in males with idiopathically low sperm counts remains indistinct. An analysis conducted by Cochrane, which reviewed six randomized controlled studies encompassing 456 participants, identified a notable enhancement in the incidence of live births and spontaneous pregnancies among pairs in which the male partner was administered FSH therapy, in stark contrast to those who received either no treatment or a placebo. However, it is important to note that the review also emphasized that the restricted number of trials and the modest sample size may diminish the definitiveness of these findings [101].

In a separate investigation focusing on men diagnosed with idiopathic oligozoospermia who exhibited normal FSH levels, significant improvements were observed in sperm retrieval rates, fertilization rates, and successful pregnancy outcomes following FSH treatment. This was particularly evident when FSH therapy was paired with a specific form of assisted reproduction technology (TESE-ICSI), compared to counterparts who underwent no treatment [102]. Moreover, a recent meta-analysis that encompassed 15 controlled studies, including 9 randomized trials and 6 non-randomized studies, involving a collective total of 614 men subjected to FSH treatment and 661 either not receiving treatment or given a placebo, demonstrated that men with idiopathic infertility reported superior pregnancy outcomes, whether through natural conception or assisted reproductive technologies, post FSH therapy. Additionally, this analysis revealed no significant variances in initial FSH levels between the cohort receiving treatment and those that did not [103].

Selective Estrogen Receptor Modulators and Aromatase Inhibitors

Selective estrogen receptor modulators (SERMs) diminish the impact of estradiol, consequently liberating GnRH and facilitating the release of pituitary gonadotropins, which augments the stimulation of the testes. The enzyme aromatase converts testosterone and androstenedione into estradiol and estrone. Like SERMs, aromatase inhibitors also mitigate estradiol's inhibitory feedback on the hypothalamic–pituitary–testicular (HPT) axis [104, 105]. An exhaustive examination of 11 randomized controlled trials underscored significant enhancements in sperm quality, including improvements in concentration and motility, as well as a higher rate of spontaneous pregnancies among males afflicted with unexplained infertility and oligoasthenoteratozoospermia who received antiestrogen treatment in comparison to those who did not [104]. Furthermore, an additional review involving 16 studies, both controlled and uncontrolled, focusing on males with idiopathic normogonadotropic oligozoospermia, disclosed elevated levels of sperm concentration, total sperm count, LH, FSH, and total testosterone following treatment with selective estrogen receptor modulators [106]. In a more constrained, randomized study that observed 46 patients with nonobstructive azoospermia and cryptozoospermia, where 22 were administered letrozole and the remaining 22 a placebo for a duration of 6 months, the cohort receiving letrozole exhibited significant improvements in sperm parameters and hormone levels. This included increases in sperm concentration and motility, as well as in FSH, LH, and testosterone levels, accompanied by a reduction in estradiol. However, the body of evidence on this subject is inconsistent and diverse, rendering it challenging to reach definitive conclusions. Additionally, there is a notable lack of standardized protocols regarding the duration of treatment, the dosage and type of antiestrogenic therapy administered, and the initial characteristics of the patients involved [107].

The utilization of pharmaceutical approaches for addressing testicular dysfunction prior to the implementation of procedures such as ICSI or TESE remains a contentious issue, as current medical guidelines do not advocate for their application [74, 108]. Notably, the safety profile of these drugs, when employed beyond their initial approval parameters, is still pending verification in male patients. Furthermore, there is a notable lack of consensus regarding the optimum pharmaceutical agent for such treatments, coupled with significant ambiguity surrounding their effects on fertility outcomes. In addition, treatments aimed at modulating estrogen levels have been associated with adverse events, including an elevated risk of thromboembolic diseases and gynecomastia. These conditions not only detrimentally influence a male's sexual wellness, encompassing both desire and the capability to sustain an erection, but may also precipitate adverse long-term effects on bone mineral density [109–111]. Despite these issues, certain medical centers proceed with the use of these pharmacological interventions under specific conditions, such as cases characterized by normal FSH levels that signify a primary impediment in sperm production and instances of inexplicably low sperm count. The objective in such scenarios is to augment FSH levels to stimulate spermatogenesis and enhance testosterone concentrations in the testes before engaging in ART [112]. There exists an imperative requirement for comprehensive, multicentric randomized controlled trials (RCTs) in the forthcoming period to determine the efficacy of these pharmacological interventions conclusively.

Antioxidant Therapy

Men with infertility exhibit higher levels of seminal reactive oxygen species compared to their fertile counterparts, which contributes to spermatic dysfunction and damage [113]. Medical professionals frequently prescribe antioxidant supplements as a form of treatment, although the scientific evidence supporting their efficacy is inconsistent, with a notable number of studies being inadequately structured. The precise mechanism through which these supplements exert their effects and their optimal type remains to be elucidated [114]. To date, no research has definitively confirmed that antioxidants enhance natural conception rates, even though they have been shown to safeguard spermatozoa in laboratory environments [115]. A comprehensive review has suggested that antioxidants might improve the chances of pregnancy and live births among men with subfertility who are undergoing assisted reproductive technologies. However, the identification of the specific agents and the appropriate dosages that are effective remains undetermined [116]. Compounds such as carnitines and vitamins C and E have shown potential, with various studies demonstrating their ability to improve sperm quality or increase pregnancy rates [117, 118]. Nevertheless, further investigations are essential to establish the safety and effectiveness of antioxidants in the treatment of low sperm count, as well as to determine the optimal dosage. The selection of treatments should be guided by the clinical judgment of the healthcare provider in conjunction with the patient's preferences. Additionally, zinc, folate, and certain herbal remedies are favored for their potential to enhance the quality of semen, though their use should be approached with caution pending further substantiating evidence [119].

Surgical Sperm Retrieval Techniques

For individuals diagnosed with obstructive azoospermia, there exist methods such as sperm extraction from the epididymis or directly from the testicles. The former method is typically less invasive in nature [120]. Epididymal sperm retrieval techniques encompass microsurgical epididymal sperm aspiration (MESA), percutaneous epididymal sperm aspiration (PESA), and surgical reconstruction. In cases of nonobstructive azoospermia (NOA), it becomes imperative to extract sperm directly from the testicles in order to locate active sperm-producing areas for intracytoplasmic sperm injection (ICSI); this can be achieved through TESA (a minimally invasive fine-needle aspiration technique) or TESE/micro-TESE (a surgical procedure entailing an incision in the scrotum to biopsy the testicles, sometimes under microscopic guidance, for the identification of productive seminiferous tubules) [121]. Research encompassing over 21,000 men with NOA indicates that TESE/micro-TESE procedures exhibit a success rate of up to 50% in sperm retrieval, independent of the subject's age or hormonal levels [122]. Presently, no precise method exists to predict the likelihood of successful sperm recovery in NOA patients prior to undergoing these operations. However, specific genetic abnormalities, such as AZFa/AZFb deletions or XX male syndrome, are recognized as exceptions for TESE owing to their detrimental effects on sperm production. Investigations into NOA attributable to Klinefelter syndrome (KS) have demonstrated encouraging outcomes, with success rates of up to 50% in sperm retrieval and comparable success rates in pregnancy and childbirth following TESE-ICSI, regardless of the patient's age, testicular dimensions, or hormonal profile [123]. Recorded instances of TESE-ICSI involving sperm from men with KS have led to the birth of healthy offspring, with chromosomal abnormality risks equating to those observed in men without KS [124]. The influence of sperm cryopreservation on reproductive capabilities remains a topic of inquiry. Although cryopreservation may elevate the proportion of immotile or nonviable sperm within a sample, conclusive evidence indicating its negative impact on conception and live birth rates post-TESE-ICSI is yet to be established [125]. Risks associated with TESE encompass the potential development of an intratesticular hematoma and fibrosis. Recent findings disclose a reduction in total serum testosterone levels in men with NOA 6 months post-TESE, with normalization periods ranging between 18 and 26 months, underscoring the necessity for hypogonadism monitoring post-procedure in these patients [126].

Stem Cell Therapy as an Emerging Treatment

Stem Cell Therapy represents the frontier of regenerative medicine, offering unprecedented opportunities to restore organ function lost due to disease or injury [127]. In primary hypogonadism, the focus is on regenerating Leydig cells or enhancing their functionality to resume normal testosterone production [128].

Mechanism This therapy utilizes stem cells' inherent ability to differentiate into various cell types, including Leydig cells in the testes. These stem cells can be derived from multiple sources, such as adipose tissue or bone marrow. Once introduced into the patient's body, the stem cells migrate to the testes and potentially differentiate into Leydig cells or repair the existing impaired cells, thus restoring their testosterone-producing capacity [129].

Current Research The scientific community's interest in stem cell therapy for hypogonadism has grown, with multiple preclinical studies illustrating its potential. Research has shown that stem cell therapy can lead to the regeneration of Leydig cells and a subsequent increase in testosterone levels in animal models [128, 130]. Clinical trials in humans, however, are still required to fully understand the therapy's effectiveness, optimal cell types, and administration routes [131].

Considerations Despite its potential, stem cell therapy's applicability in primary hypogonadism management is still under investigation. Issues such as the source of stem cells, ensuring their safe and ethical use, and long-term viability and integration within the testes need to be thoroughly addressed through rigorous scientific investigation [131].

Conclusion

In conclusion, managing male infertility and primary hypogonadism demands a holistic approach, encompassing precise diagnostic processes, genetic insights, lifestyle considerations, and a spectrum of treatment options ranging from pharmacological interventions to cutting-edge ART and emerging regenerative therapies. Ongoing research and clinical advancements are imperative to unravel the complexities of male infertility, aiming to enhance therapeutic efficacy, offer personalized treatment plans, and, ultimately, fulfill the aspirations of parenthood for affected individuals.

References

1. Ross A, Bhasin S. Hypogonadism: its prevalence and diagnosis. Urol Clin North Am. 2016;43(2):163–76. https://doi.org/10.1016/j.ucl.2016.01.002.
2. Nieschlag E, Behre HM, Kliesch S, Nieschlag S. Andrology: male reproductive health and dysfunction. Springer; 2023.
3. Jasuja GK, Bhasin S, Reisman JI, Berlowitz DR, Rose AJ. Ascertainment of testosterone prescribing practices in the VA. Med Care. 2015;53(9):746–52.
4. Araujo AB, Esche GR, Kupelian V, O'Donnell AB, Travison TG, Williams RE, et al. Prevalence of symptomatic androgen deficiency in men. J Clin Endocrinol Metabol. 2007;92(11):4241–7. https://doi.org/10.1210/jc.2007-1245.
5. Bhasin S, Pencina M, Jasuja GK, Travison TG, Coviello A, Orwoll E, et al. Reference ranges for testosterone in men generated using liquid chromatography tandem mass spectrometry in a community-based sample of healthy nonobese young men in the Framingham heart study and applied to three geographically distinct cohorts. J Clin Endocrinol Metabol. 2011;96(8):2430–9. https://doi.org/10.1210/jc.2010-3012.
6. Mohr BA, Bhasin S, Link CL, O'Donnell AB, McKinlay JB. The effect of changes in adiposity on testosterone levels in older men: longitudinal results from the Massachusetts male aging study. Eur J Endocrinol. 2006;155(3):443–52. https://doi.org/10.1530/eje.1.02241.
7. Wu FC, Tajar A, Beynon JM, Pye SR, Silman AJ, Finn JD, et al. Identification of late-onset hypogonadism in middle-aged and elderly men. N Engl J Med. 2010;363(2):123–35.
8. Orwoll E, Lambert LC, Marshall LM, Phipps K, Blank J, Barrett-Connor E, et al. Testosterone and estradiol among older men. J Clin Endocrinol Metabol. 2006;91(4):1336–44. https://doi.org/10.1210/jc.2005-1830.
9. Tajar A, Huhtaniemi IT, O'Neill TW, Finn JD, Pye SR, Lee DM, et al. Characteristics of androgen deficiency in late-onset hypogonadism: results from the European Male Aging Study (EMAS). J Clin Endocrinol. 2012;97(5):1508–16.
10. Casarini L, Huhtaniemi IT, Simoni M, Rivero-Müller A. Endocrinology of the testis and male reproduction endocrinology. In: Gonadotropin receptors. Cham: Springer; 2017. p. 123–68.
11. Tajar A, Forti G, O'Neill TW, Lee DM, Silman AJ, Finn JD, et al. Characteristics of secondary, primary, and compensated hypogonadism in aging men: evidence from the European Male Ageing Study. J Clin Endocrinol Metab. 2010;95(4):1810–8. https://doi.org/10.1210/jc.2009-1796.
12. Hohl A, Ronsoni MF. Male hypogonadism. In: Endocrinology and diabetes: a problem oriented approach. Springer; 2022. p. 139–55.
13. Santi D, Corona G. Primary and secondary hypogonadism. In: Simoni M, Huhtaniemi IT, editors. Endocrinology of the testis and male reproduction. Cham: Springer; 2017. p. 687–747.
14. Salonia A, Rastrelli G, Hackett G, Seminara SB, Huhtaniemi IT, Rey RA, et al. Paediatric and adult-onset male hypogonadism. Nat Rev Dis Primers. 2019;5(1):38. https://doi.org/10.1038/s41572-019-0087-y.
15. Singh S, Ilyayeva S. Androgen insensitivity syndrome. In: StatPearls. Treasure Island: StatPearls; 2024.
16. Ide H, Akehi Y, Fukuhara S, Ohira S, Ogawa S, Kataoka T, et al. Summary of the clinical practice manual for late-onset hypogonadism. Int J Urol. 2023;30(5):422–30. https://doi.org/10.1111/iju.15160.
17. Groth KA, Skakkebæk A, Høst C, Gravholt CH, Bojesen A. Clinical review: Klinefelter syndrome–a clinical update. J Clin Endocrinol Metab. 2013;98(1):20–30. https://doi.org/10.1210/jc.2012-2382.
18. Lanfranco F, Kamischke A, Zitzmann M, Nieschlag E. Klinefelter's syndrome. Lancet. 2004;364(9430):273–83. https://doi.org/10.1016/s0140-6736(04)16678-6.
19. Linden MG, Bender BG, Robinson A. Sex chromosome tetrasomy and pentasomy. Pediatrics. 1995;96(4 Pt 1):672–82.

20. Visootsak J, Graham JM Jr. Klinefelter syndrome and other sex chromosomal aneuploidies. Orphanet J Rare Dis. 2006;1:42. https://doi.org/10.1186/1750-1172-1-42.
21. Zitzmann M, Bongers R, Werler S, Bogdanova N, Wistuba J, Kliesch S, et al. Gene expression patterns in relation to the clinical phenotype in Klinefelter syndrome. J Clin Endocrinol Metab. 2015;100(3):E518–23. https://doi.org/10.1210/jc.2014-2780.
22. Aksglaede L, Juul A. Testicular function and fertility in men with Klinefelter syndrome: a review. Eur J Endocrinol. 2013;168(4):R67–76. https://doi.org/10.1530/eje-12-0934.
23. Basaria S. Male hypogonadism. Lancet. 2014;383(9924):1250–63. https://doi.org/10.1016/s0140-6736(13)61126-5.
24. Forti G, Corona G, Vignozzi L, Krausz C, Maggi M. Klinefelte's syndrome: a clinical and therapeutical update. Sex Dev. 2010;4(4–5):249–58. https://doi.org/10.1159/000316604.
25. Fechner PY, Marcantonio SM, Jaswaney V, Stetten G, Goodfellow PN, Migeon CJ, et al. The role of the sex-determining region Y gene in the etiology of 46, XX maleness. J Clin Endocrinol Metab. 1993;76(3):690–5. https://doi.org/10.1210/jcem.76.3.8383144.
26. Hughes IA. Disorders of sex development: a new definition and classification. Best Pract Res Clin Endocrinol Metab. 2008;22(1):119–34. https://doi.org/10.1016/j.beem.2007.11.001.
27. Balsera AM, Estévez MN, Beltrán EB, Sánchez-Giralt P, García LG, Moreno TH, et al. Distinct mechanism of formation of the 48, XXYY karyotype. Mol Cytogenet. 2013;6(1):25. https://doi.org/10.1186/1755-8166-6-25.
28. Ferlin A, Arredi B, Speltra E, Cazzadore C, Selice R, Garolla A, et al. Molecular and clinical characterization of Y chromosome microdeletions in infertile men: a 10-year experience in Italy. J Clin Endocrinol Metab. 2007;92(3):762–70. https://doi.org/10.1210/jc.2006-1981.
29. Simoni M, Bakker E, Eurlings MC, Matthijs G, Moro E, Müller CR, et al. Laboratory guidelines for molecular diagnosis of Y-chromosomal microdeletions. Int J Androl. 1999;22(5):292–9. https://doi.org/10.1046/j.1365-2605.1999.00193.x.
30. Stouffs K, Gheldof A, Tournaye H, Vandermaelen D, Bonduelle M, Lissens W, et al. Sertoli cell-only syndrome: behind the genetic scenes. Biomed Res Int. 2016;2016:6191307. https://doi.org/10.1155/2016/6191307.
31. Hopps CV, Mielnik A, Goldstein M, Palermo GD, Rosenwaks Z, Schlegel PN. Detection of sperm in men with Y chromosome microdeletions of the AZFa, AZFb and AZFc regions. Hum Reprod. 2003;18(8):1660–5. https://doi.org/10.1093/humrep/deg348.
32. Krausz C, Hoefsloot L, Simoni M, Tüttelmann F. EAA/EMQN best practice guidelines for molecular diagnosis of Y-chromosomal microdeletions: state-of-the-art 2013. Andrology. 2014;2(1):5–19. https://doi.org/10.1111/j.2047-2927.2013.00173.x.
33. Miller WL, Auchus RJ. The molecular biology, biochemistry, and physiology of human steroidogenesis and its disorders. Endocr Rev. 2011;32(1):81–151. https://doi.org/10.1210/er.2010-0013.
34. Latronico AC, Arnhold IJ. Inactivating mutations of LH and FSH receptors–from genotype to phenotype. Pediatr Endocrinol Rev. 2006;4(1):28–31.
35. Menon KM, Menon B. Structure, function and regulation of gonadotropin receptors – a perspective. Mol Cell Endocrinol. 2012;356(1–2):88–97. https://doi.org/10.1016/j.mce.2012.01.021.
36. Redman JF. Impalpable testes: observations based on 208 consecutive operations for undescended testes. J Urol. 1980;124(3):379–81. https://doi.org/10.1016/s0022-5347(17)55457-9.
37. Pirgon Ö, Dündar BN. Vanishing testes: a literature review. J Clin Res Pediatr Endocrinol. 2012;4(3):116–20. https://doi.org/10.4274/Jcrpe.728.
38. Berkowitz GS, Lapinski RH, Dolgin SE, Gazella JG, Bodian CA, Holzman IR. Prevalence and natural history of cryptorchidism. Pediatrics. 1993;92(1):44–9.
39. Mathers MJ, Sperling H, Rübben H, Roth S. The undescended testis: diagnosis, treatment and long-term consequences. Dtsch Arztebl Int. 2009;106(33):527–32. https://doi.org/10.3238/arztebl.2009.0527.
40. El Houate B, Rouba H, Sibai H, Barakat A, Chafik A, Chadli el B, et al. Novel mutations involving the INSL3 gene associated with cryptorchidism. J Urol. 2007;177(5):1947–51. https://doi.org/10.1016/j.juro.2007.01.002.

41. Ferlin A, Zuccarello D, Garolla A, Selice R, Foresta C. Hormonal and genetic control of testicular descent. Reprod Biomed Online. 2007;15(6):659–65. https://doi.org/10.1016/s1472-6483(10)60532-9.
42. Fawzy F, Hussein A, Eid MM, El Kashash AM, Salem HK. Cryptorchidism and fertility. Clin Med Insights Reprod Health. 2015;9:39–43. https://doi.org/10.4137/cmrh.S25056.
43. Myers A, Bernstein JA, Brennan ML, Curry C, Esplin ED, Fisher J, et al. Perinatal features of the RASopathies: Noonan syndrome, cardiofaciocutaneous syndrome and Costello syndrome. Am J Med Genet A. 2014;164a(11):2814–21. https://doi.org/10.1002/ajmg.a.36737.
44. Allen MJ, Sharma S. Noonan syndrome. In: StatPearls. Treasure Island: StatPearls Publishing; 2024.
45. Parizot E, Dard R, Janel N, Vialard F. Down syndrome and infertility: what support should we provide? J Assist Reprod Genet. 2019;36(6):1063–7. https://doi.org/10.1007/s10815-019-01457-2.
46. Ghanami Gashti N, Sadighi Gilani MA, Abbasi M. Sertoli cell-only syndrome: etiology and clinical management. J Assist Reprod Genet. 2021;38(3):559–72. https://doi.org/10.1007/s10815-021-02063-x.
47. Cross JJ, Berman LH, Elliott PG, Irving S. Scrotal trauma: a cause of testicular atrophy. Clin Radiol. 1999;54(5):317–20. https://doi.org/10.1016/s0009-9260(99)90562-7.
48. DaJusta DG, Granberg CF, Villanueva C, Baker LA. Contemporary review of testicular torsion: new concepts, emerging technologies and potential therapeutics. J Pediatr Urol. 2013;9(6 Pt A):723–30. https://doi.org/10.1016/j.jpurol.2012.08.012.
49. Woodruff DY, Horwitz G, Weigel J, Nangia AK. Fertility preservation following torsion and severe ischemic injury of a solitary testis. Fertil Steril. 2010;94(1):352.e4–5. https://doi.org/10.1016/j.fertnstert.2009.12.057.
50. Agarwal A, Deepinder F, Cocuzza M, Agarwal R, Short RA, Sabanegh E, et al. Efficacy of varicocelectomy in improving semen parameters: new meta-analytical approach. Urology. 2007;70(3):532–8. https://doi.org/10.1016/j.urology.2007.04.011.
51. Dabaja AA, Goldstein M. When is a varicocele repair indicated: the dilemma of hypogonadism and erectile dysfunction? Asian J Androl. 2016;18(2):213–6. https://doi.org/10.4103/1008-682x.169560.
52. Hayden RP, Tanrikut C. Testosterone and Varicocele. Urol Clin North Am. 2016;43(2):223–32. https://doi.org/10.1016/j.ucl.2016.01.009.
53. Rajfer J, Turner TT, Rivera F, Howards SS, Sikka SC. Inhibition of testicular testosterone biosynthesis following experimental varicocele in rats. Biol Reprod. 1987;36(4):933–7. https://doi.org/10.1095/biolreprod36.4.933.
54. Ternavasio-de la Vega HG, Boronat M, Ojeda A, García-Delgado Y, Ángel-Moreno A, Carranza-Rodríguez C, et al. Mumps orchitis in the post-vaccine era (1967-2009): a single-center series of 67 patients and review of clinical outcome and trends. Medicine (Baltimore). 2010;89(2):96–116. https://doi.org/10.1097/MD.0b013e3181d63191.
55. Iglesias P, Carrero JJ, Díez JJ. Gonadal dysfunction in men with chronic kidney disease: clinical features, prognostic implications and therapeutic options. J Nephrol. 2012;25(1):31–42. https://doi.org/10.5301/jn.2011.8481.
56. Foresta C, Schipilliti M, Ciarleglio FA, Lenzi A, D'Amico D. Male hypogonadism in cirrhosis and after liver transplantation. J Endocrinol Investig. 2008;31(5):470–8. https://doi.org/10.1007/bf03346393.
57. Rochira V, Zirilli L, Orlando G, Santi D, Brigante G, Diazzi C, et al. Premature decline of serum total testosterone in HIV-infected men in the HAART-era. PLoS One. 2011;6(12):e28512. https://doi.org/10.1371/journal.pone.0028512.
58. Simon B, Lee SJ, Partridge AH, Runowicz CD. Preserving fertility after cancer. CA Cancer J Clin. 2005;55(4):211–28; quiz 63-4. https://doi.org/10.3322/canjclin.55.4.211.
59. DeBaun MR. Hydroxyurea therapy contributes to infertility in adult men with sickle cell disease: a review. Expert Rev Hematol. 2014;7(6):767–73. https://doi.org/10.1586/17474086.2014.959922.

60. Trottmann M, Becker AJ, Stadler T, Straub J, Soljanik I, Schlenker B, et al. Semen quality in men with malignant diseases before and after therapy and the role of cryopreservation. Eur Urol. 2007;52(2):355–67. https://doi.org/10.1016/j.eururo.2007.03.085.
61. Ankley GT, Cavallin JE, Durhan EJ, Jensen KM, Kahl MD, Makynen EA, et al. A time-course analysis of effects of the steroidogenesis inhibitor ketoconazole on components of the hypothalamic-pituitary-gonadal axis of fathead minnows. Aquat Toxicol. 2012;114-115:88–95. https://doi.org/10.1016/j.aquatox.2012.02.012.
62. Hu GX, Lian QQ, Lin H, Latif SA, Morris DJ, Hardy MP, et al. Rapid mechanisms of glucocorticoid signaling in the Leydig cell. Steroids. 2008;73(9–10):1018–24. https://doi.org/10.1016/j.steroids.2007.12.020.
63. Markovina S, Weschenfelder DC, Gay H, McCandless A, Carey B, DeWees T, et al. Low incidence of new biochemical hypogonadism after intensity modulated radiation therapy for prostate cancer. Pract Radiat Oncol. 2014;4(6):430–6. https://doi.org/10.1016/j.prro.2014.02.004.
64. Lee SH, Shin CH. Reduced male fertility in childhood cancer survivors. Ann Pediatr Endocrinol Metab. 2013;18(4):168–72. https://doi.org/10.6065/apem.2013.18.4.168.
65. Delli Paoli E, Di Chiano S, Paoli D, Lenzi A, Lombardo F, Pallotti F. Androgen insensitivity syndrome: a review. J Endocrinol Investig. 2023;46(11):2237–45. https://doi.org/10.1007/s40618-023-02127-y.
66. Gottlieb B, Beitel LK, Nadarajah A, Paliouras M, Trifiro M. The androgen receptor gene mutations database: 2012 update. Hum Mutat. 2012;33(5):887–94. https://doi.org/10.1002/humu.22046.
67. Markouli M, Michala L. Fertility potential in 5α-reductase type 2 deficient males. J Pediatr Urol. 2023;19(1):108–14. https://doi.org/10.1016/j.jpurol.2022.09.002.
68. Handelsman DJ. Androgen misuse and abuse. Endocr Rev. 2021;42(4):457–501.
69. Gormley GJ, Stoner E, Rittmaster RS, Gregg H, Thompson DL, Lasseter KC, et al. Effects of finasteride (MK-906), a 5α-reductase inhibitor, on circulating androgens in male volunteers*. J Clin Endocrinol Metabol. 1990;70(4):1136–41. https://doi.org/10.1210/jcem-70-4-1136.
70. Kurada S, Veeraraghavan G, Kaswala D, Hansen J, Cohen D, Kelly C, et al. Low testosterone in non-responsive coeliac disease: a case series, case–control study with comparisons to the National Health and Nutrition Examination Survey. Dig Liver Dis. 2016;48(10):1155–61. https://doi.org/10.1016/j.dld.2016.06.006.
71. Pye SR, Huhtaniemi IT, Finn JD, Lee DM, O'Neill TW, Tajar A, et al. Late-onset hypogonadism and mortality in aging men. J Clin Endocrinol Metab. 2014;99(4):1357–66. https://doi.org/10.1210/jc.2013-2052.
72. Wang C, Nieschlag E, Swerdloff R, Behre HM, Hellstrom WJ, Gooren LJ, et al. Investigation, treatment and monitoring of late-onset hypogonadism in males: ISA, ISSAM, EAU, EAA and ASA recommendations. Eur J Endocrinol. 2008;159(5):507–14.
73. Fode M, Salonia A, Minhas S, Burnett AL, Shindel AW. Late-onset hypogonadism and testosterone therapy–a summary of guidelines from the American Urological Association and the European Association of Urology. Eur Urol Focus. 2019;5(4):539–44.
74. Minhas S, Bettocchi C, Boeri L, Capogrosso P, Carvalho J, Cilesiz NC, et al. European Association of Urology guidelines on male sexual and reproductive health: 2021 update on male infertility. Eur Urol. 2021;80(5):603–20. https://doi.org/10.1016/j.eururo.2021.08.014.
75. Sharma A, Minhas S, Dhillo WS, Jayasena CN. Male infertility due to testicular disorders. J Clin Endocrinol Metabol. 2021;106(2):e442–e59.
76. Carnegie C. Diagnosis of hypogonadism: clinical assessments and laboratory tests. Rev Urol. 2004;6(Suppl 6):S3–8.
77. Lotti F, Maggi M. Ultrasound of the male genital tract in relation to male reproductive health. Hum Reprod Update. 2015;21(1):56–83. https://doi.org/10.1093/humupd/dmu042.
78. Yu YD, Hong YK. A case of cryptorchidism with ipsilateral congenital unilateral absence of the vas deferens and contralateral renal agenesis. Case Rep Urol. 2016;2016:2379793. https://doi.org/10.1155/2016/2379793.

79. Fleseriu M, Hashim IA, Karavitaki N, Melmed S, Murad MH, Salvatori R, et al. Hormonal replacement in hypopituitarism in adults: an endocrine society clinical practice guideline. J Clin Endocrinol Metab. 2016;101(11):3888–921. https://doi.org/10.1210/jc.2016-2118.
80. Sartorius G, Spasevska S, Idan A, Turner L, Forbes E, Zamojska A, et al. Serum testosterone, dihydrotestosterone and estradiol concentrations in older men self-reporting very good health: the healthy man study. Clin Endocrinol. 2012;77(5):755–63. https://doi.org/10.1111/j.1365-2265.2012.04432.x.
81. Lehtihet M, Arver S, Bartuseviciene I, Pousette A. S-testosterone decrease after a mixed meal in healthy men independent of SHBG and gonadotrophin levels. Andrologia. 2012;44(6):405–10. https://doi.org/10.1111/j.1439-0272.2012.01296.x.
82. Brambilla DJ, Matsumoto AM, Araujo AB, McKinlay JB. The effect of diurnal variation on clinical measurement of serum testosterone and other sex hormone levels in men. J Clin Endocrinol Metab. 2009;94(3):907–13. https://doi.org/10.1210/jc.2008-1902.
83. Schoor RA, Elhanbly S, Niederberger CS, Ross LS. The role of testicular biopsy in the modern management of male infertility. J Urol. 2002;167(1):197–200.
84. Sikaris K, McLachlan RI, Kazlauskas R, de Kretser D, Holden CA, Handelsman DJ. Reproductive hormone reference intervals for healthy fertile young men: evaluation of automated platform assays. J Clin Endocrinol Metab. 2005;90(11):5928–36. https://doi.org/10.1210/jc.2005-0962.
85. Wang C, Mbizvo M, Festin MP, Björndahl L, Toskin I. Evolution of the WHO "Semen" processing manual from the first (1980) to the sixth edition (2021). Fertil Steril. 2022;117(2):237–45.
86. McLachlan RI, Rajpert-De Meyts E, Hoei-Hansen CE, de Kretser DM, Skakkebaek NE. Histological evaluation of the human testis–approaches to optimizing the clinical value of the assessment: mini review. Hum Reprod. 2007;22(1):2–16. https://doi.org/10.1093/humrep/del279.
87. Tournaye H. Management of male infertility by assisted reproductive technologies. Baillieres Best Pract Res Clin Endocrinol Metab. 2000;14(3):423–35. https://doi.org/10.1053/beem.2000.0089.
88. Inhorn MC, Patrizio P. Infertility around the globe: new thinking on gender, reproductive technologies and global movements in the 21st century. Hum Reprod Update. 2015;21(4):411–26. https://doi.org/10.1093/humupd/dmv016.
89. Oyeyipo IP, Raji Y, Bolarinwa AF. Nicotine alters male reproductive hormones in male albino rats: The role of cessation. J Hum Reprod Sci. 2013;6(1):40–4. https://doi.org/10.4103/0974-1208.112380.
90. Teskereci G, Oncel S. Effect of lifestyle on quality of life of couples receiving infertility treatment. J Sex Marital Ther. 2013;39(6):476–92. https://doi.org/10.1080/0092623x.2012.665817.
91. Chambers TJ, Richard RA. The impact of obesity on male fertility. Hormones (Athens). 2015;14(4):563–8. https://doi.org/10.14310/horm.2002.1621.
92. Ameratunga D, Gebeh A, Amoako A. Obesity and male infertility. Best Pract Res Clin Obstet Gynaecol. 2023;90:102393. https://doi.org/10.1016/j.bpobgyn.2023.102393.
93. Legro RS, Kunselman AR, Meadows JW, Kesner JS, Krieg EF, Rogers AM, et al. Time-related increase in urinary testosterone levels and stable semen analysis parameters after bariatric surgery in men. Reprod Biomed Online. 2015;30(2):150–6. https://doi.org/10.1016/j.rbmo.2014.10.014.
94. Belan M, Duval K, Jean-Denis F, Ainmelk Y, Carranza-Mamane B, Pesant M-H, et al. Anthropometric and lifestyle changes in male partners of infertile couples in which the women is obese are associated with pregnancy-preliminary results. Can J Diabetes. 2015;39(6):530.
95. Håkonsen LB, Thulstrup AM, Aggerholm AS, Olsen J, Bonde JP, Andersen CY, et al. Does weight loss improve semen quality and reproductive hormones? Results from a cohort of severely obese men. Reprod Health. 2011;8:1–8.
96. Mir J, Franken D, Andrabi SW, Ashraf M, Rao K. Impact of weight loss on sperm DNA integrity in obese men. Andrologia. 2018; https://doi.org/10.1111/and.12957.

97. Ibañez-Perez J, Santos-Zorrozua B, Lopez-Lopez E, Matorras R, Garcia-Orad A. An update on the implication of physical activity on semen quality: a systematic review and meta-analysis. Arch Gynecol Obstet. 2019;299(4):901–21. https://doi.org/10.1007/s00404-019-05045-8.
98. Corona G, Rastrelli G, Maggi M. The pharmacotherapy of male hypogonadism besides androgens. Expert Opin Pharmacother. 2015;16(3):369–87. https://doi.org/10.1517/14656566.2015.993607.
99. Rastrelli G, Corona G, Mannucci E, Maggi M. Factors affecting spermatogenesis upon gonadotropin-replacement therapy: a meta-analytic study. Andrology. 2014;2(6):794–808. https://doi.org/10.1111/andr.262.
100. Dwyer AA, Raivio T, Pitteloud N. Gonadotrophin replacement for induction of fertility in hypogonadal men. Best Pract Res Clin Endocrinol Metab. 2015;29(1):91–103. https://doi.org/10.1016/j.beem.2014.10.005.
101. Attia AM, Abou-Setta AM, Al-Inany HG. Gonadotrophins for idiopathic male factor subfertility. Cochrane Database Syst Rev. 2013;2013(8):Cd005071. https://doi.org/10.1002/14651858.CD005071.pub4.
102. Cocci A, Cito G, Russo GI, Falcone M, Capece M, Timpano M, et al. Effectiveness of highly purified urofollitropin treatment in patients with idiopathic azoospermia before testicular sperm extraction. Urologia. 2018;85(1):19–21. https://doi.org/10.5301/uj.5000253.
103. Santi D, Granata AR, Simoni M. FSH treatment of male idiopathic infertility improves pregnancy rate: a meta-analysis. Endocr Connect. 2015;4(3):R46–58. https://doi.org/10.1530/ec-15-0050.
104. Chua ME, Escusa KG, Luna S, Tapia LC, Dofitas B, Morales M. Revisiting oestrogen antagonists (clomiphene or tamoxifen) as medical empiric therapy for idiopathic male infertility: a meta-analysis. Andrology. 2013;1(5):749–57. https://doi.org/10.1111/j.2047-2927.2013.00107.x.
105. Del Giudice F, Busetto GM, De Berardinis E, Sperduti I, Ferro M, Maggi M, et al. A systematic review and meta-analysis of clinical trials implementing aromatase inhibitors to treat male infertility. Asian J Androl. 2020;22(4):360–7. https://doi.org/10.4103/aja.aja_101_19.
106. Cannarella R, Condorelli RA, Mongioì LM, Barbagallo F, Calogero AE, La Vignera S. Effects of the selective estrogen receptor modulators for the treatment of male infertility: a systematic review and meta-analysis. Expert Opin Pharmacother. 2019;20(12):1517–25. https://doi.org/10.1080/14656566.2019.1615057.
107. Cavallini G, Biagiotti G, Bolzon E. Multivariate analysis to predict letrozole efficacy in improving sperm count of non-obstructive azoospermic and cryptozoospermic patients: a pilot study. Asian J Androl. 2013;15(6):806–11. https://doi.org/10.1038/aja.2013.99.
108. Schlegel PN, Sigman M, Collura B, De Jonge CJ, Eisenberg ML, Lamb DJ, et al. Diagnosis and treatment of infertility in men: AUA/ASRM guideline part II. Fertil Steril. 2021;115(1):62–9. https://doi.org/10.1016/j.fertnstert.2020.11.016.
109. Birzniece V. Gonadal steroids and body composition, strength, and sexual function in men. N Engl J Med. 2013;369(25):2455. https://doi.org/10.1056/NEJMc1313169.
110. Sartorius GA, Ly LP, Handelsman DJ. Male sexual function can be maintained without aromatization: randomized placebo-controlled trial of dihydrotestosterone (DHT) in healthy, older men for 24 months. J Sex Med. 2014;11(10):2562–70. https://doi.org/10.1111/jsm.12550.
111. Vanderschueren D, Laurent MR, Claessens F, Gielen E, Lagerquist MK, Vandenput L, et al. Sex steroid actions in male bone. Endocr Rev. 2014;35(6):906–60. https://doi.org/10.1210/er.2014-1024.
112. Hussein A, Ozgok Y, Ross L, Rao P, Niederberger C. Optimization of spermatogenesis-regulating hormones in patients with non-obstructive azoospermia and its impact on sperm retrieval: a multicentre study. BJU Int. 2013;111(3 Pt B):E110–4. https://doi.org/10.1111/j.1464-410X.2012.11485.x.
113. Abd-Elmoaty MA, Saleh R, Sharma R, Agarwal A. Increased levels of oxidants and reduced antioxidants in semen of infertile men with varicocele. Fertil Steril. 2010;94(4):1531–4. https://doi.org/10.1016/j.fertnstert.2009.12.039.

114. Zini A, Al-Hathal N. Antioxidant therapy in male infertility: fact or fiction? Asian J Androl. 2011;13(3):374–81. https://doi.org/10.1038/aja.2010.182.
115. Lopes S, Jurisicova A, Sun JG, Casper RF. Reactive oxygen species: potential cause for DNA fragmentation in human spermatozoa. Hum Reprod. 1998;13(4):896–900. https://doi.org/10.1093/humrep/13.4.896.
116. Showell MG, Brown J, Yazdani A, Stankiewicz MT, Hart RJ. Antioxidants for male subfertility. Cochrane Database Syst Rev. 2011;2011(1):Cd007411. https://doi.org/10.1002/14651858.CD007411.pub2.
117. Ross C, Morriss A, Khairy M, Khalaf Y, Braude P, Coomarasamy A, et al. A systematic review of the effect of oral antioxidants on male infertility. Reprod Biomed Online. 2010;20(6):711–23. https://doi.org/10.1016/j.rbmo.2010.03.008.
118. Agarwal A, Sekhon LH. The role of antioxidant therapy in the treatment of male infertility. Hum Fertil (Camb). 2010;13(4):217–25. https://doi.org/10.3109/14647273.2010.532279.
119. Ramasamy R, Stahl PJ, Schlegel PN. Medical therapy for spermatogenic failure. Asian J Androl. 2012;14(1):57–60. https://doi.org/10.1038/aja.2011.63.
120. Coward RM, Mills JN. A step-by-step guide to office-based sperm retrieval for obstructive azoospermia. Transl Androl Urol. 2017;6(4):730–44. https://doi.org/10.21037/tau.2017.07.15.
121. Bernie AM, Mata DA, Ramasamy R, Schlegel PN. Comparison of microdissection testicular sperm extraction, conventional testicular sperm extraction, and testicular sperm aspiration for nonobstructive azoospermia: a systematic review and meta-analysis. Fertil Steril 2015;104(5):1099–103.e1–3. https://doi.org/10.1016/j.fertnstert.2015.07.1136.
122. Corona G, Minhas S, Giwercman A, Bettocchi C, Dinkelman-Smit M, Dohle G, et al. Sperm recovery and ICSI outcomes in men with non-obstructive azoospermia: a systematic review and meta-analysis. Hum Reprod Update. 2019;25(6):733–57. https://doi.org/10.1093/humupd/dmz028.
123. Corona G, Pizzocaro A, Lanfranco F, Garolla A, Pelliccione F, Vignozzi L, et al. Sperm recovery and ICSI outcomes in Klinefelter syndrome: a systematic review and meta-analysis. Hum Reprod Update. 2017;23(3):265–75. https://doi.org/10.1093/humupd/dmx008.
124. Nodar F, De Vincentiis S, Olmedo SB, Papier S, Urrutia F, Acosta AA. Birth of twin males with normal karyotype after intracytoplasmic sperm injection with use of testicular spermatozoa from a nonmosaic patient with Klinefelter's syndrome. Fertil Steril. 1999;71(6):1149–52. https://doi.org/10.1016/s0015-0282(99)00151-x.
125. Hessel M, Robben JC, D'Hauwers KW, Braat DD, Ramos L. The influence of sperm motility and cryopreservation on the treatment outcome after intracytoplasmic sperm injection following testicular sperm extraction. Acta Obstet Gynecol Scand. 2015;94(12):1313–21. https://doi.org/10.1111/aogs.12769.
126. Eliveld J, van Wely M, Meißner A, Repping S, van der Veen F, van Pelt AMM. The risk of TESE-induced hypogonadism: a systematic review and meta-analysis. Hum Reprod Update. 2018;24(4):442–54. https://doi.org/10.1093/humupd/dmy015.
127. Larijani B, Esfahani EN, Amini P, Nikbin B, Alimoghaddam K, Amiri S, et al. Stem cell therapy in treatment of different diseases. Acta Med Iran. 2012;50(2):79–96.
128. Zhang M, Wang J, Deng C, Jiang MH, Feng X, Xia K, et al. Transplanted human p75-positive stem Leydig cells replace disrupted Leydig cells for testosterone production. Cell Death Dis. 2017;8(10):e3123. https://doi.org/10.1038/cddis.2017.531.
129. Odeh HM, Kleinguetl C, Ge R, Zirkin BR, Chen H. Regulation of the proliferation and differentiation of Leydig stem cells in the adult testis. Biol Reprod. 2014;90(6):123. https://doi.org/10.1095/biolreprod.114.117473.
130. Jiang MH, Cai B, Tuo Y, Wang J, Zang ZJ, Tu X, et al. Characterization of Nestin-positive stem Leydig cells as a potential source for the treatment of testicular Leydig cell dysfunction. Cell Res. 2014;24(12):1466–85. https://doi.org/10.1038/cr.2014.149.
131. Li L, Papadopoulos V. Advances in stem cell research for the treatment of primary hypogonadism. Nat Rev Urol. 2021;18(8):487–507. https://doi.org/10.1038/s41585-021-00480-2.

Chapter 7
Management of Secondary Hypogonadism in Men with NOA

Christopher C. K. Ho, Sang Thanh Le, and Murat Gül

Introduction

About 1 in 6 couples are affected by infertility. About 50% of cases are caused by male factor infertility [1]. Azoospermia is defined as the absence of spermatozoa in the ejaculate and is considered the most extreme form of male factor infertility. Azoospermia can be classified as either nonobstructive azoospermia (NOA) or obstructive azoospermia (OA). NOA is due to an impairment of spermatogenesis, while OA is seen when there is an occlusion of the genital ductular system.

Etiology and Prevalence

The etiology of NOA is conventionally categorized by the anatomical position of the cause: pre-testicular or testicular. Pre-testicular NOA (or secondary hypogonadism) arises due to deficiency of the pituitary hormones so that a structurally normal testis is not stimulated effectively to produce sperm, and this is usually secondary to hypothalamic–pituitary disorders. Prevalence of NOA has been estimated to be 1 in 100 men [2].

C. C. K. Ho (✉)
Department of Urology, School of Medicine, Taylor's University, Subang Jaya, Selangor, Malaysia

S. T. Le
Department of Urology, Cho Ray Hospital, Ho Chi Minh City, Vietnam

M. Gül
Department of Urology, Selçuk University School of Medicine, Konya, Türkiye

Department of Andrology, Selçuk University School of Medicine, Konya, Türkiye

W. Zohdy et al. (eds.), *Non-Obstructive Azoospermia*,
https://doi.org/10.1007/978-3-031-99431-9_7

Human Chorionic Gonadotropin (hCG), FSH, and GnRH

The preferred medication for men wishing to maintain normal intra-testicular testosterone production and re-establish spermatogenesis is hCG. hCG acts by directly stimulating the LH receptors on the Leydig cells. To enhance spermatogenesis, recombinant FSH or hMG can be added. The hCG/hMG combination has shown superiority over single treatment with hCG regarding spermatogenesis, with success rates of 60% vs. 40%, respectively [3]. FSH (or an FSH analogue) is usually started after normalizing testosterone levels with hCG [4]. According to the EAU guidelines, in order to reach a normal testosterone level in blood, an hCG dose of 1500–5000 IU is given intramuscularly or subcutaneously twice weekly, while an FSH regimen of 150 IU is given three times weekly intramuscularly or subcutaneously [5]. If this regimen is continued for 6 months, the success rate (defined as sperm in the ejaculate) is ~80%. However, to maximize the chances of achieving spermatogenesis, the course of therapy can be extended for up to 2 years [6]. An alternative regimen, with a similar success rate, but more expensive, is the administration of GnRH in a pulsatile manner [7]. The most convenient route for GnRH administration is a bi-hourly dose regimen of 5–20 μg over 12–24 months via a subcutaneous pump infusion. There are also other FSH preparations like highly purified urinary FSH preparations (hpFSH) (e.g., urofollitropin) and recombinant FSH (rFSH).

One study recruited ten men with hypogonadotropic hypogonadism and divided them into two groups: a human gonadotropins (150 IU of HMG and 1500 IU of HCG, three times/week) group and a pure FSH (150 IU, three times/week) and testosterone (250 mg of T, once/week) group [8]. Five patients first received HMG–HCG and then pure FSH in addition to testosterone, while the other five men started with pure FSH plus testosterone, for 24 months each. HMG–HCG triggered spermatogenesis after 24 months in all patients. The combination of pure FSH and testosterone did not trigger spermatogenesis, and the sperm count significantly decreased to $0.3 \pm 0.1 \times 10^6$/mL after 3 months and 0 after 6 months. Plasma testosterone levels increased in both treatments, but they increased significantly more after treatment with pure FSH and testosterone (35.3 ± 5.2 nmol/L) compared with HMG–HCG (20.4 ± 5.2 nmol/L; $P < 0.05$) [9]. These results support the theory that testosterone stimulation via LH is crucial for spermatogenesis, which probably cannot be achieved with FSH alone.

hMG, which contains FSH, stimulates spermatogenesis, but only after intratesticular testosterone is brought into the normal range with hCG stimulation. Therefore, hMG needs to be given only after hCG administration [10]. The dose is 75 IU two to three times weekly until pregnancy is achieved. HMG treatment is usually continued until pregnancy has been achieved and maintained for 3 months. After that, it can be withdrawn, and spermatogenesis can be maintained by continued administration of hCG [11].

Besides spermatogenesis, the combination of hCG/hMG therapy can induce pubertal development, increase physical strength, double the testicular volume, and normalize testosterone level [12–14]. When treated with hCG plus hMG, 64.9–89.2% of patients had spermatozoa in the ejaculate with an average treatment duration of 9.2–10.5 months [15–17].

GnRH Pump Treatment

A portable infusion pump administers pulses of GnRH into the subcutaneous tissue of the abdominal wall every 2 h, with doses ranging from 100 to 400 ng/kg. This treatment lasts approximately 4 months and is usually shorter than gonadotropin therapy. However, GnRH usage is costly and interferes with the patient's everyday life.

In a recent meta-analysis, response to medical therapy resulting in at least one spermatozoon in the ejaculate as a result of gonadotropin and GnRH therapy occurred in 75% (69–81) and 75% (60–85) of patients, respectively. Combined pregnancy rate for the gonadotropin and GnRH study groups were 30% and 50%, respectively, with a minority of the pregnancies requiring ART [18].

Other Medical Treatments (SERMs, Aromatase Inhibitors)

Selective Estrogen Receptor Modulators

Since the 1970s, when Paulson and colleagues published their studies, clomiphene citrate has emerged as an off-label treatment option for male infertility. Its antiestrogenic properties influence the pituitary, resulting in elevated serum levels of FSH and LH. This mechanism positions clomiphene as a potentially beneficial therapy for individuals presenting with low testosterone levels and subnormal sperm counts, particularly in cases where gonadotropin levels are low to normal . However, clomiphene citrate will not be effective in severe hypogonadotropic hypogonadism because these cases usually have pituitary failure [19–21]. Despite widespread utilization by urologists, particularly in instances of simple idiopathic infertility, where patients exhibit low normal testosterone levels and sperm counts, robust evidence supporting its efficacy in this context remains scarce [22].

Approved in the 1970s for breast cancer treatment, tamoxifen citrate stands as another oral selective estrogen receptor modulator (SERM) [23]. While predominantly prescribed for women, its off-label use in men's health is because of its action as an estrogen antagonist within the hypothalamus and pituitary gland [24]. Tamoxifen operates by inhibiting estrogen's negative feedback at these sites, thereby facilitating the release of LH and FSH. This release subsequently stimulates testosterone biosynthesis and spurs spermatogenesis.

Clomiphene citrate stands as a potentially safe and effective choice for long-term management of testosterone deficiency. It warrants consideration as a primary treatment option for testosterone deficiency, irrespective of the patient's fertility preservation goals [25]. However, in cases of severe hypogonadotropic hypogonadism, where pituitary failure is often present, clomiphene citrate proves to be ineffective. In contrast, tamoxifen presents with a higher incidence of adverse effects compared to clomiphene citrate, encompassing gastrointestinal discomfort, venous thromboembolic events, and other cardiovascular complications [26].

However, similar to clomiphene citrate and aromatase inhibitors, tamoxifen's application in idiopathic infertility remains contentious, with much of the existing data derived from case reports or uncontrolled studies [27, 28].

A couple of articles exploring tamoxifen's efficacy in idiopathic infertility yield mixed and conflicting results [29, 30].

Aromatase Inhibitors

Employing aromatase inhibitors (AIs) such as anastrozole or letrozole for men with idiopathic OAT or azoospermia constitutes an off-label use of these medications. The rationale behind their use lies in their ability to elevate testosterone levels, reduce estrogen levels, and inhibit the peripheral metabolism of testosterone. Reduced estrogen levels result in less inhibition of the hypothalamic–pituitary–gonadal (HPG) axis, leading to increased LH and FSH production, both pivotal for testosterone synthesis and sperm production [12]. Since a notable portion of men with low sperm concentration exhibit heightened aromatase activity, resulting in a diminished T/E ratio, AIs prove effective in restoring LH, FSH, and testosterone levels. Consequently, improvements in semen parameters and the restoration of fertility are observed. This is specifically indicated in individuals with NOA or idiopathic oligoasthenospermia, and with low testosterone levels and a T/E ratio $< 10{:}1$ [31–33]. However, the utility of AI prior to microTESE in NOA patients necessitates further investigation [34]. Furthermore, uncertainties persist regarding the clinical relevance of changes in testosterone levels and testosterone to estradiol (T:E2) ratios associated with AIs, given that certain studies have failed to demonstrate enhancements in psychological or physiological parameters or alleviation of hypogonadal symptoms alongside these alterations [35, 36]. Additionally, there are currently no specific guidelines on the dosage of AIs, with recommendations largely relying on the expertise and experience of healthcare professionals.

AIs come with potential side effects such as nausea, elevation of liver enzymes, headaches, and hot flashes [37]. It is worth noting that prolonged use of AIs has been associated with reductions in bone mineral density due to the suppression of estradiol, leading the American Urological Association (AUA) to caution against extended AI usage [13, 38].

Anabolic Steroid-Induced Secondary Hypogonadism

Testosterone, a pivotal sex hormone, alongside other androgens, plays a crucial role in the development of sexual characteristics, and facilitates muscle protein synthesis, thereby promoting muscle hypertrophy, recognized as the anabolic effect. In light of these effects, synthetic derivatives of steroid hormones have been formulated and utilized across various contexts for decades. While these drugs find application in disease treatment, they are also indiscriminately used, often without medical necessity, to enhance athletic performance and for aesthetic purposes [39–41].

The abuse of anabolic-androgenic steroids (AAS) can lead to severe disruption of the HPG axis, triggering a negative feedback loop that results in a notable reduction in testosterone synthesis and secretion by the testes. This imbalance typically manifests in clinical symptoms such as sexual impotence, decreased libido, reduced physical capacity, and sometimes depressive symptoms, a condition medically referred to as anabolic steroid-induced hypogonadism (ASIH) [42, 43].

Administration of AAS elevates serum androgen levels to supraphysiological states, leading to significant disturbances in the HPG axis and suppression of GnRH, LH, FSH, and testosterone [44]. This disruption results in decreased serum testosterone levels, characteristic of secondary hypogonadism, specifically termed ASIH, wherein testicular function is compromised, leading to subnormal or impaired testosterone synthesis and/or sperm production due to exogenous AAS administration [42]. Although AAS abuse commonly induces secondary hypogonadism (ASIH), there exists a real possibility for this condition to progress to primary hypogonadism, known as testicular failure. The pathophysiology of ASIH is multifaceted, extending beyond the mere effect of negative feedback from androgen excess. AAS abusers typically employ blends of high-dose synthetic androgens, which, in addition to endocrine disruption, can directly contribute to primary testicular failure, as evidenced by animal studies conducted by Boetcher et al., Chainy et al., and Karavolos et al. [45, 46].

hCG is a useful option for restoring endogenous testosterone production in men who have lost this ability, normalizing sexual potency, and ameliorating hypogonadism symptoms [47, 48]. Unlike other medications, hCG acts directly on the testicles, eliciting an immediate response [49, 50]. It is noteworthy that therapeutic use of hCG in men has become more prevalent, particularly due to the rise in AAS abuse and subsequent hypogonadism cases [44].

There exists compelling evidence suggesting that two factors significantly influence an individual's capacity to restore normal testosterone synthesis and reverse ASIH: the patient's age and the duration of compromised endogenous testosterone synthesis. Previous research indicates potential reversibility in younger men owing to the efficiency of their "elastic axis" in recovering GnRH pulsation and gonadotropin secretion [51, 52].

Hypogonadism emerges as a predictable outcome for AAS users, representing a significant and often overlooked issue. Moreover, this condition may underlie fertility problems, depression, decreased libido, and sexual impotence in men.

Impact of Long-Term Anabolic Androgenic Steroids (AAS)

Long-term use of supraphysiologic doses of anabolic-androgenic steroids (AAS) may cause irreversible cardiovascular toxicity, especially atherosclerotic effects and cardiomyopathy [53, 54]. Testicular atrophy and gynecomastia are well-documented sequalae when anabolic steroids are administered for long duration [55, 56]. Men exposed to long-term exogenous androgens are at higher risk of developing hepatic adenoma and adenocarcinoma [57]. Significant psychiatric symptoms, including aggression, mania, and less frequently psychosis and suicide, have been associated with anabolic steroid abuse [58]. In adolescents, anabolic steroids may lead to early closure of growth plates, leading to stunted growth [59]. Long-term anabolic steroid use may lead to kidney damage, including glomerulosclerosis and chronic kidney disease [60]. Anabolic steroid abuse can lead to severe acne and skin infections due to increased sebaceous gland activity as well as alopecia [61]. Chronic anabolic steroid use has been linked to an increased risk of liver and prostate cancers [62].

Side Effects of Gonadotropin Therapy

Outside the realm of NOA, research suggests that a significant portion, estimated between 58% and 80%, of men with idiopathic infertility, may possess FSH receptor gene polymorphisms, rendering them potentially responsive to exogenous FSH stimulation [63, 64]. Consequently, it is believed that increasing circulating FSH levels could offer benefits to these individuals. However, it is estimated that a considerable number, ranging from 10% to 18% males with idiopathic infertility, must undergo medical treatment with exogenous gonadotropins to achieve one additional pregnancy [65]. Given the costs associated with gonadotropin therapy and the limited evidence regarding its efficacy, there is an ongoing debate regarding whether FSH should be a standard treatment for males [66]. Despite encouraging outcomes in men with idiopathic infertility, there is no consensus regarding the use of gonadotropins in NOA males with spermatogenic failure, and routine treatment is not recommended [67–69].

Generally deemed safe for stimulating spermatogenesis in the context of idiopathic infertility and hypogonadotropic hypogonadism, gonadotropins are associated with minimal side effects, such as gynecomastia and temporary mastalgia, particularly in patients with excessive endogenous testosterone and estradiol levels [70, 71]. However, a previous case report detailed the development of a seminoma following prolonged FSH and hCG therapy in a 43-year-old patient with oligozoospermia. This underscores the need for cautious monitoring during hormonal therapy [72].

Determining which patients would benefit from gonadotropin therapy remains a subject of ongoing research, considering the treatment's high cost, lengthy duration, uncertainties surrounding sperm acquisition, and potential side effects. Factors such as the female partner's age should be considered when evaluating the likelihood of achieving pregnancy. Introducing this new treatment regimen also prompts questions regarding the most optimal treatment plan, sperm retrieval method, and cryopreservation technique in cases where only a minimal number of spermatozoa are present. Additionally, monitoring during treatment, potential side effects, and the future need for exogenous testosterone supplementation in males with low testosterone levels after sperm retrieval warrant careful consideration.

Failure of Medical Therapy and ART

For men with secondary hypogonadism who do not respond adequately to medical therapy to achieve pregnancy through natural conception, assisted reproductive technology (ART) is recommended [73]. Some individuals may be suitable candidates for intrauterine insemination, while others may need in vitro fertilization (IVF) or ICSI using ejaculated sperm. In cases where ejaculated sperm are undetectable, sperm-retrieval procedures should be considered. While data are limited, a minimum therapy duration of 6 months, associated with increased testicular volumes and normalization of hormones, should be given before considering retrieval [74].

For individuals experiencing ASIH, discontinuation of exogenous androgens/steroids and prevention of further use are strongly advised. The duration of spermatogenesis recovery varies among suppressed individuals [75]. For those with hypogonadism resulting from anabolic steroid abuse, administering intramuscular injections of hCG at doses of 3000 units 2–3 times per week for 3 or more months can expedite spermatogenesis recovery [76–78]. However, higher hCG doses may suppress FSH, necessitating the addition of clomiphene citrate to preserve pituitary function. Alternatively, monotherapy with clomiphene citrate may be considered, although adherence may be affected by hypogonadal symptoms [79].

Following infertility therapy completion, most hypogonadal men benefit from lifelong hormonal therapy to manage symptoms associated with clinical testosterone deficiency [80]. These individuals may continue medical therapy to maintain reproductive potential, such as gonadotropin replacement therapy or clomiphene citrate, or transition to testosterone replacement therapy (TRT). While TRT results in relapse to infertility, it is more cost-effective than gonadotropin replacement therapy and has been extensively studied for long-term use [81, 82]. However, the risks and benefits of long-term TRT should be thoroughly discussed before initiating therapy.

Summary

In addressing secondary hypogonadism among men with NOA, a multifaceted approach combining medical therapy and ART is crucial. While surgical sperm extraction paired with ART offers a pathway to parenthood, it does not resolve the underlying pathology. In contrast, personalized medical treatment tailored to specific patients can yield comparable results, obviating the need for invasive interventions. Moreover, for couples unable to conceive naturally, even with medical management, these therapies may enhance success rates of surgical sperm extraction or facilitate less invasive ART interventions like intrauterine insemination (IUI). Thus, a comprehensive medical evaluation is essential for optimizing fertility outcomes in all affected men.

References

1. Agarwal A, Mulgund A, Hamada A, et al. A unique view on male infertility around the globe. Reprod Biol Endocrinol. 2015;13:37. https://doi.org/10.1186/s12958-015-0032-1.
2. Jarow JP, Espeland MA, Lipshultz LI. Evaluation of the azoospermic patient. J Urol. 1989;142(1):62–5. https://doi.org/10.1016/s0022-5347(17)38662-7.
3. Yang L, Zhang SX, Dong Q, et al. Application of hormonal treatment in hypogonadotropic hypogonadism: more than ten years experience. Int Urol Nephrol. 2012;44(2):393–9. Epub 2011 Oct 12
4. Schlegel PN, Sigman M, Collura B, et al. Diagnosis and treatment of infertility in men: AUA/ASRM guideline part I. J Urol. 2021;205:36–43.
5. Dohle GR (Chair), Arver S, Bettocchi C, Jones TH, Kliesch S, Dohle GR, et al. EAU guidelines panel on male hypogonadism, Edn. Presented at the EAU Annual Congress Paris 2012: Arnhem, The Netherlands.
6. George B, Bantwal G. Endocrine management of male subfertility. Indian. J Endocrinol Metab. 2013;17(Suppl1):S32–4. PMID: 24251201; PMCID: PMC3830347
7. Pitteloud N, Hayes FJ, Dwyer A, et al. Predictors of outcome of long-term GnRH therapy in men with idiopathic hypogonadotropic hypogonadism. J Clin Endocrinol Metab. 2002;87(9):4128–36.
8. Foresta C, Bettella A, Spolaore D, Merico M, Rossato M, Ferlin A. Suppression of the high endogenous levels of plasma FSH in infertile men are associated with improved Sertoli cell function as reflected by elevated levels of plasma inhibin B. Hum Reprod. 2004;19:1431–7.
9. Shiraishi K, Ohmi C, Shimabukuro T, Matsuyama H. Human chorionic gonadotrophin treatment prior to microdissection testicular sperm extraction in non-obstructive azoospermia. Hum Reprod. 2012;27:331–9.
10. Shinjo E, Shiraishib K, Matsuyama H. The effect of human chorionic gonadotropin-based hormonal therapy on intratesticular testosterone levels and spermatogonial DNA synthesis in men with non-obstructive azoospermia. Andrology. 2013;1:929–35.
11. Steger K, Aleithe I, Behre H, Bergmann M. The proliferation of spermatogonia in normal and pathological human seminiferous epithelium: an immunohistochemical study using monoclonal antibodies against Ki-67 protein and proliferating cell nuclear antigen. Mol Hum Reprod. 1998;4:227–33.
12. Schaison G, Young J, Pholsena M, Nahoul K, Couzinet B. Failure of combined follicle-stimulating hormone-testosterone administration to initiate and/or maintain spermatogenesis in men with hypogonadotropic hypogonadism. J Clin Endocrinol Metab. 1993;77:1545–9.

13. Sokol RZ. Endocrinology of male infertility: Evaluation and treatment. Semin Reprod Med. 2009;27:149–58.
14. Sokol RZ. Male factor infertility. In: Lobo RA, Mishell Jr DR, Paulson RJ, Shoupe D, editors. Infertility, contraception, and reproductive endocrinology. 4th ed. Malden: Blackwell Science; 1997. p. 547–66.
15. Homayoun A, Asghar D, Darab M, Mohammad AH. Gonadotropins in infertile men with idiopathic hypogon-adotropic hypogonadism. Int J Fertil Steril. 2008;2:113–4.
16. Yang L, Zhang SX, Dong Q, Xiong ZB, Li X. Application of hormonal treatment in hypogonadotropic hypogonadism: more than ten years experience. Int Urol Nephrol. 2012;44:393–9.
17. Ho CC, Tan HM. Treatment of the hypogonadal infertile male-a Review. Sex Med Rev. 2013 May;1(1):42–9.
18. Rastrelli G, Corona G, Mannucci E, Maggi M. Factors affecting spermatogenesis upon gonadotropin-replacement therapy: a meta-analytic study. Andrology. 2014;2(6):794–808.
19. Paulson DF. Clomiphene citrate in the management of male hypofertility: predictors for treatment selection. Fertil Steril. 1977;28(11):1226–9.
20. Ross LS, Kandel GL, Prinz LM, Auletta F. Clomiphene treatment of the idiopathic hypofertile male: high-dose, alternate-day therapy. Fertil Steril. 1980;33(6):618–23.
21. Pasqualotto FF, Pasqualotto EB. Is there a special subgroup of males with adult-onset idiopathic hypogonadotrophic hypogonadism who may respond with increases in sperm concentration after clomiphene citrate? Fertil Steril. 2007;88(1):249.
22. Ko EY, Siddiqi K, Brannigan RE, Sabanegh ES Jr. Empirical medical therapy for idiopathic male infertility: a survey of the American Urological Association. J Urol. 2012;187(3):973–8. https://doi.org/10.1016/j.juro.2011.10.137.
23. Goetz MP. The development of endoxifen for breast cancer. Clin Adv Hematol Oncol. 2018;16(2):102–5.
24. Tsourdi E, Kourtis A, Farmakiotis D, Katsikis I, Salmas M, Panidis D. The effect of selective estrogen receptor modulator administration on the hypothalamic-pituitary-testicular axis in men with idiopathic oligozoospermia. Fertil Steril. 2009;91(4 Suppl):1427–30. https://doi.org/10.1016/j.fertnstert.2008.06.002.
25. Krzastek SC, Smith RP. Non-testosterone management of male hypogonadism: an examination of the existing literature. Transl Androl Urol. 2020;9(Suppl 2):S160–70. https://doi.org/10.21037/tau.2019.11.16.
26. Wibowo E, Pollock PA, Hollis N, Wassersug RJ. Tamoxifen in men: a review of adverse events. Andrology. 2016;4(5):776–88. https://doi.org/10.1111/andr.12197.
27. Garg H, Kumar R. Empirical drug therapy for idiopathic male infertility: what is the new evidence? Urology. 2015;86(6):1065–75. https://doi.org/10.1016/j.urology.2015.07.030.
28. Shah T, Shin D. Empiric medical therapy for idiopathic male infertility. In: Male infertility: contemporary clinical approaches, andrology, ART and antioxidants; 2020. p. 873–82.
29. Kotoulas IG, Cardamakis E, Michopoulos J, Mitropoulos D, Dounis A. Tamoxifen treatment in male infertility. I. Effect on spermatozoa. Fertil Steril. 1994;61(5):911–4. https://doi.org/10.1016/s0015-0282(16)56705-3.
30. AinMelk Y, Belisle S, Carmel M, Jean-Pierre T. Tamoxifen citrate therapy in male infertility. Fertil Steril. 1987;48(1):113–7. https://doi.org/10.1016/s0015-0282(16)59299-1.
31. Santen RJ. Feedback control of luteinizing hormone and follicle-stimulating hormone secretion by testosterone and estradiol in men: physiological and clinical implications. Clin Biochem. 1981;14(5):243–51. https://doi.org/10.1016/s0009-9120(81)90964-4.
32. Raman JD, Schlegel PN. Aromatase inhibitors for male infertility. J Urol. 2002;167(2 Pt 1):624–9. https://doi.org/10.1016/S0022-5347(01)69099-2.
33. Saylam B, Efesoy O, Cayan S. The effect of aromatase inhibitor letrozole on body mass index, serum hormones, and sperm parameters in infertile men. Fertil Steril. 2011;95(2):809–11. https://doi.org/10.1016/j.fertnstert.2010.09.021.
34. Schlegel PN. Aromatase inhibitors for male infertility. Fertil Steril. 2012;98(6):1359–62. https://doi.org/10.1016/j.fertnstert.2012.10.023.

35. Loves S, de Jong J, van Sorge A, Telting D, Tack CJ, Hermus A, Westerterp K, de Boer H. Somatic and psychological effects of low-dose aromatase inhibition in men with obesity-related hypogonadotropic hypotestosteronemia. Eur J Endocrinol. 2013;169(5):705–14. https://doi.org/10.1530/EJE-13-0190.
36. Helo S, Ellen J, Mechlin C, Feustel P, Grossman M, Ditkoff E, McCullough A. A randomized prospective double-blind comparison trial of clomiphene citrate and Anastrozole in raising testosterone in hypogonadal infertile men. J Sex Med. 2015;12(8):1761–9. https://doi.org/10.1111/jsm.12944.
37. Gregoriou O, Bakas P, Grigoriadis C, Creatsa M, Hassiakos D, Creatsas G. Changes in hormonal profile and seminal parameters with use of aromatase inhibitors in management of infertile men with low testosterone to estradiol ratios. Fertil Steril. 2012;98(1):48–51. https://doi.org/10.1016/j.fertnstert.2012.04.005.
38. Mulhall JP, Trost LW, Brannigan RE, Kurtz EG, Redmon JB, Chiles KA, Lightner DJ, Miner MM, Murad MH, Nelson CJ, Platz EA, Ramanathan LV, Lewis RW. Evaluation and management of testosterone deficiency: AUA guideline. J Urol. 2018;200(2):423–32. https://doi.org/10.1016/j.juro.2018.03.115.
39. Burnett-Bowie SA, McKay EA, Lee H, Leder BZ. Effects of aromatase inhibition on bone mineral density and bone turnover in older men with low testosterone levels. J Clin Endocrinol Metab. 2009;94(12):4785–92. https://doi.org/10.1210/jc.2009-0739.
40. Evans NA. Current concepts in anabolic-androgenic steroids. Am J Sports Med. 2004;32(2):534–42. https://doi.org/10.1177/0363546503262202.
41. Pope HG Jr, Wood RI, Rogol A, Nyberg F, Bowers L, Bhasin S. Adverse health consequences of performance-enhancing drugs: An Endocrine Society scientific statement. Endocr Rev. 2014;35(3):341–75. https://doi.org/10.1210/er.2013-1058.
42. Sagoe D, Molde H, Andreassen CS, Torsheim T, Pallesen S. The global epidemiology of anabolic-androgenic steroid use: a meta-analysis and meta-regression analysis. Ann Epidemiol. 2014;24(5):383–98. https://doi.org/10.1016/j.annepidem.2014.01.009.
43. Hartgens F, Kuipers H. Effects of androgenic-anabolic steroids in athletes. Sports Med. 2004;34(8):513–54. https://doi.org/10.2165/00007256-200434080-00003.
44. Wu FCW, Tajar A, Beynon JM, Pye SR, Silman AJ, Finn JD, O'Neill TW, Bartfai G, Casanueva FF, Forti G, Giwercman A, Han TS, Kula K, Lean MEJ, Pendleton N, Punab M, Boonen S, Vanderschueren D, Labrie F, Huhtaniemi IT. Identification of late-onset hypogonadism in middle-aged and elderly men. N Engl J Med. 2010;363(2):123–35. https://doi.org/10.1056/NEJMoa091110125.
45. Vilar Neto JDO, da Silva CA, Lima AB, Caminha JDSR, Pinto DV, Alves FR, Araújo JS, Daher EDF. Disorder of hypothalamic-pituitary-gonadal axis induced by abusing of anabolicandrogenic steroids for short time: a case report. Andrologia. 2018;50(9):e13107. https://doi.org/10.1111/and.13107.
46. Boettcher M, Kosmehl T, Braunbeck T. Low-dose effects and biphasic effect profiles: Is trenbolone a genotoxicant? Mutat Res. 2011;723(2):152–7. https://doi.org/10.1016/j.mrgentox.2011.04.012.
47. Chainy GB, Samantaray S, Samanta L. Testosterone-induced changes in testicular antioxidant system. Andrologia. 1997;29(6):343–9. https://doi.org/10.1111/j.1439-0272.1997.tb00328.x.
48. Karavolos S, Reynolds M, Panagiotopoulou N, McEleny K, Scally M, Quinton R. Male central hypogonadism secondary to exogenous androgens: a review of the drugs and protocols highlighted by the online community of users for prevention and/or mitigation of adverse effects. Clin Endocrinol. 2015;82(5):624–32. https://doi.org/10.1111/cen.12641.
49. Gill GV. Anabolic steroid induced hypogonadism treated with human chorionic gonadotropin. Postgrad Med J. 1998;74(867):45–6. https://doi.org/10.1136/pgmj.74.867.45.
50. Habous M, Giona S, Tealab A, Aziz M, Williamson B, Nassar M, Abdelrahman Z, Remeah A, Abdelkader M, Binsaleh S, Muir G. Clomiphene citrate and human chorionic gonadotropin are both effective in restoring testosterone in hypogonadism: a shortcourse randomized study. BJU Int. 2018;122(5):889–97. https://doi.org/10.1111/bju.14401.

51. Coviello AD, Matsumoto AM, Bremner WJ, Herbst KL, Amory JK, Anawalt BD, Sutton PR, Wright WW, Brown TR, Yan X, Zirkin BR, Jarow JP. Low-dose human chorionic gonadotropin maintains intratesticular testosterone in normal men with testosterone-induced gonadotropin suppression. J Clin Endocrinol Metab. 2005;90(5):2595–602. https://doi.org/10.1210/jc.2004-0802.
52. Toscano V, Balducci R, Adamo MV, Manca Bitti ML, Sciarra F, Boscherini B. Response to a single dose of human chorionic gonadotropin in prepubertal boys. J Clin Endocrinol Metab. 1983;57(2):421–4. https://doi.org/10.1210/jcem-57-2-421.
53. Rahnema CD, Lipshultz LI, Crosnoe LE, Kovac JR, Kim ED. Anabolic steroid-induced hypogonadism: Diagnosis and treatment. Fertil Steril. 2014;101(5):1271–9. https://doi.org/10.1016/j.fertnstert.2014.02.002.
54. Moretti E, Collodel G, La Marca A, Piomboni P, Scapigliati G, Baccetti B. Structural sperm and aneuploidies studies in a case of spermatogenesis recovery after the use of androgenic anabolic steroids. J Assist Reprod Genet. 2007;24(5):195–8. https://doi.org/10.1007/s10815-005-9002-4.
55. Thiblin I, Petersson A. Pharmacoepidemiology of anabolic androgenic steroids: a review. Fundam Clin Pharmacol. 2005;19(1):27–44. https://doi.org/10.1111/j.1472-8206.2004.00299.x.
56. Baggish AL, Weiner RB, Kanayama G, Hudson JI, Lu MT, Hoffmann U, Pope HG. Cardiovascular toxicity of illicit anabolic-androgenic steroid use. Circulation. 2017;135(21):1991–2002. https://doi.org/10.1161/CIRCULATIONAHA.116.026945.
57. Handelsman DJ. Clinical pharmacology of anabolic steroids. Br J Pharmacol. 2013;154(3):502–21. https://doi.org/10.1038/bjp.2013.220.
58. Kanayama G, Hudson JI, Pope HG. Long-term psychiatric and medical consequences of anabolic–androgenic steroid abuse: a looming public health concern? Drug Alcohol Depend. 2008;98(1–2):1–12. https://doi.org/10.1016/j.drugalcdep.2008.05.004.
59. Socas L, Zumbado M, Pérez-Luzardo O, Ramos A, Pérez C, Hernández JR, Boada LD. Hepatocellular adenomas associated with anabolic androgenic steroid abuse in bodybuilders: a report of two cases and a review of the literature. Br J Sports Med. 2005;39(5):e27.
60. Pope HG, Wood RI, Rogol A, Nyberg F, Bowers L, Bhasin S. Adverse health consequences of performance-enhancing drugs: an Endocrine Society scientific statement. Endocr Rev. 2014;35(3):341–75.
61. Maravelias C, Dona A, Stefanidou M, Spiliopoulou C. Adverse effects of anabolic steroids in athletes. a constant threat. Toxicol Lett. 2005;158(3):167–75.
62. Herlitz LC, Markowitz GS, Farris AB, Schwimmer JA, Stokes MB, Kunis C, Colvin RB, D'Agati VD. Development of focal segmental glomerulosclerosis after anabolic steroid abuse. J Am Soc Nephrol. 2010;21(1):163–72.
63. Nieschlag E, Vorona E. Mechanisms in endocrinology: Medical consequences of doping with anabolic androgenic steroids: effects on reproductive functions. Eur J Endocrinol. 2015;173(2):R47–58. https://doi.org/10.1530/EJE-15-0080.
64. Hartgens F, Kuipers H. Effects of androgenic-anabolic steroids in athletes. Sports Med. 2004;34(8):513–54.
65. Selice R, Garolla A, Pengo M, Caretta N, Ferlin A, Foresta C. The response to FSH treatment in oligozoospermic men depends on FSH receptor gene polymorphisms. Int J Androl. 2011;34(4):306–12. https://doi.org/10.1111/j.1365-2605.2010.01086.x.
66. Simoni M, Santi D, Negri L, Hoffmann I, Muratori M, Baldi E, Cambi M, Marcou M, Greither T, Baraldi E, Tagliavini S, Carra D, Lombardo F, Gandini L, Pallotti F, Krausz C, Rastrelli G, Ferlin A, Menegazzo M, Pignatti E, et al. Treatment with human, recombinant FSH improves sperm DNA fragmentation in idiopathic infertile men depending on the FSH receptor polymorphism p.N680S: a pharmacogenetic study. Hum Reprod. 2016;31(9):1960–9. https://doi.org/10.1093/humrep/dew167.

67. Santi D, Granata AR, Simoni M. FSH treatment of male idiopathic infertility improves pregnancy rate: a meta-analysis. Endocr Connect. 2015;4(3):R46–58. https://doi.org/10.1530/EC-15-0050.
68. Simoni M, Santi D. FSH treatment of male idiopathic infertility: time for a paradigm change. Andrology. 2020;8(3):535–44. https://doi.org/10.1111/andr.12746.
69. Tharakan T, Salonia A, Corona G, Dhillo W, Minhas S, Jayasena C. The role of hormone stimulation in men with nonobstructive azoospermia undergoing surgical sperm retrieval. J Clin Endocrinol Metab. 2020;105(12):dgaa556. https://doi.org/10.1210/clinem/dgaa556.
70. Minhas S, Bettocchi C, Boeri L, Capogrosso P, Carvalho J, Cilesiz NC, Cocci A, Corona G, Dimitropoulos K, Gül M, Hatzichristodoulou G, Jones TH, Kadioglu A, Martínez Salamanca JI, Milenkovic U, Modgil V, Russo GI, Serefoglu EC, Tharakan T, Verze P, et al. European Association of Urology Guidelines on male sexual and reproductive health: 2021 update on male infertility. Eur Urol. 2021;80(5):603–20. https://doi.org/10.1016/j.eururo.2021.08.014.
71. Caroppo E, Colpi GM. Hormonal treatment of men with nonobstructive azoospermia: what does the evidence suggest? J Clin Med. 2021;10(3):387. https://doi.org/10.3390/jcm10030387.
72. Attia AM, Abou-Setta AM, Al-Inany HG. Gonadotrophins for idiopathic male factor subfertility. Cochrane Database Syst Rev. 2013;8
73. Fraietta R, Zylberstejn DS, Esteves SC. Hypogonadotropic hypogonadism revisited. Clinics (Sao Paulo, Brazil). 2013;68(Suppl 1):81–8. https://doi.org/10.6061/clinics/2013(sup01)09.
74. Fukagai T, Kurosawa K, Sudo N, Aso T, Sugawara S, Naoe M, Sakamoto H, Yoshida H. Bilateral testicular tumors in an infertile man previously treated with follicle-stimulating hormones. Urology. 2005;65(3):592. https://doi.org/10.1016/j.urology.2004.09.017.
75. Resorlu B, Abdulmajed MI, Kara C, Unsal A, Aydos K. Is intracytoplasmic sperm injection essential for the treatment of hypogonadotrophic hypogonadism? A comparison between idiopathic and secondary hypogonadotrophic hypogonadism. Hum Fertil (Camb). 2009;12(4):204–8. https://doi.org/10.3109/14647270903331139.
76. Practice Committee of the American Society for Reproductive Medicine. Electronic address: asrm@asrm.org. Management of nonobstructive azoospermia: a committee opinion. Fertil Steril. 2018;110(7):1239–45. https://doi.org/10.1016/j.fertnstert.2018.09.012.
77. Liu PY, Swerdloff RS, Christenson PD, Handelsman DJ, Wang C, Hormonal Male Contraception Summit Group. Rate, extent, and modifiers of spermatogenic recovery after hormonal male contraception: an integrated analysis. Lancet (London, England). 2006;367(9520):1412–20. https://doi.org/10.1016/S0140-6736(06)68614-5.
78. Menon DK. Successful treatment of anabolic steroid-induced azoospermia with human chorionic gonadotropin and human menopausal gonadotropin. Fertil Steril. 2003;79(Suppl 3):1659–61. https://doi.org/10.1016/s0015-0282(03)00365-0.
79. Turek PJ, Williams RH, Gilbaugh JHI, Lipshultz LI. The reversibility of anabolic steroid-induced azoospermia. J Urol. 1995;153(5):1628–30.
80. Coward RM, Rajanahally S, Kovac JR, Smith RP, Pastuszak AW, Lipshultz LI. Anabolic steroid induced hypogonadism in young men. J Urol. 2013;190(6):2200–5. https://doi.org/10.1016/j.juro.2013.06.010.
81. Ramasamy R, Armstrong JM, Lipshultz LI. Preserving fertility in the hypogonadal patient: an update. Asian J Androl. 2015;17(2):197–200. https://doi.org/10.4103/1008-682X.142772.
82. Mao JF, Xu HL, Duan J, Chen RR, Li L, Li B, Nie M, Min L, Zhang HB, Wu XY. Reversal of idiopathic hypogonadotropic hypogonadism: a cohort study in Chinese patients. Asian J Androl. 2015;17(3):497–502. https://doi.org/10.4103/1008-682X.145072.

Chapter 8
Follow-Up and Monitoring of Adolescents with Delayed Puberty, Testicular Dysgenesis Syndrome

Angelo Alessandro Marino, Massimiliano Timpano, and Islam Fathy

Definition and Epidemiology of Delayed Puberty

Puberty is defined as the period of the initial process of change leading to reproduction, and it is characterized by maturation of the genital organs, development of secondary sexual characteristics, growth acceleration and psychological changes. As indicated in this definition, puberty is the result of a variegate and highly coordinated interaction between different inhibitory and stimulatory systems, central and peripheral, which increase or decrease their activity during the transitional period from prepuberty to adulthood.

Puberty is characterized by two typical events: adrenarche and gonadarche.

Adrenarche, which represents the first event of puberty, involves the maturation of the adrenal cortex with an increase in the secretion of adrenal androgens—dehydroepiandrosterone (DHEA), dehydroepiandrosterone sulfate (DHEAS), androstenedione—and leads to the appearance of sexual hair (pubarche).

Gonadarche involves the growth and maturation of the gonads, and it is associated with increased secretion of sex steroids, with the onset of folliculogenesis and subsequently ovulation in females and spermatogenesis in males.

A. A. Marino (✉)
ANDROS Day Surgery Clinic, Reproductive Medicine Unit, Palermo, Italy
e-mail: angelo.marino@clinicaandros.it

M. Timpano
MediCare – Center for Male and Female Sexual and Reproductive Health, Turin, Italy

I. Fathy
Faculty of Medicine, Department of Andrology, Cairo University, Cairo, Egypt

Armed Forces College of Medicine, Cairo, Egypt

W. Zohdy et al. (eds.), *Non-Obstructive Azoospermia*,
https://doi.org/10.1007/978-3-031-99431-9_8

The increase in gonadal steroidogenesis and the completion of gametogenesis during gonadarche are induced by the secretion of the pituitary gonadotropins luteinizing hormone (LH) and follicle-stimulating hormone (FSH). This increased secretion is determined by gonadotropin-releasing hormone (GnRH), a decapeptide, produced by the widespread neuronal network located in the medial preoptic area and in the arcuate nucleus of the hypothalamus. The hypothalamus represents a phylogenetically ancient and stable component of the Central Nervous System (CNS), which has undergone minimal variations throughout the evolution of mammals both in its general organization and in its connections with other brain areas.

The number of neurons secreting GnRH in humans is relatively low, ranging from 1000 to 1500 [1]. GnRH supervises the gonadotropic secretion and plays a critical role in the activation of the gonadarche.

GnRH secretion is pulsatile: the frequency and amplitude of GnRH pulses with a periodicity of 60–100 min are crucial for the regulation of the entire hypothalamic–pituitary–gonadal (HPG) axis.

Classical studies conducted in rhesus monkeys with experimentally induced hypothalamic lesions have shown that the continuous administration of exogenous GnRH fails to restore normal pituitary gonadotropic secretion, unlike intermittent administration. This demonstrates that it is not the amount of total GnRH that determines the activation of the HPG axis but rather its secretion pattern [2].

GnRH production is negatively controlled by gonadal steroids (negative feedback effectors) that act directly on GnRH-secreting neurons. The neuronal mechanisms by which steroids control the release of GnRH are still largely unknown. Interesting research indicates that steroids act indirectly on GnRH-secreting neurons, through activation and/or inhibition of other neurons. In particular, Kisspeptin neurons, located in the arcuate and anteroventral periventricular nucleus of the hypothalamus, appear to be of greatest importance in this process. The hormone secreted by these neurons, Kisspeptin-1, also known as metastin (META), is a 54-aminoacid peptide encoded by the *Kiss1* gene; it was first identified in the human placenta [3, 4] and regulates the activity of the GnRH pulse-generator, participating in the early events of pubertal maturation [5].

Nowadays, kisspeptins are considered the main activator of GnRH neurons, interplaying with other neuronal patterns secreting, in a pulsatile manner, neurokinin B (NKB) and dynorphin (Dyn). This neuronal network, located in the arcuate nucleus of the hypothalamus, is known as the term KNDy (for Kiss1, NKB, and Dyn) and will be analyzed below.

Furthermore, the GnRH-secreting neuronal network is regulated by other neuromodulators, which act as activators (glutamate, melanocortins) or as repressors (Gamma-aminobutyric acid-GABA, Neuropeptide Y (NPY). During the pubertal transition, the action of the activators increases and that of the repressors decreases.

Recent evidence highlights the importance of the proopiomelanocortin (POMC) system, whose melanocortins are the products, in the stimulatory action on GnRH-secreting neurons, a process that seems to be mediated by Kiss-1 neurons. In fact, a direct connection between Kiss-1, GnRH-secreting, and melanocortin neurons has been demonstrated in the arcuate nucleus of pubertal female rats [6]. Furthermore, the important role of semaphorin 3 (SEMA3) in the connection between the melanocortin pathway and the GnRH pulse generator has recently been suggested [7].

Indeed, the GnRH pulse generator can be considered the final junction point of multiple neuronal and nonneuronal interconnections [8].

These interactions also involve peripheral mediators. It is well known that the onset of puberty is influenced by body weight. Conditions of energy deficiency, such as those observed in chronic malnutrition, anorexia, or strenuous physical exercise, result in a delay in the onset of puberty. On the contrary, obesity is frequently associated with an early onset of puberty. In this regard, the early onset of puberty, a process underway in all industrialized countries, has been linked to the dramatic increase in childhood obesity observed in the same countries. It has been hypothesized that a critical fat mass (also known as the critical body weight of Frisch) is required to determine the activation of the hypothalamic GnRH pulse generator [9].

Once again, Kiss-1 neurons play a role as key system regulators: conditions of negative energy balance suppress the activity of these neurons, reducing the concentration of kisspeptins [10]. Furthermore, in pre-pubertal rats, with a condition of undernutrition, the administration of kisspeptin restores the onset of puberty [11].

In the same manner, conditions of early-onset obesity induced in female rats have been associated with an increase in the activity of Kiss-1 neurons determining an earlier accelerated frequency of the GnRH pulse generator [12].

Nevertheless, the metabolic control of the pubertal transition is a very complex mechanism not completely elucidated. As described in a significant recent review [13], experimental studies have highlighted the importance, in the onset of puberty, of the mammalian target of rapamycin (mTOR) and the AMP activated protein kinase (AMPK), regulators of the energy state, through the modulation of food intake and thermogenesis. Based on the studies conducted on mice, it has been hypothesized that mTOR and AMPK act reciprocally depending on the energy state: in case of overnutrition, mTOR prevails on AMPK enhancing the activity of Kiss-1 neurons and leading to early puberty; in case of undernutrition, AMPK predominates and mTOR is inhibited, leading to suppression of Kiss-1 neurons and consequently to delayed puberty.

The relation, described above, between the metabolism/body fat composition and the central neuropeptide pathways, however, requires the action of peripheral mediators. Among these peripheral regulators of the HPG axis, leptin is thought to be the most important. Leptin is a metabolic hormone produced by white adipocytes. It has been demonstrated that mice without leptin or leptin receptors have a pubertal arrest and become infertile [14]. Further evidence of the role of leptin in pubertal maturation comes from studies in women. In detail, leptin concentrations increase from stage 1 to stage 5 of Tanner classification of breast development.

Nevertheless, the action of leptin on GnRH-secreting neurons appears not to be direct but mediated: leptin activates proopiomelanocortin and inhibits NPY neurons. In particular, the suppression leptin-mediated of NPY, which has a repressive function on the onset of puberty, seems to be crucial for the permissive effect of leptin on the activation of the "gonadostat." The important role of the inhibitory effect of NPY is demonstrated by the huge increase of this neuropeptide in conditions of malnutrition or negative energy balance [15].

Returning to the analysis of the physiology of the HPG axis, at puberty, the activation of the hypothalamic GnRH-secreting pulse generator determines the release of GnRH into the pituitary portal venous system through which it is transported to the anterior region of the pituitary where it stimulates the production and secretion of LH and FSH.

The first endocrine event of puberty is the increase in LH during the night, first, and during daytime, second. Interestingly, the pattern of secretory pulses of LH is very similar to that of GnRH, thus allowing an easier method of study, since the dosage of LH is much simpler than that of GnRH. When the complete maturity of the HPG axis is reached, in males, LH stimulates the production of testosterone by the Leydig cells while FSH acts on the Sertoli cells inducing spermatogenesis.

If we look at the chronobiology of the HPG axis activation, this begins during fetal life around 20th week of gestation. The secretion of pituitary gonadotropins increases until the 24th week of gestation and then undergoes a drastic reduction due to the negative feedback provided by placental steroids. After birth, an increase in gonadotropic secretion occurs (the so-called mini-puberty) due to the reduction in estrogen concentration typical of the postpartum period. FSH increases more in girls and stimulates follicular growth while LH in boys stimulates the Leydig cells to produce testosterone. After this initial spurt, the negative feedback mechanisms begin to function and become fully active after 9–12 months in boys and 24–36 months in girls, thus reducing the levels of gonadotropins, which remain low until the axis is reactivated at puberty. The biological mechanisms responsible for the quiescence of the hypothalamic "gonadostat," during the pre-pubertal period, are not fully understood, and it is hypothesized that peripheral and central mediators may inhibit the "gonadostat."

This is what happens at the central level.

What are, instead, the modifications that occur in the testis? In the pre-pubertal testis, during the transitional age, many events occur, in particular the proliferation of Sertoli cells and the initial increase in testicular volume. Recently, it has been demonstrated that the growth hormone (GH)-insulin-like growth factor 1 (IGF1) system acts as a promoter of the proliferation of Sertoli cells, increasing the production of AMH and inhibin B in synergy with FSH [16]. The testicular volume is 2 ml at the beginning of the gonadarche. During the transitional phase, the testicular volume is 3 ml and reaches 4 ml at the beginning of puberty. The testicular volume of 4 ml is considered the gold standard for identifying the pubertal onset in males and occurs between 9 and 14 years.

In females, instead, puberty normally occurs between 8 and 13 years.

The typical features of puberty in males are driven by androgens and are the following:

- Growth of the external genitalia and associated glands, with the onset of spermatogenesis.
- Body growth (direct and growth hormone-mediated action) and increase in muscle mass (anabolic action).
- Appearance of secondary male characteristics, enlargement of the penis, enlargement of the larynx, lengthening and thickening of the vocal cords, the appearance of hair on the face, trunk, legs, and pubis.
- Inhibition of the growth of mammary glands.
- Stimulation of sebaceous gland activity.

Passing through the physiology to the pathology, delayed puberty is defined as the absence of pubertal signs, in particular increase in testicular volume ($\geq$ 4 ml) in males and telarche and menarche in females, at an age 2–2.5 standard deviations higher than the normal population.

The limit of age for defining delayed puberty is set at 14 years for boys and 13 years for telarche and 16 years for menarche, in girls.

Delayed puberty is a condition that affects around 2.5% of the adolescents, mainly boys.

The definition of delayed puberty does not consider the velocity of pubertal progression. Indeed, frequently, patients may have a reduced velocity of pubertal development with a testicular volume of 4–6 ml and increased morning testosterone levels compared to the prepubertal status.

Genetic Basis Regulating the Onset of Puberty

In the last century, the onset of puberty has moved toward a progressive anticipation. The reasons for this effect are not fully understood but the increase in body mass, the improvement in socioeconomics factors, and the ubiquitous presence of environmental endocrine disruptors certainly play an important role. Genetic factors appear to be the primary contributors to both early and delayed puberty, among other potential influences [17]. This thought derives from the observation that the onset of puberty has a high grade of concordance within families, ethnic groups and monozygotic compared with dizygotic twins. This evidence suggests that around 60–80% of the variation in pubertal starting is under genetic determinants [18]. Nevertheless, despite the identification of genes involved in specific conditions of delayed puberty such as Kallmann syndrome and hypogonadotropic hypogonadism, the genetic alterations responsible for the onset of puberty in the general population are not well understood. This derives from the fact that puberty involves a multitude of different genetic traits whose interaction system is currently under investigation. Furthermore, as previously indicated, environmental factors impact the timing of puberty influencing the expression of specific genes.

In order to simplify a complex topic, such as the genetic basis of the onset of puberty, we can identify two main fields of analysis: the central activation and regulation of the HPG axis and the involvement of metabolic systems influencing the body fat composition.

With regard to the central activation and regulation of the HPG axis, the single genes that have been correlated with specific features of delayed puberty are genes encoding the gonadotropin-releasing hormone receptor (*GnRHR*) and genes encoding the G-protein-coupled receptor 54 (*GPR54*), which is the receptor for kisspeptins [19]. GPR54 is now identified as the KISS-1 receptor, KISS1R.

The mutations in the GnRH receptor, leading to reduced activity of GnRH, have been associated with hypogonadotropic hypogonadism, a pathological condition that causes delayed puberty and which will be analyzed subsequently.

Kisspeptins, as already mentioned, appear to have a crucial role in the activation of the HPG axis and mutations with loss of function in their receptor have been associated with pubertal alterations, even if these mutations are very rare in humans [20].

Furthermore, kisspeptin coexists and interacts with other neuropeptides that are neurokinin B and dynorphin, in a cluster of neurons known as KNDy, strictly connected with the GnRH-secreting neurons and modulating the onset of puberty. To date, the majority of the evidence comes from studies in rodents and suggests a stimulatory effect sorted by neurokinin B and an inhibitory effect sorted by dynorphin on kisspeptins secretion [21].

Furthermore, the KNDy neurons are under the regulation of the negative feedback sorted by the estrogens and testosterone. The loss-of-function mutations in the gene encoding neurokinin B (*TAC3*) and in its receptor (*TACR3*) have been found in patients with pubertal failure [22].

Concerning the genetic analyses conducted on the metabolic/body fat composition pathways, recently, great attention has been paid to defective mutations in the leptin (*LEP*) and leptin receptor (*LEPR)* genes. Nevertheless, no association was found between the *LEP* and *LEPR* polymorphisms and delayed puberty [23].

Regarding the melanocortin system, which controls appetite, food intake, and energy expenditure mainly through melanocortin 4 receptor (MC4R), genetic studies have been focused on the other melanocortin receptor (MC3R), which is highly expressed in the brain and contributing to sexual development and linear growth. In a recent study, it has been demonstrated that humans with mutations in the *MC3R* gene have a later onset of puberty, reduced linear growth, and circulating IGF1 levels [24].

In order to have a general view of the different genetic variants involved in the onset of puberty, large genome-wide association studies (WGA) have been conducted mainly investigating the differences in the age of menarche in healthy girls. A recent WGA study involving 370,000 women identified 389 independent signals, which can explain 7.4% of variability in the age of menarche. Many of these signals also have an effect in delaying the voice breaking in males [25].

Another recent observation in male delayed puberty is the mutations in IGSF1, a member of the immunoglobulin superfamily, which can determine a late increase in testosterone levels [26]. IGSF1 seems to play a role in the transmigration of GnRH-secreting neurons from the olfactory placode to the hypothalamus: pathogenic mutations could therefore reduce the number of these neurons, reducing GnRH secretion.

In conclusion, the genetic inheritance of the timing of puberty is far from being a complete understanding. We have some pieces of a mosaic (genes involved in the activation of "gonadostat," in GnRH neuronal development, body fat composition, and metabolism), but the complete vision of the entire process is still missing.

We have to clearly understand that alterations in the age of puberty may determine long-term consequences, from infertility to psychological development. Therefore, an in-depth knowledge of the biological and regulatory mechanisms of the pubertal transition is essential not only in terms of increased theoretical knowledge but also because it can allow the preparation of specific and early treatments, with a clear improvement in the quality of life of the patients.

Causes of Delayed Puberty in Males

Constitutional Delay of Growth and Puberty (CDGP)

Constitutional delay of growth and puberty (CDGP), also known as self-limited delayed puberty, represents the most frequent cause of delayed puberty [27], and it can be considered the extreme value of normal variation in pubertal onset rather than a true pathological condition. This definition also includes conditions in which a delayed pubertal progression occurs.

Skeletal maturation is slowed down, and final adult height is generally at the lower limit of the genetic height potential.

We must also consider that the diagnosis of CDGP is very often underestimated as many adolescents with a nonsevere condition are not evaluated by endocrinologists.

It is estimated that up to 63% of boys with delayed puberty have CDGP [28]. In another important series, this proportion was higher, 82% in boys versus 56% in girls [29]. Generally, gonadotropins are low, and, for this reason, the differential diagnosis with "true" hypogonadotropic hypogonadism is challenging.

Generally, the family history is strongly positive for CDGP. The majority of patients with CDGP have a first-degree relative with delayed puberty (63% in boys and 69% in girls) [29]. In many cases, the modality of inheritance is highly complex, and can be autosomal-dominant, autosomal-recessive and X-linked, with a prevalence of autosomal-dominant transmission [30].

The identification of genes involved in CDGP is very difficult because this condition may be considered a variant of normality, therefore, it can be assumed that genetic mutation may be present also in the general population, not being exclusive to CDGP.

As shown in the first paragraph of this chapter, the onset of puberty is under the influence of multiple factors (genetic, nutritional, endocrine, neurological) that synergistically cooperate to activate the GnRH pulse generator. Among others, genetic disorders are the most common.

In an important study of 2018 [31], the genetic inheritance of CDGP and congenital hypogonadotropic hypogonadism (CHH), the two most frequent causes of delayed puberty, were compared. The analysis was conducted on 116 probands with CHH, 72 probands with CDGP, and ethnically matched controls from the Exome Aggregation Consortium. Single-gene mutations were observed in 51% of CHH probands, a much higher percentage than in patients with CDGP (7%) or controls (18%). In the same manner, mutations in more than one gene were more common in CHH patients (15%) than in CDGP patients (1.4%) and in controls (2%). These results indicate a strong difference in the genetic transmission mode of the two different conditions and may open new possibilities for differential diagnosis in patients with delayed puberty. The consciousness that is not the presence of a single-gene mutation responsible for CDGP represents a challenge to clarify the genetic basis of this frequent condition.

Furthermore, recent technological advancements, especially next-generation sequencing (NGS), are widening the genetic diagnostic possibilities even if, until now, the complete genetic interplay is far from being entirely understood.

Hypergonadotropic Hypogonadism

This clinical feature, manifesting as delayed puberty, is characterized by an increase in pituitary gonadotropins due to primary gonadal failure. The elevation of FSH and LH indicates that the HPG axis is normally functioning, and it is the consequence of the lack of production of sex steroids by the gonads (absence of the negative feedback).

This condition is relatively uncommon in boys (7%) and much more frequent in girls (26%) [28]. The etiology includes sex chromosomal abnormalities that can determine an anomalous gonadal differentiation (gonadal dysgenesis), other congenital pathologies, or acquired injuries (chemotherapy, radiotherapy, bilateral testicular torsion, vanishing testis, autoimmunity, infections).

Klinefelter Syndrome

Among males, the most frequent chromosomal aberration leading to gonadal failure is Klinefelter syndrome (KS), a chromosomal abnormality characterized by a 47, XXY karyotype, which may be diagnosed before or after puberty.

KS is the most frequent sex chromosome aneuploidy (1/600). The prevalence is 0.1–0.2% in the general male population and 2–3% in the infertile male population. Due to the extremely variable phenotype, the diagnosis is often not made early: only 25% of adult men with KS receive a diagnosis, and less than 10% of patients are diagnosed before puberty. Very often the diagnosis is made during the infertility diagnostic work-up.

In 80–90% of cases, the syndrome is characterized by a 47, XXY karyotype. In the remaining 10–20% of cases, 46, XX/47, XXY mosaicisms and more serious sex chromosome aneuploidies with karyotypes 48, XXXY, 48, XXYY, 49, XXXXY, or structural abnormalities of the X chromosomes are found.

Indeed, it is a matter of debate whether the reproductive potential of pre-pubertal children with KS is already compromised.

Germ cell degeneration may be caused by a negative effect of the extra X chromosome during chromosome segregation. It is unclear whether germ cell development is normal in the early embryo. In infants not affected by KS, up to the age of 6 months, the hypothalamic–pituitary–gonadal axis is significantly activated, and there is a production of FSH, LH, and, consequently, of testosterone and inhibin B at pubertal or adult levels. This is the so-called "mini-puberty," which has already been described.

After this period, hormone levels decrease to very low levels until the moment of pubertal reactivation.

The same phenomenon is observed in KS newborns, but with lower testosterone values than newborns with normal karyotype, indicating an altered functionality of the Leydig cells [32].

Subsequently, during childhood, in KS subjects, the supernumerary X chromosome seems to have reduced effects on testis development (only a reduced number of spermatogonia is observed) and the levels of testosterone, SHBG, FSH, LH, inhibin B, AMH, and E2 are normal.

During puberty, an increase in plasma testosterone levels is observed. Initially, the testes increase in volume (up to 6 ml) due to the proliferation of Sertoli cells and interstitial cells. This event is quickly followed by

- Rapid decline in germ cells.
- Hyalinization of the seminiferous tubules.
- Sertoli cell degeneration.
- Leydig cell hyperplasia.

The degeneration of the interstitial stroma is accompanied by a reduction in testicular volume up to pre-pubertal dimensions (2–3 ml).

It is unclear whether the increase in plasma or intratesticular concentrations of testosterone during puberty is the cause of the rapid destruction of the seminiferous tubules.

In terms of clinical presentation, the syndrome is characterized by the symptomatic triad:

- Hypergonadotropic hypogonadism with delayed puberty.

- Gynecomastia.
- Infertility.

In addition to the aforementioned gynecomastia, present in 30% of the cases, the other main phenotypic characteristics are the following: tall stature, feminized physique, impaired IQ (in average 15 points less than the general population), reduced chest hairs, small testes (<4 ml), and distribution of pubic hair similar to that of a female partner, sparse beard hair, and low frontal hairline.

Learning disabilities, increased height, delayed language development, and reduced penis size are frequently present in children with KS.

In adults, azoospermia and infertility are present in over 99% of the patients. In case of fertility desire, in adults with KS, both conventional testicular sperm extraction (TESE) or microdissection testicular sperm extraction (micro-TESE) followed by intracytoplasmic sperm injection (ICSI) are feasible. In a recent meta-analysis, the sperm recovery rate in adults with KS was approximately 40% [33]. Focal spermatogenesis in adult KS results from self-correcting 46 XY spermatogonia, which probably arise from 47, XXY spermatogonia that undergo erroneous self-renewal with loss of one X chromosome.

One of the most debated issues in peri-pubertal boys affected by KS is whether to propose fertility preservation. This problem is growing because the amount of diagnosis of KS during gestation is expected to increase due to noninvasive prenatal testing. Many more parents than in the past will be faced with the difficult situation of having to manage the future fertility of their children with KS.

As previously described, massive apoptosis of spermatogonia occurs at the onset of puberty and the fibrosis is a sequential process that initiates after the germ cell loss.

It remains questionable whether to propose sperm retrieval in adolescents KS and cryopreserve the spermatozoa recovered or to propose sperm retrieval in adult patients when they desire a child. In some reports, a reduction in sperm recovery rate has been observed in advanced age: 31% in patients between 20 and 45 years versus 45% in patients between 15 and 19 years [34]. On the contrary,in the meta-analysis by Corona et al. [33], already cited, no influence of age on sperm recovery rate was observed.

However, in the most recent study on the prospective of fertility preservation in adolescents with KS [35], spermatozoa after TESE were found in only one out of 20 adolescents (5.0%) (aged 12–16 years) compared to 48.1% (13 out of 27) in adult patients (aged 18–41 years). By analyzing the testicular biopsies, in the same study, only 30% of peripubertal KS had residual germ cells albeit in very limited numbers. The results of this study suggest that testicular damage, with germ cell loss, occurs much earlier than expected. This data was confirmed in a large real-life study, in which the sperm retrieval rate was not influenced by the patient's age [36]. The rationale that is the basis of this finding is that progressive fibrosis of the seminiferous tubules is not ubiquitous and tubules with normal residual activity can be observed even in adulthood. Nevertheless, in a recent major meta-analysis, younger age was associated with better sperm retrieval [37], making it even more difficult to draw a definitive conclusion.

Concerning hormonal markers predictive of sperm retrieval, also in this case the results are contradictory: in the study by Rohayem et al. [34], higher serum testosterone (≥7.5 nmol/L) and lower serum LH levels (≤17.5 IU/L) have been correlated with better sperm recovery; in the study by Van Saen et al. [35], instead, this effect was not observed and no cutoff was proposed.

In the cited meta-analysis by Majzoub et al. [37], higher testosterone and lower LH and FSH values were significantly associated with positive sperm retrieval.

It is also a matter of debate whether prior treatment with testosterone may impact sperm retrieval. Current evidence does not justify postponing clinically indicated androgen treatment in adolescent boys with KS for fear of reducing their future fertility and TESE prospects [34].

Thus, returning to the initial question "fertility preservation in adolescents or pre-ICSI sperm recovery?", we can conclude that, in relation to the documented depletion of germ cells that precedes the progressive hyalinization of the seminiferous tubules, it is not advisable to cryopreserve sperm in order to preserve future fertility in peripubertal patients with KS.

Gonadal Dysgenesis

Partial gonadal dysgenesis (PGD) and mixed gonadal dysgenesis (MGD) determine testicular dysgenesis, and they are associated with a partial testicular differentiation in patients with a 46,XY or 45,X0/46,XY karyotype. The external genitalia are ambiguous, and a combination of Wolffian and Müllerian ducts is present. Only 1/3 of the newborns are classified as male. The presence of the Y chromosome increases the risk of gonadoblastoma and dysgerminoma. Gonadectomy during childhood is recommended. Gonadal dysgenesis represents the most severe form of testicular dysgenesis syndrome, which will be discussed in the last paragraph of the chapter.

Sex Reversal or 46,XX Males

Among the rarer causes of congenital hypergonadotropic hypogonadism, it is worth mentioning the condition of sex reversal or male 46,XX, occurring in 1/20.000 male newborns. At birth, the external genitalia are male, with hypospadias in some cases. The young patients may be referred to the doctors for delayed puberty and some degree of gynecomastia. On clinical examination, the testes are located in the scrotum, and are small in size. Despite the absence of the Y chromosome, testicular development occurs due to the presence of the *SRY* (*Sex-Determining Region Y*) gene, encoding for the testis-determining factor (TDF), as a result of translocation between the X and Y chromosome, during paternal meiosis.

Partial Androgen Insensitivity Syndrome (PAIS)

Furthermore, partial androgen insensitivity syndrome (PAIS) should be mentioned. This syndrome is due to mutations in the *androgen receptor* (*AR*) gene located on the X chromosome (Xq11.2q12). The karyotype is 46,XY. In this condition, the phenotype is male with a deficit in the virilization process. These patients may present with gynecomastia, hypospadias, cryptorchidism, and azoospermia. The pubic hair is normal, while facial and chest hair is severely reduced.

Acquired Hypergonadotropic Hypogonadism

Chemotherapy and radiotherapy are the most frequent causes of acquired hypergonadotropic hypogonadism. The spermatogenic cell line is more sensitive to irradiation than the Leydig cells: low-dose irradiation >1–2 Gy is sufficient to cause damage to spermatogenesis, unlike what happens for the steroidogenic function of the Leydig cells where a dose of 12 Gy is necessary. Concerning chemotherapy, alkylating agents (such as cyclophosphamide, ifosfamide, procarbazine, cisplatin, and chlorambucil) are the most capable of causing delayed puberty.

Hypogonadotropic Hypogonadism (HH)

Hypogonadotropic hypogonadism is a clinical condition characterized by low plasma gonadotropin levels and low testosterone levels in males, with the consequent absence of pubertal signs.

This definition does not include the temporal immaturity of the HPG axis that instead refers to the constitutional delay of growth and puberty that has already been discussed. Therefore, the conditions of hypogonadotropic hypogonadism that will be discussed in this paragraph refer to the failure of the functionality of the HPG axis.

Hypogonadotropic hypogonadism can be classified into

- Functional HH in case of chronic diseases, undernutrition, or intensive exercise that exerts an inhibitory effect on the HPG axis. Functional hypogonadotropic hypogonadism represents approximately 16–20% of cases of delayed puberty [28].
- Permanent HH, which affect 15% of females and 8% of males according to the study by Festa et al. [38], or 9% of females and 7% of males according to the

study by Varimo et al. [29]. Permanent HH may be congenital (CHH) or acquired. CHH is present in 4% of boys and 6% of girls with delayed puberty and represents the main cause of permanent HH.

Functional HH (FHH)

This feature may be considered a hypothalamic dysfunction, which occurs as a consequence of a systemic illness. There are a lot of general diseases that may exert an effect on the GnRH hypothalamic pulse generator, leading to delayed or arrested puberty: anorexia nervosa, hypothyroidism, diabetes mellitus, cystic fibrosis, inflammatory bowel disease, celiac disease, hemochromatosis, juvenile rheumatoid arthritis, sickle cell disease, and prolonged treatment with glucocorticoids [39].

Among these chronic pathologies, anorexia nervosa, a chronic psychiatric disorder, potentially life-threatening, is the most associated with delayed puberty and can be considered an example of the complex interactions, central and peripheral, involving the hypothalamus.

Anorexia nervosa affects approximately 1–2% of the population and 0.3% of adolescents. This condition is characterized by decreased caloric intake, weight loss, abnormal body image, intense fear of weight gain, and often strenuous physical exercise. Anorexia nervosa has symptoms similar to those of another eating disorder, bulimia nervosa but with some important differences in eating behaviors. Patients affected by bulimia eat an excessive amount of food in a short period of time (binge eating) followed by self-induced vomiting, the use of laxatives or thyroid hormones for preventing weight gain. Furthermore, the body mass index (BMI) of bulimic patients is normal or slightly above the optimal levels, whereas the BMI of anorexic patients is typically below 18.5 kg/m^2.

Anorexia nervosa is much more common in females (90%) than in males. The biological mechanism underlying the HH is not fully understood. Certainly, there is a suppression of the HPG axis that precedes the weight loss and can be maintained despite the weight gain. The pattern of gonadotropic secretion is similar to that of a pre-pubertal status with nonpulsatile, low-amplitude, low-frequency secretion pattern. Low estradiol and testosterone levels, as consequence of low gonadotropins levels, may increase the risk of osteopenia and osteoporosis in both sexes.

Another condition frequently associated with delayed or arrested puberty in both sexes is strenuous physical exercise. Runners, ballerinas, and wrestlers are the most frequently affected athletes. The loss of body weight and fat mass in male wrestlers adversely affects the hypothalamic GnRH pulse generator, leading to a reduction in testicular function. Impaired hypothalamic functional activity may be reversible, within months, after cessation of agonistic physical activity.

Congenital Hypogonadotropic Hypogonadism (CHH)

CHH accounts for 24% to 85% of permanent HH [38]. It can be divided into anosmic CHH and normosmic CHH. The main cause of anosmic CHH is Kallmann syndrome, which affects 1 out of 7500 male newborns and 1 out of 75,000 female newborns and represents 50% of the cases of CHH. It is a condition, often with X-linked transmission, characterized by agenesis of the hypothalamic nuclei producing GnRH that is associated with hypoplasia of the olfactory lobes. In normosmic CHH, on the other hand, an isolated gonadotropin deficiency is found, secondary to the inability of GnRH-secreting neurons to migrate from the olfactory placode to the hypothalamus during embryonic development.

The most frequent mutations involve the *ANOS1* gene, formerly *KAL1,* located on chromosome Xp22.3 and are typically associated with Kallmann syndrome. This gene encodes Anosmin 1, an extracellular protein implicated in cell adhesion and migration of GnRH neurons from the olfactory bulb to the hypothalamus.

Other frequent mutations correlated with CHH, not X-linked, but with an autosomal inheritance dominant pattern, are those involving fibroblast growth factor receptor 1 (*FGFR1*) and chromodomain helicase DNA binding protein 7 (*CHD7*). These mutations are present in both Kallmann syndrome and normosmic CHH. *FGFR1* encodes a tyrosine kinase receptor implicated in several mechanisms mainly related to cell migration and proliferation. Current evidence supports the interaction between anosmin-1 and FGFR1, where anosmin-1 plays a role as a co-ligand activator enhancing the signaling activity of FGFR1 [40].

CHD7 gene, located in 8q12.1, is responsible for CHARGE syndrome (1 in 8500 to 10,000 newborns), a rare genetic disorder commonly diagnosed during the prenatal or neonatal period due to the identification of numerous dysmorphic and congenital anomalies. It is characterized by coloboma, heart defects, atresia of the choanae, restriction of growth and development, genital abnormalities (micropenis and/or cryptorchidism), and ear abnormalities (ears sticking out or lacking lobes associated with hearing problems that can lead to deafness). The expression of the protein encoded by *CHD7* has been identified in the hypothalamus and in the olfactory bulb, highlighting its possible role in the HPG axis.

In addition to the X-linked or autosomal-dominant forms, there is also an autosomal-recessive inheritance pattern of CHH. The most frequent recessive mutations affect three genes: *GNRHR* (with more than 60 families identified), *KISS1R* (with 27 families identified), and *TACR3* (with 20 families identified) [38]. The clinical features associated with these mutations are those typical of normosmic CHH. The G-protein-coupled receptor, encoded by *GNRHR*, when mutated, impairs the release of pituitary gonadotropins induced by GnRH. At a higher level, mutations in *KISS1R*, encoding the G-protein-coupled receptor of kisspeptin and *TACR3*, encoding the neurokinin receptor, impair the functionality of the complex neuronal network KNDy in the hypothalamic arcuate nucleus responsible for the regulation of GnRH-secreting neurons.

Nevertheless, the majority of cases of CHH are sporadic.

Clinically, patients with Kallmann syndrome have anosmia, a eunuchoid appearance (limbs long relative to the body, with an overall normal stature) and marked sexual infantilism. Other clinical manifestations include synkinesis, present in 75% of patients [41] and renal agenesis, observed in 30% of patients [38]. Nevertheless, the heterogeneity of clinical findings, in the presence of the same mutation, highlights the role of epigenetic modulations in gene expression.

Other clinical manifestations of CHH present at birth are micropenis, described in 20–40% of newborns with Kallmann syndrome; cryptorchidism, evident in 30–50% of patients with CHH.

Another congenital condition that can be associated with HH and, consequently, with delayed puberty is the adrenal hypoplasia congenita, a rare pathological condition that affects the adrenal cortex and leads to adrenal insufficiency and HH. It is an X-linked condition caused by mutations in the *NR0B1* (*DAX1*) gene, whose encoded protein has been identified in the hypothalamus, pituitary, adrenal glands, and gonads. Symptoms typically appear at 6–8 weeks of age; other typical symptoms of adrenal insufficiency are present during childhood. Delayed adrenarche is present, and, in some cases, when associated with a partial or complete HH, also delayed gonadarche.

Among other genetic syndromes associated with delayed puberty and HH, it is worthy mentioning Prader–Willi syndrome. This is a rare genetic neurological condition with an estimated birth prevalence of 1/15,000–30,000. The clinical features of the syndrome are hypotonia, short stature, hyperphagia, childhood obesity, mental retardation, poor verbal, and social skills that persist throughout life. It is often caused by a 15q11-q13 deletion transmitted by the father, or by maternal disomy or, very rarely, by imprinting defects in the same region.

Acquired Hypogonadotropic Hypogonadism

Permanent acquired hypogonadotropic hypogonadism is due to organic causes that directly impact the hypothalamus or the pituitary gland.

Intracranial tumors are the most important cause of permanent acquired HH because they suppress gonadotropin secretion, acting at the hypothalamic level. Deficiencies of other pituitary hormones may be present. There is also the action of antineoplastic treatments (radiotherapy and/or chemotherapy) that can lead to gonadotropin deficiency.

Among intracranial tumors, the most frequent is the craniopharyngioma (10% of CNS neoplasms in children) with intrasellar or suprasellar localization. It arises from the remnants of Rathke's pouch. Its clinical presentation varies between 5 and 20 years of age. The clinical features of craniopharyngioma are delayed puberty, decreasing growth velocity, headache, changes in vision, fatigue, and polyuria. Diagnosis of craniopharyngioma is carried out by neurological examination, hormonal dosages (in particular pituitary hormones), X-rays, computed tomography

(CT), and magnetic resonance imaging (MRI). Treatment is surgical, with different outcomes on the basis of size and localization. Radiotherapy may be useful as an adjunctive treatment.

Other intracranial tumors that can be associated with delayed puberty are germ cell tumors, epidermoid or dermoid cysts, prolactinomas, and optic gliomas. Germ cell tumors, which account for approximately 6.5% of intracranial tumors in children [42], generally present with diabetes insipidus and other manifestations of deficiency of pituitary hormones. Germ cell tumors originate from the hypothalamus or pineal gland. The tumoral markers β-hCG and α-fetoprotein show elevated serum concentration. Radiotherapy is the treatment of choice.

Thalassemia major may impair the HPG axis at the pituitary level. Patients affected by this pathology, indeed, are treated with frequent transfusions, and this could cause an iron overload in the pituitary gland that alters the functionality of gonadotropin secretion. This negative effect is nowadays mitigated by adequate iron chelation therapy.

Hyperprolactinemia

Hyperprolactinemia directly inhibits the action of GnRH-secreting neurons, resulting in delayed or arrested puberty, growth retardation, weight gain, and galactorrhea. Indeed, the condition of delayed puberty should trigger an evaluation for hyperprolactinemia in children (strong recommendation), as established by the recent international consensus statement of the Pituitary Society [43].

Hyperprolactinemia is often the consequence of prolactinomas, which can be distinguished into microprolactinomas (<10 mm) or macroprolactinomas (>10 mm).

Dynamic gadolinium-based MRI is recommended for the initial diagnosis of prolactinoma. MRI should be always proposed for values of prolactin above 200 ng/ml [43] because, in these cases, prolactinoma represents the most common cause. For moderately elevated values of prolactin (40–200 ng/ml), MRI may be proposed after the exclusion of other causes such as concomitant medications, stress, hypothyroidism, renal dysfunctions, and liver disease. Furthermore, for these serum prolactin levels (40–200 ng/ml), especially in the absence of specific symptoms of hyperprolactinemia, macroprolactin, which is biologically inactive, should be measured. In fact, most of the circulating prolactin has a molecular weight of 23 kDa (monomeric bioactive prolactin), but "big" prolactin (dimeric isoform, molecular weight of 40–60 kDa), with a reduced bioactivity, and "big-big" prolactin (polymeric isoform, molecular weight >150kDa), also known as macroprolactin, with very limited bioavailability and bioactivity, may also be present. In a percentage of hyperprolactinemic patients ranging from 10 to 25%, macroprolactin can be detected in the serum [43]. However, it is important to remark that in any case the clinical evaluation must be carried out on the basis of the characteristics of each individual patient.

Among the medications, special attention should be paid to antipsychotics, antidepressants, domperidone, and metoclopramide. Psychotropic drugs cause hyperprolactinemia because they have an anti-dopaminergic effect. Dopamine is the main inhibitor of prolactin secretion. Psychotropic drugs bind to dopamine receptors on pituitary lactotrophic pituitary cells, blocking them and therefore ultimately preventing the dopamine inhibitory action on prolactin.

The treatment of hyperprolactinemia is based on dopamine agonists, which reduce serum levels of prolactin and the size of the adenoma. Cabergoline is the first-choice treatment for its tolerability, long half-life, and high efficacy. Bromocriptine and quinagolide are second-choice treatments.

Differential Diagnosis

The evaluation of children with problems related to pubertal development first requires a detailed collection of the **medical history**, with particular attention to the family history.

The timing of anamnestic collection is crucial in every field of medicine but it is absolutely essential for problems correlated with delayed puberty, as the medical history can significantly influence the subsequent diagnostic and therapeutic approach.

As previously decribed, a positive family history of delayed puberty is highly suggestive of constitutional delay of growth and puberty. Indeed, the majority of patients with this condition have a first-degree relative with delayed puberty (63% for boys and 69% for girls) [29].

On the other hand, if one parent has CHH, hormonal evaluation during minipuberty is recommended, and it should be followed by a genetic study if a specific parental mutation is known.

In addition to the family history, specific questions about the child's personal history should be asked. Specifically, it is necessary to ask whether the patient exhibits signs of pubertal development and at what age they appeared, whether he is undergoing or has undergone medical treatments for other pathologies, whether he has had previous treatments (surgical or medical) for cryptorchidism, whether he has anosmia or other neurological problems, and whether adrenarche has occurred.

A detailed assessment of thyroid function and the presence of systemic diseases, such as celiac disease and inflammatory bowel disease, is necessary. Furthermore, given the relevant impact on the GnRH pulse generator, a specific assessment of body weight and its eventual fluctuations, eating behavior, and strenuous physical exercise is mandatory to role out anorexia nervosa. Care should be taken to the history of hematological diseases (in particular, beta-thalassemia) for the risks associated with hemosiderosis leading to permanent HH, or to the history of neoplastic pathologies and related treatments (particularly, chemotherapy and/or radiotherapy), which can cause, depending on the site, HH or hypergonadotropic hypogonadism. The presence of neurologic signs and/or symptoms (diplopia, vomiting, headache) is suggestive of intracranial tumors.

Furthermore, parents should be asked if any signs of concern were present at birth that could guide the diagnosis: for example, evidence of micropenis or cryptorchidism, which are suggestive of CHH.

After taking the clinical history, the physical examination includes the evaluation of the presence of testes in the scrotum, testicular volume, measured using the Prader orchidometer and, where necessary, ultrasound and assessment of pubertal stage, through the analysis of auxological parameters (weight, height, BMI, bone age) that must be reported on growth curves and interpreted on the basis of the parental target. In particular, assessing bone age is important for evaluating the degree of delay, the subsequent pubertal progression and estimating the final adult height.

Another aspect that should be considered is the growth spurt that in males occurs when testicular volume reaches 10–12 ml [44]. If there is a lack of harmonious correspondence between growth spurt and pubertal development, it is more common to be in the presence of an endocrine disorder or malnutrition, secondary to a chronic disease. Malnutrition during childhood modulates the timing of sexual development in both sexes, and it can reduce the growth velocity and cause delayed puberty. Thus, a careful evaluation of nutritional status and lean and fat mass is also necessary, given their correlation with adequate pubertal development.

Longitudinal monitoring of patients, through serial growth measurements and assessments of pubertal development using specific nomograms, is essential to determine the progression of puberty and growth velocity. After taking the medical history and performing the physical examination, laboratory tests should be carried out: FSH, LH, testosterone, DHEA, androstenedione, inhibin B, TSH, free T_4 and prolactin to evaluate the HPG axis and thyroid function. Furthermore, screening for celiac disease should be performed.

In case of significant hyperprolactinemia (>200 ng/ml), MRI is always recommended [43]. Instead, for moderately elevated values of prolactin (40–200 ng/ml), macroprolactin should be dosed and MRI may be recommended after ruling out stress, concomitant drugs (particularly, antipsychotics, antidepressants, domperidone, metoclopramide), renal insufficiency, liver diseases, and hypothyroidism.

Elevated basal gonadotropins account for hypergonadotropic hypogonadism. In this case, a karyotype is indicated to identify Klinefelter syndrome or another rarer gonadal dysgenesis. When gonadotropin levels are low, the differential diagnosis between CDGP and HH may be difficult.

This distinction is very important, especially for the related therapeutic and prognostic implications. Family history, in this context, is very helpful for correlation with CDGP. Furthermore, bone age represents another crucial step in the differential diagnosis. The diagnosis of CDGP is more frequent in boys shorter than their chronological age but with a height consistent with bone age and pubertal development. This correspondence is not present in permanent hypogonadotropic hypogonadism (PHH). Moreover, in CDGP there is a delay in adrenarche.

Nevertheless, in many cases, a more in-depth evaluation of the hypothalamic–pituitary axis and gonadal function with appropriate dynamic stimulation tests is necessary.

Among these stimulation tests, the most used are the hCG test and the GnRH test, although neither has demonstrated high selective diagnostic efficacy.

hCG stimulation test is indicated in case of non-palpable testes or when testosterone levels are particularly low. The modalities of stimulation with hCG vary (from daily injections for 5 days to biweekly injections for several weeks) as well as the used dosages (at least 5.000 UI, not exceeding 15.000 UI in total or 3.000 UI per single injection). The assessment of androgens (testosterone, DHEA, androstenedione) should be carried out within 24 h of the last administration. The other classically used stimulation test is the GnRH test, which evaluates the gonadotropin response induced by GnRH (with 100 μg of GnRH).

Recently, a retrospective cohort study showed that testicular volume (cutoff level 1.1 ml, sensitivity 100%, and specificity 91%), GnRH-induced LH (cutoff 4.3 IU/L, sensitivity 100%, and specificity 75%), and inhibin B levels (cutoff 61 ng/L, sensitivity 90%, and specificity 83%) are the best predictive markers to distinguish prepubertal boys with CDGP from those with CHH [29]. In the same study, a growth velocity > 3 cm/year was more frequent in boys with CDGP or CHH than in boys with functional HH, with a sensitivity of 50% and a specificity of 80%. It has been hypothesized that patients with slow growth (<3 cm/year) may have a chronic disease responsible for functional HH more frequently than prepubertal patients with growth ≥3 cm/year.

In Table 8.1, the key points for the differential diagnosis between CDGP, FHH, PHH, and hypergonadotropic hypogonadism are reported.

Figure 8.1 provides a logical, simple and intuitive diagnostic algorithm.

Table 8.1 Key diagnostic points in delayed puberty

	CDGP	FHH	PHH	Hypergonadotropic hypogonadism
Family history	++	–	–	–
Bone age concordant with pubertal development	+	+	–	–
Adrenarche	–	+	+	±
Basal FSH/LH	Low	Low	Low	High
Inhibin B	Normal	Normal/low	Low	Low
GnRH test	Positive (LH >4.3 UI/L)	Prepubertal	Prepubertal	Not indicated
Karyotype	–	–	±	±
Concomitant disease	–	+	–	–
Cryptorchidism	–	–	+	+
Malnutrition	–	+	–	–
Anosmia/hyposmia	–	–	+	–

CDGP constitutional delay of growth and puberty, *FHH* functional hypogonadotropic hypogonadism, *PHH* permanent hypogonadotropic hypogonadism

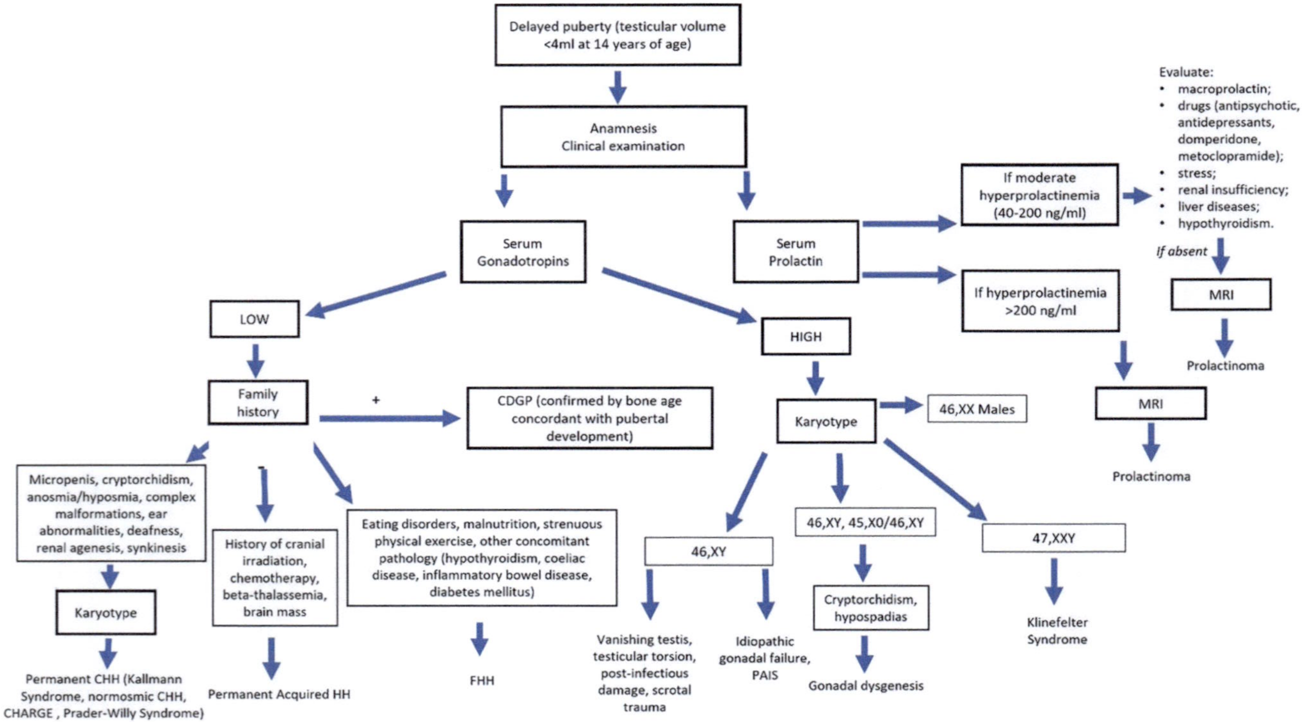

Fig. 8.1 Diagnostic algorithm for delayed puberty in males. *CDGP* constitutional delay of growth and puberty, *HH* hypogonadotropic hypogonadism, *CHH* congenital hypogonadotropic hypogonadism, *FHH* functional hypogonadotropic hypogonadism, *PAIS* partial androgen insensitivity syndrome, *MRI* magnetic resonance imaging

Follow-Up and Management of Delayed Puberty in Males

In this paragraph, we briefly and schematically outline the therapeutic approach and clinical management of male patients with delayed puberty.

For patients with CDGP, the most common cause of delayed puberty, longitudinal observations for evaluating the pubertal progression represent the most appropriate "treatment." Nevertheless, in case of psychological problems and/or in the absence of a correct differential diagnosis between CDGP and HH, the treatment of choice both for delayed and slowly progressing puberty is testosterone, which, when used at low dosages, increases growth velocity and does not compromise adult height. There are different methods of administration of testosterone: the classic, well-tolerated, regimen involves monthly administration of intramuscular depot testosterone enanthate at a low dosage (50–75 mg) for 6 months. After at least 2 months of a medication-free period, a clinical evaluation is carried out, followed by the assay of testosterone. If testosterone levels are still low (a sign of failed gonadarche activation), a second treatment period of 6 months is indicated. After this second step, it is generally possible to distinguish patients with CDGP from those with permanent HH: in the first ones, natural pubertal progression is observed with an increase in testicular volume and testosterone levels, demonstrating the integrity of the HPG axis. In these patients, treatment with testosterone is useful as a trigger of the pubertal onset due to the positive feedback of steroids on the hypothalamus, but it can be discontinued.On the other hand, in patients with permanent HH, the triggering action of exogenous testosterone cannot be expressed due to the failure of the HPG axis. In this condition, testosterone treatment should be continued, with slow increases for a period of 3–4 years, until serum levels typical of adulthood are reached (Fig. 8.2). In adulthood, a shift to different testosterone formulations (transdermal gel and patches) may be considered. Testosterone treatment should be discontinued if fertility is desired. In this case, a treatment with both gonadotropins should be started for the induction of spermatogenesis.In patients with hypergonadotropic hypogonadism, hormone replacement therapy

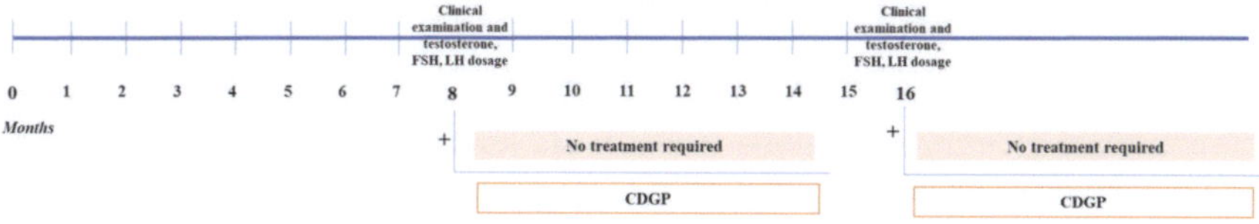

Fig. 8.2 Follow-up and treatment management of male patients with low gonadotropin levels and delayed puberty. During treatment, clinical assessments are carried out at eighth and 16th months. If clinical assessments are negative (no response to treatment), testosterone treatment should be continued. If clinical assessments are positive (good response to treatment), treatment may be discontinued and the diagnosis of CDGP is made. *CDGP* constitutional delay of growth and puberty, *HH* hypogonadotropic hypogonadism

will obtain pubertal induction and progression. In the case of the desire for fertility, induction of spermatogenesis with gonadotropins has no place. In patients affected by Klinefelter syndrome, as debated in the specific paragraph, a search for testicular spermatogenic foci may be proposed. In case of failure to retrieve sperm from the genital tract, heterologous assisted reproductive technology (ART) treatments are the unique, viable option.

Among other new treatment options, topical treatments (transdermal gels and patches) are not currently used for pubertal induction because optimal dosing regimens have not been established. To date, no randomized controlled trials have been published on these new treatment formulations. Nevertheless, recently, some evidence, coming from small-case studies, supports the use of transdermal testosterone treatments.In a pilot study, in patients with CDGP, the induction of puberty was adequately obtained with short-term transdermal testosterone gel treatment (10 mg daily 2%) compared to conventional treatment (intramuscular testosterone 50 mg/monthly) [45].Furthermore, the same authors published in 2022 [46] a retrospective study, including 246 male patients with delayed puberty and demonstrated that height velocity, LH value, and testicular enlargement were significantly increased in patients treated with transdermal testosterone gel compared to conventional intramuscular treatment. Another information that can be drawn from this study is that pubertal progression also occurs in patients who received no treatment (control group). Moreover, this topical treatment may be useful for the differential diagnosis between CDGP and permanent HH.

Recently, new attention has been focused on long-acting testosterone undecanoate administered every 3 months. A recent prospective randomized small-case trial, including patients with slow pubertal progression (inclusion criteria: morning testosterone levels 0.5–3 nmol/L and testicular volume $\leq$ 6 ml), compared six intramuscular injections of testosterone enanthate 75 mg/month with two intramuscular injections of testosterone undecanoate 250 mg/3 months. The primary outcome was testicular volume $\geq$ 8 ml (representing mid-puberty close to peak height velocity) 12 months after the start of treatment [47]. Results showed that 86% of patients treated with testosterone undecanoate reached the primary outcome versus 100% in the testosterone enanthate group. This difference was not significant, and the authors conclude that both treatments may be beneficial in patients with delayed puberty or slow pubertal progression. This is also evident when analyzing endocrine markers. Indeed, testosterone levels reached an optimal level in both groups after 12 months of treatment (1.6 nmol/L at baseline and 10.1 nmol/L at 12 months in the testosterone undecanoate group and 2.7 nmol/l at baseline and 11.7 nmol/l in the testosterone enanthate group); in the same manner, LH levels increased during treatment reaching the same level after 12 months (1.0 mUI/ml at baseline and 2.6 mUI/ml after 12 months, in the testosterone undecanoate group and 1.0 mUI/ml at baseline and 2.54 mUI/ml in the testosterone enanthate group). The same trend was observed for FSH.

In conclusion, we can affirm that further larger randomized controlled trials are needed to evaluate the efficacy and tolerability of new testosterone formulations in inducing puberty. It is important to reassure the boys and their families that, with the correct diagnosis, the best treatment choice allows patients to have a good overall quality of life, with a low impact on adulthood.

For what concerns fertility, in HH patients, normal spermatogenesis may be achieved with the use of both gonadotropins, stopping the treatment with testosterone.

It is much more difficult to follow up on the fertility desire in patients with hypergonadotropic hypogonadism. In KS patients, TESE or microTESE may be proposed, knowing that the spermatozoa retrieval rate is significantly lower than in patients with normal karyotype.

Definition and Features of Testicular Dysgenesis Syndrome (TDS)

Definition of TDS and Clinical Presentation

TDS encompasses a spectrum of male reproductive disorders, including cryptorchidism (undescended testes), hypospadias (abnormal urethral opening on the penis), impaired spermatogenesis leading to reduced semen quality, and an elevated risk of testicular cancer [48]. These conditions are thought to be manifestations of testicular developmental disorders, resulting from a combination of genetic and environmental factors, notably including exposure to endocrine disruptors. Patients with a 45,X0/46,XY karyotype, exhibiting intersex phenotype and testicular dysgenesis, often present with several of these conditions concomitantly, exemplifying the most severe form of TDS. The etiology of the syndrome is related to both fetal development and external influences, including maternal exposure to certain chemicals known to interfere with the endocrine system.

The developmental disturbances underlying TDS symptoms share several common risk factors, such as small birth weight and a history of being small for gestational age [49]. These factors not only contribute to the individual manifestations of TDS but also link them to each other, highlighting the common pathophysiological basis of these disorders. Epidemiological data underscore strong correlations among these conditions, suggesting a unified syndrome rather than isolated incidents. For instance, countries with high incidences of testicular cancer also report increased rates of cryptorchidism, hypospadias, and poor semen quality, further supporting the interconnected nature of the syndrome. While genetic abnormalities can lead to these disorders, the majority of cases have uncleared causes, suggesting a significant role for environmental and lifestyle factors, including endocrine disruptors. Recent studies have demonstrated that fetal exposure to high doses of certain chemicals, such as dibutyl phthalate, can induce a TDS-like phenotype in animal models, highlighting the potential environmental contribution to the etiology of the syndrome.

Epidemiological Evidence

Epidemiological evidence supporting the TDS hypothesis comes from various studies and data sources, indicating an increase in TDS-related disorders over recent decades [50]. Notably, a rise in the incidence of testicular cancer, cryptorchidism (undescended testis), hypospadias (abnormal urethral opening), and impaired spermatogenesis have been reported, suggesting a common etiological pathway linked to developmental disturbances during fetal life.

A compelling aspect of the epidemiological evidence is the birth cohort effect, demonstrating that individuals born in more recent years are at a higher risk for these conditions. This effect is particularly pronounced in testicular cancer and sperm quality, underscoring the potential impact of environmental changes over time on male reproductive health. Additionally, there are significant geographical variations in the incidence rates of TDS components, with certain regions exhibiting higher rates of testicular cancer and other TDS-related disorders. For instance, countries like Denmark have reported a high incidence of testicular cancer and poor semen quality, whereas Finland shows comparatively lower rates, suggesting that environmental factors may play a critical role in the manifestation of TDS.

Moreover, the co-occurrence of TDS features within individuals, such as an increased risk of testicular cancer in men with a history of cryptorchidism or poor semen quality, further supports the notion of a shared developmental origin. This interrelation emphasizes the need for a broader understanding of risk factors, including potential genetic and environmental contributors to TDS.

Etiology and Risk Factors

The etiology of TDS is multifaceted, encompassing both genetic predispositions and a range of environmental factors [51].

Genetic factors play a crucial role in the manifestation of TDS. Specific genetic abnormalities, including karyotype variations such as 45,X0/46,XY, often present with a severe form of TDS, highlighting the genetic basis of this syndrome. However, for the majority of TDS cases, the precise genetic contributions remain unclear. This uncertainty underscores the complexity of TDS etiology, where both genetic susceptibilities and environmental influences converge.

Environmental factors, particularly exposure to endocrine-disrupting chemicals (EDCs), have been implicated in the increasing prevalence of TDS-related disorders. EDCs, including substances such as phthalates, have shown the potential to disrupt the hormonal balance necessary for normal testicular development. Fetal exposure to high doses of specific EDCs, such as dibutyl phthalate, has been experimentally linked to a TDS-like phenotype in animal models, reinforcing concerns about the environmental contributions to TDS.

Key categories include

1. Phthalates: Used as plasticizers in PVC plastics, cosmetics, and personal care products. Dibutyl phthalate has been specifically mentioned for its potential role in inducing TDS-like conditions in animal models.
2. Polychlorinated biphenyls (PCBs): Industrial chemicals previously used in electrical equipment, paints, and building materials. Although banned in many countries, PCBs persist in the environment and have been linked to various health issues, including potentially TDS-related disorders.
3. Pesticides: Certain pesticides have anti-androgenic properties that might contribute to the development of TDS. Studies have suggested a potential link between exposure to pesticides and an increased risk of cryptorchidism and hypospadias.
4. Bisphenol A (BPA): Found in polycarbonate plastics and epoxy resins, BPA is used in food and beverage packaging, water bottles, and as an internal coating on metal products. It has estrogenic activity and has been associated with various health problems, including potential impacts on male reproductive health.
5. Persistent organic pollutants (POPs): A large group of substances, including certain pesticides (DDT), industrial chemicals (PCBs), and by-products, that resist environmental degradation. Exposure to POPs has been linked to adverse reproductive health effects.

These substances can disrupt endocrine signaling pathways critical for testicular development, potentially leading to the various components of TDS. The association between exposure to endocrine disruptors and the development of TDS in humans is supported by both epidemiological data and findings from animal studies. However, direct evidence of causality in humans is difficult to establish due to ethical and methodological constraints.

Lifestyle factors also contribute to the increasing prevalence of TDS. Epidemiological evidence suggests that lifestyle and environmental factors, potentially exacerbated by global industrialization and the proliferation of EDCs, play a significant role in the etiology of TDS. These factors include maternal lifestyle choices and exposure to pollutants and chemicals capable of interfering with the endocrine system during critical periods of fetal development.

Pathophysiology of TDS

The TDS hypothesizes that a cluster of male reproductive disorders, including cryptorchidism, hypospadias, impaired spermatogenesis, and an elevated risk of testicular cancer, originates from disruptions in the normal development of the testes during fetal life [52]. These conditions, which collectively impact the male reproductive system, share a developmental foundation, suggesting a unified pathophysiological mechanism behind their occurrence.

The developmental disturbances leading to TDS are thought to arise from a complex interplay of genetic vulnerabilities and environmental exposures, including maternal exposure to certain chemicals capable of interfering with the endocrine system. Such exposures during critical periods of fetal development are hypothesized to lead to hormonal imbalances, particularly affecting the normal actions of estrogens and androgens, which are crucial for the proper development of male reproductive organs.

One of the central aspects of pathophysiology of TDS involves hormonal imbalances resulting from these environmental exposures. For instance, exposure to substances with estrogenic or anti-androgenic activities during fetal development may disrupt the normal hormonal milieu necessary for the differentiation and growth of male reproductive organs. This disruption can lead to a spectrum of developmental abnormalities, from mild undescended testes (cryptorchidism) to more severe forms of genital malformation, such as hypospadias, and potentially to the impaired formation of germ cells, resulting in compromised spermatogenesis and an increased risk of testicular cancer later in life.

Endocrine disruptors can impact the pathophysiology of TDS through several hormonal mechanisms:

1. Androgen receptor (AR) antagonism: Many endocrine disruptors act as anti-androgens, blocking the action of testosterone and dihydrotestosterone (DHT) at the androgen receptor level. This antagonism can lead to impaired masculinization and development of the male reproductive tract, contributing to conditions such as hypospadias and cryptorchidism.
2. Estrogen receptor activation: Some endocrine disruptors exhibit estrogenic activity, binding to estrogen receptors and mimicking the effects of endogenous estrogens. This can disrupt the hormonal balance critical for male reproductive development, potentially leading to TDS components like impaired spermatogenesis.
3. Interference with steroidogenesis: Endocrine disruptors can affect the synthesis of steroid hormones by impacting enzymes involved in the biosynthesis of testosterone and other sex steroids. This disruption can result in lowered testosterone levels, affecting testicular development and function.
4. Thyroid hormone disruption: Some endocrine disruptors interfere with thyroid hormone synthesis, transport, and action. Since thyroid hormones play a role in fetal brain development and growth, their disruption can indirectly affect reproductive development and contribute to TDS.
5. Disruption of hormone signaling pathways: Endocrine disruptors can interfere with hormone signaling pathways, including those involving GnRH, LH, and FSH. These disruptions can lead to altered testicular function and development.
6. Insulin-like factor 3 (INSL3) production disruption: INSL3 is critical for testicular descent during fetal development. Endocrine disruptors may impair the production or action of INSL3, contributing to cryptorchidism.

The actions of endocrine disruptors on these hormonal mechanisms disrupt the delicate endocrine balance necessary for normal testicular development and function, potentially leading to the various manifestations of TDS.

Hormonal Features

Hormonally, individuals with TDS may exhibit altered levels of sex steroids, which may reflect the underlying testicular dysgenesis. Additionally, there may be abnormalities in the levels of other hormones related to gonadal function, such as inhibin B and FSH, which further indicate disturbances in testicular development and function.

Variability in Severity and Presentation

The severity and presentation of TDS can vary widely among individuals. Some individuals may present with only one of the conditions, such as isolated hypospadias or cryptorchidism, while others may exhibit multiple manifestations, including severe impairment of spermatogenesis and an increased risk of developing testicular cancer. This variability suggests a spectrum of disease severity within the syndrome, possibly influenced by genetic, environmental, and lifestyle factors. The interrelation among the TDS components also indicates that the presence of one manifestation could increase the risk of developing others. For instance, individuals with a history of cryptorchidism are known to have an elevated risk of testicular cancer and may also experience impaired fertility.

Diagnostic Criteria

Diagnostic criteria for TDS are not universally established due to the multifaceted nature of the syndrome and the variability in its clinical manifestations. This complexity presents significant challenges in diagnosing TDS, necessitating a multidisciplinary approach that considers the potential interconnectivity among the various conditions encompassed by TDS [51].

Cryptorchidism and hypospadias are typically diagnosed based on physical examination at or shortly after birth. Cryptorchidism involves the absence of one or both testes from the scrotum, while hypospadias is characterized by the abnormal position of the urethral orifice. These conditions can often be identified through routine pediatric examinations.

The diagnosis of impaired spermatogenesis usually requires a semen analysis, which assesses sperm count, motility, and morphology. According to the World Health Organization (WHO), a sperm count below 16 million sperm per milliliter of semen is considered indicative of oligozoospermia, a form of impaired spermatogenesis [53].

Testicular cancer is diagnosed through a combination of physical examination, ultrasonography, and serum tumor marker tests (such as alpha-fetoprotein, human chorionic gonadotropin, and lactate dehydrogenase). In some cases, a biopsy may be necessary to confirm the diagnosis. Testicular cancer may present as a palpable mass in the testis or as a painless enlargement of the testicle.

One of the key challenges in diagnosing TDS stems from its broad spectrum of clinical manifestations and the fact that individuals may present with one or multiple conditions associated with the syndrome. The variability in severity and presentation among affected individuals further complicates diagnosis and management. Additionally, the latent nature of some TDS components, such as impaired spermatogenesis and testicular cancer, which may not manifest until later in life, underscores the need for vigilant monitoring and early detection strategies in individuals at risk.

Short-Term and Long-Term Impacts on Male Fertility and Overall Health

- Impacts on fertility: The spectrum of conditions that characterize TDS can significantly affect male fertility. Impaired spermatogenesis, one of the TDS components, directly impacts sperm count and quality, leading to potential difficulties in conceiving. Cryptorchidism, if left untreated, can also result in reduced fertility due to the higher temperatures to which the undescended testes are exposed, affecting sperm production and quality.
- Impacts on general health: Beyond fertility issues, TDS encompasses conditions with broader health implications. Testicular cancer, although treatable, requires early diagnosis and intervention. Moreover, the psychological and physiological impacts of dealing with TDS components, such as undergoing surgeries for cryptorchidism or hypospadias, can affect overall well-being and quality of life.

Psychosocial Implications of TDS for Affected Individuals

- Psychological impact: The diagnosis and treatment of TDS components, especially when involving surgical interventions or dealing with infertility issues, can have significant psychological effects on affected individuals. These can include anxiety, depression, and issues with body image and sexual identity, especially when the disorders impact genital appearance or function.
- Social and relationship impact: Fertility issues related to TDS can strain relationships, impacting not just the affected individual but also their partner. The societal stigma associated with reproductive disorders can lead to feelings of isolation and reduced self-esteem, further exacerbating mental health challenges.

Management and Treatment Strategies

Management and treatment strategies for TDS and its manifestations—cryptorchidism, hypospadias, impaired spermatogenesis, and testicular cancer—involve a multidisciplinary approach tailored to the individual patient's condition and needs. Given the complexity of TDS, treatment plans often require collaboration among pediatric endocrinologists, urologists, andrologists, and oncologists. Here, we outline the current treatment options for the various manifestations of TDS and discuss potential future directions in management, including preventive strategies.

Current Treatment Options

- Cryptorchidism: Treatment typically involves hormonal therapy (e.g., human chorionic gonadotropin or GnRH analogs) to stimulate testicular descent or surgical intervention (orchidopexy) to physically relocate the undescended testis into the scrotum. The goal is to perform these interventions early to reduce the risk of impaired fertility and testicular cancer.
- Hypospadias: Surgical repair, ideally performed during early childhood, aims to correct the urethral opening and, if necessary, address any associated penile curvature (chordae). Timing of surgery is crucial to promote optimal outcomes in terms of cosmetic appearance, functionality, and psychological development.
- Impaired spermatogenesis: Treatment is often symptomatically focused on enhancing fertility, including ART, in particular ICSI for men with severely compromised semen quality. Lifestyle modifications and treatment of underlying conditions may also be recommended.
- Testicular cancer: Depending on the stage and type, treatment may include orchiectomy (removal of the affected testis), radiation therapy, chemotherapy, or a combination of these approaches. Surveillance is critical for early-stage cancer, while advanced disease may require more aggressive treatment.

Future Directions in Management

- Early detection and surveillance: Enhanced screening for early markers of TDS, such as subtle alterations in testicular development or hormonal imbalances, could facilitate timely intervention.
- Preventive strategies: Given the hypothesized environmental component of TDS, strategies aimed at reducing exposure to potential endocrine disruptors during critical periods of fetal development may be effective in preventing or mitigating the syndrome. Public health initiatives could focus on minimizing exposure to known or suspected harmful substances.
- Genetic and biomarker research: Advances in understanding the genetic underpinnings of TDS may lead to targeted therapies or preventive measures for individuals at high risk. Research on biomarkers for early detection of testicular maldevelopment or dysfunction could also transform the management of TDS.

References

1. Casoni F, Malone SA, Belle M, Luzzati F, Collier F, Allet C, Hrabovszky E, Rasika S, Prevot V, Chédotal A, Giacobini P. Development of the neurons controlling fertility in humans: new insights from 3D imaging and transparent fetal brains. Development. 2016;143(21):3969–81.
2. Belchetz PE, Plant TM, Nakai Y, Keogh EJ, Knobil E. Hypophysial responses to continuous and intermittent delivery of hypopthalamic gonadotropin-releasing hormone. Science. 1978;202(4368):631–3.
3. Hori A, Honda S, Asada M, Ohtaki T, Oda K, Watanabe T, Shintani Y, Yamada T, Suenaga M, Kitada C, Onda H, Kurokawa T, Nishimura O, Fujino M. Metastin suppresses the motility and growth of CHO cells transfected with its receptor. Biochem Biophys Res Commun. 2001;286(5):958–63.
4. Ohtaki T, Shintani Y, Honda S, Matsumoto H, Hori A, Kanehashi K, Terao Y, Kumano S, Takatsu Y, Masuda Y, Ishibashi Y, Watanabe T, Asada M, Yamada T, Suenaga M, Kitada C, Usuki S, Kurokawa T, Onda H, Nishimura O, Fujino M. Metastasis suppressor gene KiSS-1 encodes peptide ligand of a G-protein-coupled receptor. Nature. 2001;411(6837):613–7.
5. Dungan HM, Clifton DK, Steiner RA. Minireview: kisspeptin neurons as central processors in the regulation of gonadotropin-releasing hormone secretion. Endocrinology. 2006;147(3):1154–8.
6. Manfredi-Lozano M, Roa J, Ruiz-Pino F, et al. Defining a novel leptin-melanocortin-kisspeptin pathway involved in the metabolic control of puberty. Mol Metab. 2016;5(10):844–57.
7. Giacobini P, Parkash J, Campagne C, Messina A, Casoni F, Vanacker C, Langlet F, Hobo B, Cagnoni G, Gallet S, et al. Brain endothelial cells control fertility through ovarian-steroid-dependent release of semaphorin 3A. PLoS Biol. 2014;12:e1001808.
8. Barroso A, Roa J, Tena-Sempere M. Neuropeptide control of puberty: beyond kisspeptins. Semin Reprod Med. 2019;37(4):155–65.
9. Frisch RE, Revelle R. Height and weight at menarche and a hypothesis of critical body weights and adolescent events. Science. 1970;169(3943):397–9.
10. Castellano JM, Bentsen AH, Mikkelsen JD, Tena-Sempere M. Kisspeptins: bridging energy homeostasis and reproduction. Brain Res. 2010;1364:129–38.
11. Castellano JM, Navarro VM, Fernández-Fernández R, Nogueiras R, Tovar S, Roa J, Vazquez MJ, Vigo E, Casanueva FF, Aguilar E, Pinilla L, Dieguez C, Tena-Sempere M. Changes in hypothalamic KiSS-1 system and restoration of pubertal activation of the reproductive axis by kisspeptin in undernutrition. Endocrinology. 2005;146(9):3917–25.
12. Li XF, Lin YS, Kinsey-Jones JS, O'Byrne KT. High-fat diet increases LH pulse frequency and kisspeptin-neurokinin B expression in puberty-advanced female rats. Endocrinology. 2012;153(9):4422–31.
13. Vazquez MJ, Velasco I, Tena-Sempere M. Novel mechanisms for the metabolic control of puberty: implications for pubertal alterations in early-onset obesity and malnutrition. J Endocrinol. 2019;242(2):R51–65.
14. Barash IA, Cheung CC, Weigle DS, Ren H, Kabigting EB, Kuijper JL, Clifton DK, Steiner RA. Leptin is a metabolic signal to the reproductive system. Endocrinology. 1996;137(7):3144–7.
15. Pralong FP. Insulin and NPY pathways and the control of GnRHfunction and puberty onset. Mol Cell Endocrinol. 2010;324(1–2):82–6.
16. Cannarella R, Mancuso F, Condorelli RA, Arato I, Mongioì LM, Giacone F, Lilli C, Bellucci C, La Vignera S, Calafiore R, Luca G, Calogero AE. Effects of GH and IGF1 on basal and FSH-modulated porcine sertoli cells in-vitro. J Clin Med. 2019;8(6):811.
17. Howard SR, Dunkel L. The genetic basis of delayed puberty. Neuroendocrinology. 2018;106(3):283–91.
18. Gajdos ZK, Henderson KD, Hirschhorn JN, Palmert MR. Genetic determinants of pubertal timing in the general population. Mol Cell Endocrinol. 2010;324(1–2):21–9.

19. Seminara SB, Messager S, Chatzidaki EE, Thresher RR, Acierno JS Jr, Shagoury JK, Bo-Abbas Y, Kuohung W, Schwinof KM, Hendrick AG, et al. The GPR54 gene as a regulator of puberty. N Engl J Med. 2003;349:1614–27.
20. Topaloglu AK, Tello JA, Kotan LD, Ozbek MN, Yilmaz MB, Erdogan S, et al. Inactivating KISS1 mutation and hypogonadotropic hypogonadism. N Engl J Med. 2012;366:629–35.
21. Navarro VM, Gottsch ML, Chavkin C, Okamura H, Clifton DK, Steiner RA. Regulation of gonadotropin-releasing hormone secretion by kisspeptin/dynorphin/neurokinin B neurons inthe arcuate nucleus of the mouse. J Neurosci. 2009;29(38):11859–66.
22. Topaloglu AK, Reimann F, Guclu M, et al. TAC3 and TACR3 mutations in familial hypogonadotropic hypogonadism reveal a key role for Neurokinin B in the central control of reproduction. Nat Genet. 2009;41(03):354–8.
23. Banerjee I, Trueman JA, Hall CM, Price DA, Patel L, Whatmore AJ, Hirschhorn JN, Read AP, Palmert MR, Clayton PE. Phenotypic variation in constitutional delay of growth and puberty: relationship to specific leptin and leptin receptor gene polymorphisms. Eur J Endocrinol. 2006;155(1):121–6.
24. BYH L, Williamson A, Finer S, Day FR, Tadross JA, Gonçalves Soares A, Wade K, Sweeney P, Bedenbaugh MN, Porter DT, Melvin A, Ellacott KLJ, Lippert RN, Buller S, Rosmaninho-Salgado J, Dowsett GKC, Ridley KE, Xu Z, Cimino I, Rimmington D, Rainbow K, Duckett K, Holmqvist S, Khan A, Dai X, Bochukova EG, Genes & Health Research Team, Trembath RC, Martin HC, Coll AP, Rowitch DH, Wareham NJ, van Heel DA, Timpson N, Simerly RB, Ong KK, Cone RD, Langenberg C, Perry JRB, Yeo GS, O'Rahilly S. MC3R links nutritional state to childhood growth and the timing of puberty. Nature. 2021 Nov;599(7885):436–41.
25. Day FR, Thompson DJ, Helgason H, Chasman DI, Finucane H, Sulem P, et al. Genomic analyses identify hundreds of variants associated with age at menarche and support a role for puberty timing in cancer risk. Nat Genet. 2017;49:834–41.
26. Joustra SD, Wehkalampi K, Oostdijk W, Biermasz NR, Howard S, Silander TL, Bernard DJ, Wit JM, Dunkel L, Losekoot M. IGSF1 variants in boys with familial delayed puberty. Eur J Pediatr. 2015;174(5):687–92.
27. Abitbol L, Zborovski S, Palmert MR. Evaluation of delayed puberty: what diagnostic tests should be performed in the seemingly otherwise well adolescent? Arch Dis Child. 2016;101(8):767–71.
28. Sedlmeyer IL, Palmert MR. Delayed puberty: analysis of a large case series from an academic center. J Clin Endocrinol Metab. 2002a;87(4):1613–20.
29. Varimo T, Miettinen PJ, Känsakoski J, Raivio T, Hero M. Congenital hypogonadotropic hypogonadism, functional hypogonadotropism or constitutional delay of growth and puberty? An analysis of a large patient series from a single tertiary center. Hum Reprod. 2017;32(1):147–53.
30. Sedlmeyer IL, Hirschhorn JN, Palmert MR. Pedigree analysis of constitutional delay of growth and maturation: determination of familial aggregation and inheritance patterns. J Clin Endocrinol Metab. 2002b;87:5581–6.
31. Cassatella D, Howard SR, Acierno JS, Xu C, Papadakis GE, Santoni FA, Dwyer AA, Santini S, Sykiotis GP, Chambion C, Meylan J, Marino L, Favre L, Li J, Liu X, Zhang J, Bouloux PM, Geyter C, Paepe A, Dhillo WS, Ferrara JM, Hauschild M, Lang-Muritano M, Lemke JR, Flück C, Nemeth A, Phan-Hug F, Pignatelli D, Popovic V, Pekic S, Quinton R, Szinnai G, L'Allemand D, Konrad D, Sharif S, Iyidir ÖT, Stevenson BJ, Yang H, Dunkel L, Pitteloud N. Congenital hypogonadotropic hypogonadism and constitutional delay of growth and puberty have distinct genetic architectures. Eur J Endocrinol. 2018;178(4):377–88.
32. Lahlou N, Fennoy I, Carel JC, Roger M. Inhibin B and anti-Müllerian hormone, but not testosterone levels, are normal in infants with nonmosaic Klinefelter syndrome. J Clin Endocrinol Metab. 2004;89(4):1864–8.
33. Corona G, Pizzocaro A, Lanfranco F, Garolla A, Pelliccione F, Vignozzi L, Ferlin A, Foresta C, Jannini EA, Magi M, et al. Sperm recovery and ICSI outcomes in Klinefelter syndrome: a systematic review and metaanalysis. Hum Reprod Update. 2017;23:265–75.

34. Rohayem J, Fricke R, Czeloth K, Mallidis C, Wistuba J, Krallmann C, Zitzmann M, Kliesch S. Age and markers of Leydig cell function, but not of Sertoli cell function predict the success of sperm retrieval in adolescents and adults with Klinefelter's syndrome. Andrology. 2015;3:868–75.
35. Van Saen D, Vloeberghs V, Gies I, Mateizel I, Sermon K, De Schepper J, Tournaye H, Goossens E. When does germ cell loss and fibrosis occur in patients with Klinefelter syndrome? Hum Reprod. 2018;33(6):1009–22.
36. Boeri L, Palmisano F, Preto M, Sibona M, Capogrosso P, Franceschelli A, Ruiz-Castañé E, Sarquella-Geli J, Bassas-Arnau L, Scroppo FI, Saccà A, Gentile G, Falcone M, Timpano M, Ceruti C, Gadda F, Trost L, Colombo F, Rolle L, Gontero P, Montorsi F, Sánchez-Curbelo J, Salonia A, Montanari E. Sperm retrieval rates in non-mosaic Klinefelter patients undergoing testicular sperm extraction: what expectations do we have in the real-life setting? Andrology. 2020;8(3):680–7.
37. Majzoub A, Arafa M, Clemens H, Imperial J, Leisegang K, Khalafalla K, Agarwal A, Henkel R, Elbardisi H. A systemic review and meta-analysis exploring the predictors of sperm retrieval in patients with non-obstructive azoospermia and chromosomal abnormalities. Andrologia. 2022;54(3):e14303.
38. Festa A, Umano GR, Miraglia Del Giudice E, Grandone A. Genetic evaluation of patients with delayed puberty and congenital hypogonadotropic hypogonadism: is it worthy of consideration? Front Endocrinol (Lausanne). 2020;11:253.
39. Dye AM, Nelson GB, Diaz-Thomas A. Delayed puberty. Pediatr Ann. 2018;47(1):e16–22.
40. Kim SH, Hu Y, Cadman S, Bouloux P. Diversity in fibroblast growth factor receptor 1 regulation: learning from the investigation of Kallmann syndrome. J Neuroendocrinol. 2008;20(2):141–63.
41. Tsai PS, Gill JC. Mechanisms of disease: Insights into X-linked and autosomal-dominant Kallmann syndrome. Nat Clin Pract Endocrinol Metab. 2006;2(3):160–71.
42. Yen & Jaffe's reproductive endocrinology: physiology, pathophysiology, and clinical management 9th Edition by Strauss, Barbieri, Dokras, Williams, Williams. Elsevier;2023.
43. Petersenn S, Fleseriu M, Casanueva FF, Giustina A, Biermasz N, Biller BMK, Bronstein M, Chanson P, Fukuoka H, Gadelha M, Greenman Y, Gurnell M, Ho KKY, Honegger J, Ioachimescu AG, Kaiser UB, Karavitaki N, Katznelson L, Lodish M, Maiter D, Marcus HJ, McCormack A, Molitch M, Muir CA, Neggers S, Pereira AM, Pivonello R, Post K, Raverot G, Salvatori R, Samson SL, Shimon I, Spencer-Segal J, Vila G, Wass J, Melmed S. Diagnosis and management of prolactin-secreting pituitary adenomas: a Pituitary Society international Consensus Statement. Nat Rev Endocrinol. 2023;19(12):722–40.
44. Gaudino R, De Filippo G, Bozzola E, Gasparri M, Bozzola M, Villani A, Radetti G. Current clinical management of constitutional delay of growth and puberty. Ital J Pediatr. 2022;48(1):45.
45. Chioma L, Papucci G, Fintini D, Cappa M. Use of testosterone gel compared to intramuscular formulation for puberty induction in males with constitutional delay of growth and puberty: a preliminary study. J Endocrinol Investig. 2018;41(2):259–63.
46. Mastromattei S, Todisco T, Chioma L, Ubertini G, Pattumelli MG, Fintini D, Cappa M. Efficacy of short-term induction therapy with low-dose testosterone as a diagnostic tool in the workup of delayed growth and puberty in boys. J Endocrinol Investig. 2022;45(12):2377–84.
47. Österbrand M, Fors H, Norjavaara E. Pharmacological treatment for pubertal progression in boys with delayed or slow progression of puberty: a small-scale randomized study with testosterone enanthate and testosterone undecanoate treatment. Front Endocrinol (Lausanne). 2023;14:1158219.
48. Skakkebaek NE, Rajpert-De Meyts E, Main KM. Testicular dysgenesis syndrome: an increasingly common developmental disorder with environmental aspects. Hum Reprod. 2001;16(5):972–8.
49. Virtanen HE, Rajpert-De Meyts E, Main KM, Skakkebaek NE, Toppari J. Testicular dysgenesis syndrome and the development and occurrence of male reproductive disorders. Toxicol Appl Pharmacol. 2005;207(2 Suppl):501–5.

50. Boisen KA, Kaleva M, Main KM, Virtanen HE, Haavisto AM, Schmidt IM, Chellakooty M, Damgaard IN, Mau C, Reunanen M, Skakkebaek NE, Toppari J. Difference in prevalence of congenital cryptorchidism in infants between two Nordic countries. Lancet. 2001;363(9417):1264–9.
51. Sharpe RM, Skakkebaek NE. Testicular dysgenesis syndrome: mechanistic insights and potential new downstream effects. Fertil Steril. 2008;89(2):e33–8.
52. Chen Y, Yang M, Zhuang Y. A review of endocrine disrupting chemical (EDC) regulation on testicular dysgenesis syndrome. Asian J Surg. 2023;46(5):2193–5.
53. WHO. WHO laboratory manual for the examination and processing of human semen. 6th ed. Geneva: World Health Organization; 2021.

Chapter 9
Fertility Restoration Options for Prepubertal Boys Undergoing Gonadotoxic Treatment

Christine Wyns, Jonathan Poels, and Marc Kanbar

Introduction

Fertility preservation (FP) in prepubertal boys is challenging as they do not produce sperm. Banking of immature testicular tissue (ITT) is, therefore, the only option as gonado-protective strategies remain of unproven efficacy [1]. Since its introduction to clinical practice in the early 2000s [2], ITT banking for prepubertal boys at risk of fertility loss has been gaining ground [1]. The need to offer FP was fueled by improved survival rates after childhood cancer (ranging from 78.8% to 83.3% between 2005 and 2007 in Europe [3] and from 83.2% to 87.8% between 2013 and 2019 in the USA [4] and by studies reporting infertility as one of the most significant long-term quality-of-life-altering complications in childhood cancer survivors [5, 6].

Several experimental FP programs have been established around the world [7, 8, 9, 10, 11, 12, 13, 14] to offer this FP option to patients. Reports on such programs contributed to demonstrating the short-term [15, 14] and long-term safety of the procedure [16, 17, 18, 19]. Additionally, the procedure was commonly associated with research protocols to establish clinically applicable fertility restoration strategies using banked ITT (reviewed in [1]).

To hasten the pace of research, international collaborations were recently established between different FP programs. Notably, the ORCHID-NET consortium was started in 2022 to perform larger-scale studies [20]. According to the latest survey of the consortium, over 3000 patients have banked their ITT as an FP measure. It is

C. Wyns (✉) · J. Poels · M. Kanbar
Andrology Lab, Reproductive Physiopathology Research Pole (REPR), Institut de Recherche Expérimentale et Clinique (IREC), Université Catholique de Louvain, Brussels, Belgium

Department of Gynecology-Andrology, Cliniques Universitaires Saint-Luc, Brussels, Belgium
e-mail: christine.wyns@saintluc.uclouvain.be

W. Zohdy et al. (eds.), *Non-Obstructive Azoospermia*,
https://doi.org/10.1007/978-3-031-99431-9_9

therefore important for the procedure to transition from an "experimental" to an "established" status.

However, emerging long-term follow-up data on infertility prevalence in cohorts of prepubertal boys who underwent ITT banking [16, 18, 21], as well as the latest PanCare recommendation to consider only patients at high risk of infertility (80%) [22] due to the invasive and still experimental nature of the procedure, point to the need to refine eligibility criteria for ITT cryobanking.

This chapter aims to highlight current practice in FP for prepubertal boys by presenting an overview of the procedure, including basic knowledge on therapy-induced damage to the testis in the pediatric population and useful follow-up data that may help to identify the best candidates for ITT banking. The state-of-the-art fertility restoration options with cryopreserved ITT, as well as the expected translation to clinical practice, will also be reviewed.

Banking Immature Testicular Tissue as an Experimental Strategy for Fertility Preservation

Identifying the Best Candidates for the Procedure

Acquiring a better knowledge of pediatric diseases influencing the fertility potential and testis-damaging effects of their treatments, including the most recent targeted therapies (for review, see [23, 1]), is a prerequisite to identify candidates who will most benefit from ITT banking.

Recent evidence suggests that the disease itself might lead to a lower fertility potential prior to any treatment [24, 25, 26], which places some of the patients at a higher risk of permanent infertility in adulthood. Indeed, in 56.7% of patients suffering from central nervous system cancers and 55.6% of patients with severe hematological disorders, the spermatogonia pool seemed to be reduced compared to simulated data from healthy controls [25]. The spermatogonia pool was also found to be decreased in 49% of boys with a severe hematological disease (excluding hemoglobinopathies) requiring hematopoietic stem cell transplantation [24] based on Z-score analyses (below −3 SD) [27]. In patients with a severe sickle cell disease phenotype, spermatogonia numbers were also reported to be decreased, regardless of the exposure to hydroxyurea (HU) [28].

In addition, both chemotherapy and radiotherapy damage the prepubertal testis in a dose-dependent way, leading to partial or complete depletion of the spermatogonial stem cell (SSC) population. In testicular biopsy specimens of patients who received alkylating agents, spermatogonia numbers were significantly decreased [29, 30, 31, 12].

Although to a lesser extent, testicular somatic cells, i.e., Sertoli, Leydig, and peritubular myoid cells, are also damaged following chemo- or radiotherapy, leading to a lower final number of Sertoli cells, decreased testosterone secretion [32,

33], and eventually to a suboptimal niche microenvironment and dysfunctional spermatogenesis in adulthood [34].

Chemotherapeutic agents are most often used in combination therapy, including alkylating agents (e.g., cyclophosphamide, ifosfamide, busulfan) along with platinum-based drugs (e.g., cisplatin) that are highly toxic to the testis. To harmonize alkylating agents' exposure, the cyclophosphamide equivalent dose (CED) calculation has been established [35]; CED ≥ 4000 mg/m^2 is considered at a significant risk of infertility [22].

With regard to radiotherapy, single doses as low as 0.1 Gy can alter spermatogonia morphology and decrease their numbers [36]. Doses superior to 6 Gy can lead to permanent azoospermia [37], and fractionation lowers this threshold to 2.5 Gy. In total body irradiation conditioning regimens, 10–12 Gy are typically delivered, inducing complete germ cell loss as well as Leydig cell dysfunction in children and adolescents (<18 years) [38].

Altered semen parameters were also reported after long-term treatment with HU for sickle-cell anemia during prepuberty [39] although recent evidence suggests that these alterations are similar in HU-exposed and HU non-exposed patients [40]. Hence, whether prepubertal HU exposure depletes the spermatogonia pool remains a matter of debate [28, 12, 13].

Targeted therapies including small molecule signaling inhibitors and immunotherapy are also gaining ground in the treatment of some pediatric cancers, but data on their impact on the reproductive potential is still scarce, sometimes even unknown, and limited to small clinical studies in adult populations or animal models, requiring thus further evidence to substantiate first findings [41, 42, 1].

Tyrosine kinase inhibitors (e.g., imatinib, dasatinib) are a mainstay treatment for Philadelphia chromosome-positive ALL and CML [43]. Imatinib has been shown to have a minor impact on spermatogenesis without altering reproductive hormone levels in adults treated for CML [44]. In boys and adolescents, data are scarce, but one small series ($n = 13$) suggested no impact on testosterone and inhibin B levels after a mean 18-month exposure time [45].

The impact on fertility of monoclonal antibodies used in the treatment of pediatric B-ALL, neuroblastomas, and rhabdomyosarcomas [46] and of immune checkpoint inhibitors used to treat some pediatric cancers like relapsed/refractory solid tumors, lymphomas, and melanomas remains largely unknown.

Table 9.1 summarizes the infertility risks of childhood cancer survivors according to the last PanCareLIFE Consortium and the International Late Effects of Childhood Cancer Guideline Harmonization Group recommendations [22].

Testicular Biopsy Procedure

Cryobanking of ITT as an FP procedure for prepubertal boys aims at cryopreserving the SSCs, a subpopulation of spermatogonia being the only germ cells present before the onset of spermatogenesis. It is also the only option to preserve the

Table 9.1 Risk categories of infertility according to treatment received

Risk of infertility	Criteria
High risk of infertility	High-dose alkylating agent: CED ≥ 4000 mg/m^2 Testicular radiotherapy Conditioning for HSCT
Low risk	Low-dose alkylating agents: (CED < 4000 mg/m^2) Cisplatin treatment Orchiectomy (unilateral)
No risk	All other treatment groups

Adapted from Mulder et al. [22]. *CED* cyclophosphamide equivalent dose, *HSCT* hematopoietic stem cell transplantation

reproductive potential in patients facing gonadotoxic therapy when there is no testicular sperm, either in azoospermic adolescents or in peripubertal boys if they fail to produce an ejaculate. The procedure implies a multicollaborative pathway involving the referring haemato-oncologist, a reproductive care specialist, a pediatric urologist, a liaison psychologist or psychiatrist, trained nurses, and easy access to the operative theatre to offer the best care to the patient [47, 14, 48]. Testicular tissue sampling is usually performed via an open surgical testicular biopsy, preferably prior to the start of gonadotoxic therapies. According to the most recent worldwide survey on ITT banking [20], the procedure is most often restricted to one side. However, 6/16 centers also sometimes take the tissue bilaterally to reduce the risk of not finding SSCs in the biopsies, especially in cases of disease relapse where FP is proposed after previous lower-risk gonadotoxic therapies that may already have decreased spermatogonia numbers, and in cases where the disease itself is known to induce SSC loss over time [25]. There is so far no recommendation on the size of the biopsy to be taken, ranging among centers offering the service from 5% of the total testicular volume [14] to a unilateral orchidectomy [18]. As the procedure is still considered experimental, it is widely accepted to perform the biopsy simultaneously with another procedure, e.g., placement of a central line, requiring general anesthesia [49].

It is a low-risk procedure, with, according to the largest follow-up cohort, 2.1% short-term complications, i.e., bleeding, infection, and severe pain [19], in agreement with a median of 1.9% in the survey of Duffin *et al.* [20] on current practice in worldwide FP programs. Cautious management is nevertheless recommended in patients with a bone marrow deficiency, as complication rates such as bleeding or infection might be higher. Serial ultrasound monitoring of the testes up to one year after a testicular biopsy for FP concluded to the absence of an impact on the growth of the biopsied testis versus the contralateral testis [15]. With regard to long-term risks, FSH levels above 10 IU/L, witnessing spermatogenic impairment, were found in 33% of the patients [19], which is in line with 33–45% in large cohorts of childhood cancer survivors that did not undergo a testicular tissue biopsy [50, 51]. Testosterone serum levels were well preserved in 79–87% of the patients according to the different studies [16, 17, 19]. More importantly, 29% and 33% of patients presented with definitive azoospermia after an average of 6.5 years (2.6–14 years) and 12.3 years (2.3–21 years), respectively [18, 19], which is also in line with 18–43% azoospermia rates in childhood cancer survivors [35, 52, 51].

Transport and Cryopreservation of ITT: Current Practice

Cryopreservation of testicular tissue with the aim of preserving SSCs that, compared to the small sperm cell, have different requirements to survive the procedure is mainly performed worldwide using slow-freezing. Literature is so far insufficient to recommend one protocol over another as comparative studies on cryopreservation methods used adult tissue, except for two of the studies [53, 54]. Vitrification of human ITT may be as effective as slow-freezing based on similar tissue integrity and spermatogonial survival found after thawing/warming in culture [53] and in 6 months' xenografts [54]. Although vitrification presents the advantage of not requiring sophisticated equipment, to the best of our knowledge, there are no reports on ITT vitrification in clinical FP programs.

With regard to cryoprotectants (CPAs), no difference was seen between dimethyl sulfoxide (DMSO) and ethylene glycol after cryopreservation of ITT from cryptorchid patients on spermatogonia survival as well as on testosterone and inhibin production, respectively, as markers of the function of Leydig and Sertoli cells [55]. The latest survey on current practice shows that DMSO is used at concentrations of 0.7 M, 1.4 M, or 1.5 M as a permeating CPA by most centers (15/16) and that non-permeating CPAs such as sucrose 0.1 M or/and human serum albumin 5–10% are added by some teams. Usually, small fragment sizes of less than 5 mm^3 are cryopreserved [20].

Cryopreservation of testicular cell suspensions is an alternative, but tissue digestion may compromise cell survival and interactions as well as limit the options for future fertility restoration [56, 49].

Currently, a limited number of centers worldwide have the expertise or logistics to cryopreserve ITT. Hence, several national networks, e.g., German Androprotect network [57], international networks, e.g., Nordfertil for Finland, Iceland, and Sweden [12], and North American coordinated network [13] have been developed aimed at transporting the tissue within and between countries and centralizing the cryopreservation procedure. Data on tissue quality when delaying its freezing are so far reassuring. Indeed, based on a study using human adult testicular tissue, the integrity of the tissue and cell survival including spermatogonia numbers were maintained after storage at 4 °C up to 72 h in Dulbecco's Modified Eagle Medium [58]. Additionally, storage of prepubertal non-human primate testicular tissue for 24 h at 4 °C before xenografting did not worsen graft development [59].

Options for Fertility Restoration Using Cryostored ITT

Elevated rates of permanent azoospermia ranging between 29% and 33% after gonadotoxic therapies in cohorts of prepubertal boys that participated in an FP program [18, 19] point to the importance of offering these patients a method to restore their fertility in adulthood using frozen ITT.

Three approaches have been proposed: autotransplantation of SSCs, autografting of testicular tissue, and in vitro maturation (IVM) by cell or organ culture (Fig. 9.1). The choice between methods mainly relies on the risk of malignant cell contamination of the tissue because of the possibility of inducing disease relapse in the patient following transplantation of tissue or unproperly selected cells. This risk was illustrated by the development of tumors or generalized leukemia in all animals following xenotransplantation of both fresh and cryopreserved testicular tissue from leukemic rats [60]. Furthermore, as few as 20 leukemic cells also induced disease relapse after transplantation of testicular cells in 3 of 5 rats [61]. Recently, studies have evaluated the presence of cancer cell contamination in testicular biopsies from prepubertal patients with hematological malignancies, revealing cancer cells in 39% of cases [62] and higher detection rates using PCR technologies [63]. These observations underscore the critical importance of ensuring that testicular cells or tissue are free of cancer cells prior to transplantation in patients with a history of

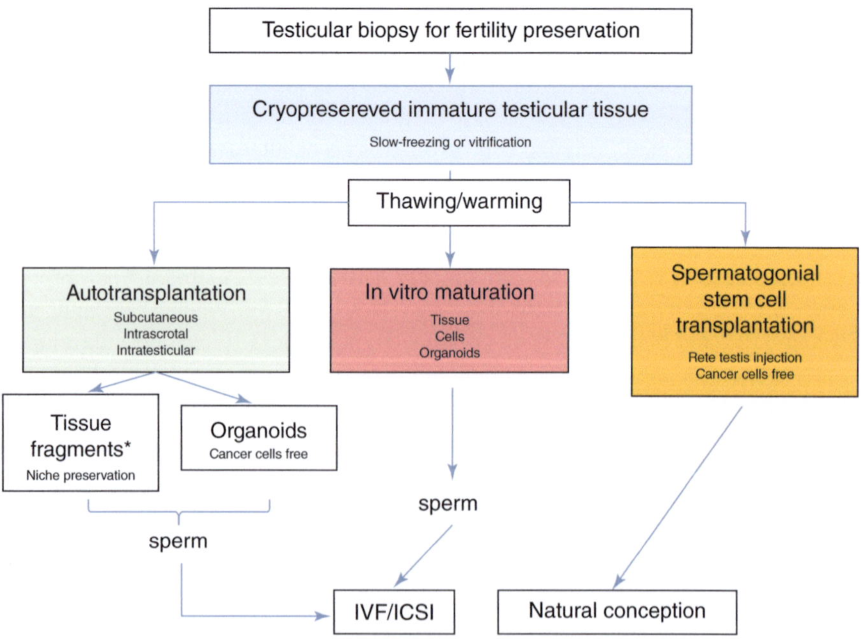

Fig. 9.1 Options for fertility restoration using the cryopreserved ITT. * Only in cases of absence of benign diseases or cancers with a low risk of cancer cell contamination in the testis. *IVF* in vitro fertilization, *ICSI* intracytoplasmic sperm injection

cancer, especially for hematological or metastatic malignancies. While cell sorting techniques on human samples were unsuccessful (for review, see [62]), innovative strategies able to eliminate cancer cells involving the isolation and culture of SSCs before their reintroduction into patients have been explored but further confirmation of their efficacy is needed [64].

Hence, if there is a high risk of cancer cell contamination or if cancerous cells are present in the tissue, IVM to produce spermatozoa ex vivo should be favored. If this risk is low (non-metastatic solid tumors) or null (benign diseases), then autografting or SSC transplantation without the need for a prior effective cell sorting can both be considered [21].

Ultimately, the definitive validation of the effectiveness of SSC cryopreservation and the safety of fertility restoration methods will be obtained from the implementation of pilot clinical trials [56].

Autografting of ITT

Testicular tissue grafting offers the significant advantage of transplanting SSCs while preserving their intact niche and original microenvironment. This approach supports SSC development by promoting essential cellular interactions. Numerous studies have evaluated autologous grafting of ITT in various animal species. Complete spermatogenesis has been achieved after the transplantation of slow-frozen ITT in mice [65, 66, 67], rabbits [67], and pigs [68, 69], as well as vitrified ITT in pigs [68, 70] and birds [71].

Healthy offspring have been obtained in mice, birds, and pigs after intracytoplasmic sperm injection of sperm isolated from cryopreserved ITT grafts [70, 71, 65, 67].

Recently, a proof-of-concept study conducted by Fayomi *et al.* [72] reported the birth of a healthy baby monkey, obtained from sperm developed in autografts of ITT into castrated male hosts. Twelve months after the transplantation, the researchers observed spermatogenesis in all grafts, displaying an exceptional recovery rate of 100%, and the presence of spermatids and elongated spermatozoa in more than 70% of the seminiferous tubules. It is of note that grafting in the scrotum led to an increased final weight of the grafts compared to the back. These findings indicate that ITT can be successfully transplanted into different locations of the body, thus likely offering flexible options for future clinical interventions aimed at restoring fertility. Moreover, no significant differences were observed between fresh and frozen-thawed tissue fragments, suggesting that cryopreservation is a viable method for tissue preservation with a view to future transplantation.

So far, no allo- or autotransplantation of human ITT has been performed [20]. However, a few studies have assessed the impact of cryopreservation and subsequent xenotransplantation on human ITT [54, 73, 74, 75, 76]. Xenografting in mice was used as an evaluation tool, as, due to the risk of zoonotic disease transmission, this strategy cannot be considered for clinical application. Increasing spermatogonia loss was noted in xenografts over time, with recovery rates of 14.5% after 3 weeks and 3.7% after 6 months [75, 76]. Such low survival rates were observed regardless of the cryopreservation method (automated/controlled or non-controlled slow-freezing or vitrification) as well as in fresh grafts [54, 73, 74, 75, 76], suggesting that the transplantation procedure itself may play a significant role. Leydig cells also seemed to be preserved, as witnessed by testosterone impregnation of the mice and by markers of steroidogenic activity [54, 76]. However, SSC differentiation typically only reached the pachytene spermatocyte stage [54, 74, 76]. Additionally, structures resembling spermatids were observed histologically, but no specific markers could be identified through immunohistochemistry, suggesting an abnormal differentiation capacity of frozen and transplanted SSCs [76]. An insufficient in vivo maturation period, as indicated by the prolonged expression of anti-Müllerian hormone (AMH) by Sertoli cells after 9 months of human ITT xenografting [73] and/or the phylogenetic distance between mice and humans, may explain incomplete and abnormal spermatogenesis. The sizes of the grafts may also influence the outcome. While in non-human primates, tissue fragments that led to offspring ranged from 9 to 20 mm^3 [72], the average size (5 mm^3) of human tissue frozen in clinical FP programs is smaller [20]. As no studies compared graft sizes, the question arises of the need to optimize the procedure for small grafts. In this regard, lessons learned from the transplantation of fresh ITT are helpful. Since hypoxia resulting from avascular grafting may cause loss of germ cells [77] and induces the formation of reactive oxygen species that accumulate in cells and cause cell death, attempts to mitigate this loss of germ cells by supporting molecules such as FSH, testosterone, or antioxidants were made, but were not successful [78, 73]. However, encapsulating mouse ITT in an alginate matrix containing nanoparticles loaded with anti-necrotic molecules has shown very promising results, significantly improving tissue integrity and germ cell survival [79]. Additionally, supplementing the encapsulated tissue with a combination of nanoparticles containing Vascular Endothelial Growth Factor (VEGF) and Platelet-Derived Growth Factor (PDGF) to accelerate the graft neovascularization and decrease hypoxic damage increased the vascular maturity and induced accelerated maturation of the vascular network in grafts [80].

Spermatogonial Stem Cell Transplantation

Cryopreserving SSCs before cancer treatment and reintroducing them into their original microenvironment after remission is a promising strategy to restart spermatogenesis and restore natural fertility in patients. In animal models, transplantation of cryopreserved and thawed SSCs into the testes of sterile males has successfully initiated spermatogenesis. Notably, SSCs from mice and rats have been shown to produce functional sperm and lead to the birth of healthy offspring [81, 82]. The potential of the technique was also demonstrated in non-human primates where preimplantation embryos were obtained using sperm produced after SSC allo-transplantation [83]. However, in murine models, the colonization efficiency was poor, relying on the number of SSCs transplanted [84] and a reduced spermatogenic efficiency post-transplantation was also observed, likely due to cryopreservation-induced alterations in cell membranes [85]. Although outcomes of autologous transplantation in humans have not been reported, studies with human SSCs have indicated that cryopreserved SSCs can colonize seminiferous tubules and proliferate in infertile mice testes [86].

The first ex vivo study on injection methods into human testicles showed that only ultrasound-guided injection into the rete testis effectively filled the rete testis and neighboring seminiferous tubules, although the success rate was only 33% with limited cell diffusion into adjacent tubules [87]. The method was deemed most effective for SSC transplantation, allowing optimal infiltration and injection of substantial volumes. More recently, the exploration of alternative injection sites for human SSC transplantation, including the deferential canal, epididymis head, rete testis, and blind perfusion confirmed the superiority of rete testis infusion based on histology and CT scans [88] with further validation of its effectiveness using a radioactive cell suspension and imaging techniques [89].

In Vitro Maturation of Testicular Cells or Tissue

In vitro maturation of cryopreserved ITT is a process that should reproduce both the maturation of the SSC niche, as it naturally occurs during the 2- to 4-year pubertal transition period in boys before the onset of spermarche, and the spermatogenic process involving the differentiation of the SSCs into competent mature sperm cells. Numerous methods have been reported, including 2D cell culture, 3D culture systems for cells with or without supporting scaffolds, culture of isolated seminiferous tubules in a chitosan bioreactor, and organotypic culture at the air–liquid interface on inserts or on agarose pillars (for review, see [1]). The 3D culture was favored as it better mimics the spatial organization of the SSC niche and could favor cell interactions. Further optimization was obtained by replacing the static supply of culture media components with a dynamic supply using microfluidic systems that improved the efficiency of murine spermatogenesis [90], and by applying polydimethylsiloxane covers (PC) on piglet tissue cultured on agarose pillars that reduced tissue core degeneration [91].

Successful IVM of ITT was so far only achieved in rodents with the generation of mice offspring with reproductive competence using sperm obtained after organotypic culture at the gas–liquid interface of fetal tissue [92] and rat offspring after oocyte intracytoplasmic injection of round spermatid developed in organotypic culture under a PC chip [93].

With regard to human tissue, most studies used adult tissue or cryptorchid tissue due to the scarcity of normal prepubertal testicular tissue for research purposes (for review, see [1]). Five groups performed organotypic cultures of human ITT, with the main observations being a progressive loss of spermatogonia over the culture period and incomplete maturation of the SSC niche [94, 95, 96, 97, 98]. While in most attempts there was no differentiation [94, 95, 97] or a blockage at the spermatocyte stage [96, 98], the highest achievement is the development of haploid germ cells, although in low amounts precluding any further characterization of the spermatids [99]. So far, no culture media components or culture system has allowed the completion of human spermatogenesis. Systematic approaches to identify culture requirements will only be possible in a collaborative effort, as, for obvious reasons, access to human ITT for research purposes is very limited.

Perspectives with Advanced Fertility Restoration Approaches

Recent advancements in research on testicular tissue preservation and fertility restoration have highlighted promising alternative methods to restore fertility. Among these innovations, the generation of organoids with selected testicular cells to eliminate cancer cells and scaffolds to support SSC growth is particularly noteworthy, both for in vitro use allowing a reduced reliance on animal models in the context of research [100] and for in vivo transplantation offering the support of still unknown blood-carried growth factors or molecules required for the completion of a normal spermatogenesis process.

In the near future, 3D bioprinting with expanded testicular cells [101] can be a promising approach for the generation of testicular organoids to precisely restore the native testicular organization, which is a prerequisite for spermatogenesis [102].

Restoring fertility with pluripotent stem cell-derived germline stem cells is another strategy to be further explored, as it was recently shown in mice that the entire male germ-cell development process can be reconstituted in vitro, leading to the production of fertilization-competent spermatids and spermatozoa [103].

Research Gaps

While there is room for optimizing cryopreservation procedures, research should focus on providing patients who have reached adulthood with a fertility restoration approach adapted to the content and quality of banked tissue or cell suspensions. In this regard, well-designed clinical pilot trials for tissue auto-transplantation are expected in the near future for patients who were administered gonadotoxic therapy for a benign condition and present a non-obstructive azoospermia and a negative testicular surgical sperm retrieval procedure. Research questions remain on the size of tissue fragments to be transplanted and on the avascular transplantation procedure, as the hypoxic damage to the grafted tissue should be minimized. Future research should therefore focus on optimizing transplantation protocols and on understanding the underlying biological mechanisms that support the survival and functionality of ITT grafts. For banked tissue carrying the risk of cancer cell contamination, there is an urgent need to find solutions to select testicular cells and obtain cancer-cell-free cell suspensions or to develop tissue purging methods to eliminate cancer cells. Effective post-sorting purity and post-purging checks should be performed before cell or tissue transplantation can be considered. Alternatively, research should aim at better understanding SSC niche interactions and cell requirements to achieve effective in vitro generation of competent and safe spermatozoa for further use in assisted reproductive technology with oocyte intracytoplasmic sperm injection. This translates into four main steps: defining a clinical grade medium for firstly achieving the SSC niche maturation and secondly the subsequent SSC differentiation into mature sperm, assessing the quality of the gametes produced in vitro, including genetic and epigenetic investigation, and proving their fertilization potential. Single-cell RNA sequencing experiments could further help to understand cell behavior and specific requirements in culture [104].

Conclusion

In vivo and in vitro approaches to restore fertility in patients with cryostored ITT are still under investigation. Encouraging preclinical data from non-human primates on cell and tissue auto-transplantation suggest that pilot clinical trials may be feasible in the short to medium term. Initially, such interventions could benefit patients who have undergone gonadotoxic treatments for non-malignant conditions such as sickle cell anemia, β-thalassemia, or aplastic anemia, as well as those diagnosed with non-metastasizing solid tumors, such as sarcomas or neuroblastomas.

Advances in the generation of cancer-cell-free testicular organoids, development of cancer cell purging methods for testicular tissue prior to autotransplantation, and IVM of ITT are paving the way toward safe infertility treatments for patients previously affected by hematological or metastasizing malignancies. Nevertheless, the clinical implementation of fertility restoration strategies requires extensive research and validation through small-scale pilot studies to ensure both efficacy and long-term safety.

References

1. Wyns C, Kanbar M, Giudice MG, Poels J. Fertility preservation for prepubertal boys: lessons learned from the past and update on remaining challenges towards clinical translation. Hum Reprod Update. 2021;27:433–59.
2. Bahadur G, Chatterjee R, Ralph D. Testicular tissue cryopreservation in boys. Ethical and legal issues: case report. Hum Reprod. 2000;15:1416–20.
3. Gatta G, Botta L, Rossi S, Aareleid T, Bielska-Lasota M, Clavel J, Dimitrova N, Jakab Z, Kaatsch P, Lacour B, et al. Childhood cancer survival in Europe 1999-2007: results of EUROCARE-5–a population-based study. Lancet Oncol. 2014;15:35–47.

4. Siegel RL, Miller KD, Fuchs HE, Jemal A. Cancer statistics, 2021. CA Cancer J Clin. 2021;71:7–33.
5. Hudson MM. Reproductive outcomes for survivors of childhood cancer. Obstet Gynecol. 2010;116:1171–83.
6. Schover LR. Motivation for parenthood after cancer: a review. J Natl Cancer Inst Monogr. 2005:2–5. https://doi.org/10.1093/jncimonographs/lgi010.
7. Barraud-Lange V, Boissel N, Gille AS, Jean C, Sitbon L, Schubert B, Yakouben K, Fahd M, Peycelon M, Paye-Jaouen A, et al. A 10-year experience in testicular tissue cryopreservation for boys under 18 years of age: what can be learned from 350 cases? Andrology. 2024;12:385–95.
8. Braye A, Tournaye H, Goossens E. Setting up a cryopreservation programme for immature testicular tissue: lessons learned after more than 15 years of experience. Clin Med Insights Reprod Health. 2019;13:1179558119886342.
9. Ginsberg JP, Carlson CA, Lin K, Hobbie WL, Wigo E, Wu X, Brinster RL, Kolon TF. An experimental protocol for fertility preservation in prepubertal boys recently diagnosed with cancer: a report of acceptability and safety. Hum Reprod. 2010;25:37–41.
10. Heckmann L, Langenstroth-Röwer D, Pock T, Wistuba J, Stukenborg JB, Zitzmann M, Kliesch S, Schlatt S, Neuhaus N. A diagnostic germ cell score for immature testicular tissue at risk of germ cell loss. Hum Reprod. 2018;33:636–45.
11. Sadri-Ardekani H, Atala A. Testicular tissue cryopreservation and spermatogonial stem cell transplantation to restore fertility: from bench to bedside. Stem Cell Res Ther. 2014;5:68.
12. Stukenborg JB, Alves-Lopes JP, Kurek M, Albalushi H, Reda A, Keros V, Tohonen V, Bjarnason R, Romerius P, Sundin M, et al. Spermatogonial quantity in human prepubertal testicular tissue collected for fertility preservation prior to potentially sterilizing therapy. Hum Reprod. 2018a;33:1677–83.
13. Valli-Pulaski H, Peters KA, Gassei K, Steimer SR, Sukhwani M, Hermann BP, Dwomor L, David S, Fayomi AP, Munyoki SK, et al. Testicular tissue cryopreservation: 8 years of experience from a coordinated network of academic centers. Hum Reprod. 2019;34:966–77.
14. Wyns C, Curaba M, Petit S, Vanabelle B, Laurent P, Wese JF, Donnez J. Management of fertility preservation in prepubertal patients: 5 years' experience at the Catholic University of Louvain. Hum Reprod. 2011;26:737–47.
15. Uijldert M, Meissner A, de Melker AA, van Pelt AMM, van de Wetering MD, van Rijn RR, van Wely M, van der Veen F, Repping S. Development of the testis in pre-pubertal boys with cancer after biopsy for fertility preservation. Hum Reprod. 2017;32:2366–72.
16. Borgstrom B, Fridstrom M, Gustafsson B, Ljungman P, Rodriguez-Wallberg KA. A prospective study on the long-term outcome of prepubertal and pubertal boys undergoing testicular biopsy for fertility preservation prior to hematologic stem cell transplantation. Pediatr Blood Cancer. 2020:e28507. https://doi.org/10.1002/pbc.28507.
17. Braye A. Immature testicular tissue banking for fertility preservation in (pre) pubertal boys: patient enrolment and follow-up. Doctor in Medical Sciences, Vrije Universiteit Brussel; 2023
18. Delgouffe E, Braye A, Vloeberghs V, Mateizel I, Ernst C, Ferster A, Devalck C, Tournaye H, Gies I, Goossens E. Spermatogenesis after gonadotoxic childhood treatment: follow-up of 12 patients. Hum Reprod Open. 2023;2023:hoad029.
19. Kanbar M, de Michele F, Giudice MG, Desmet L, Poels J, Wyns C. Long-term follow-up of boys who have undergone a testicular biopsy for fertility preservation. Hum Reprod. 2021;36:26–39.
20. Duffin K, Neuhaus N, Andersen CY, Barraud-Lange V, Braye A, Eguizabal C, Feraille A, Ginsberg JP, Gook D, Goossens E, et al. A 20-year overview of fertility preservation in boys: new insights gained through a comprehensive international survey. Hum Reprod Open. 2024;2024:hoae010.
21. Kanbar M, Delwiche G, Wyns C. Fertility preservation for prepubertal boys: are we ready for autologous grafting of cryopreserved immature testicular tissue? Ann Endocrinol (Paris). 2022b;83:210–7.

22. Mulder RL, Font-Gonzalez A, Hudson MM, van Santen HM, Loeffen EAH, Burns KC, Quinn GP, van Dulmen-den Broeder E, Byrne J, Haupt R, et al. Fertility preservation for female patients with childhood, adolescent, and young adult cancer: recommendations from the PanCareLIFE Consortium and the International Late Effects of Childhood Cancer Guideline Harmonization Group. Lancet Oncol. 2021;22:e45–56.
23. Wyns C (2010) Fertility preservation strategies in males cryopreservation and transplantation of testicular tissue.
24. Lahtinen AK, Funke M, Krallmann C, Wyrwoll MJ, Jarisch A, Yang Y, Bjarnason R, Romerius P, Sundin M, Noren-Nystrom U, et al. Decreased spermatogonial numbers in boys with severe haematological diseases. Br J Haematol. 2024; https://doi.org/10.1111/bjh.19572.
25. Masliukaite I, Ntemou E, Feijen EAM, van de Wetering M, Meissner A, Soufan AT, Repping S, Kremer LMC, Jahnukainen K, Goossens E, et al. Childhood cancer and hematological disorders negatively affect spermatogonial quantity at diagnosis: a retrospective study of a male fertility preservation cohort. Hum Reprod. 2023; https://doi.org/10.1093/humrep/dead004.
26. Wigny KM, van Dorp W, van der Kooi AL, de Rijke YB, de Vries AC, Smit M, Pluijm SM, van den Akker EL, Pieters R, Laven JS, et al. Gonadal function in boys with newly diagnosed cancer before the start of treatment. Hum Reprod. 2016;31:2613–8.
27. Funke M, Yang Y, Lahtinen A, Benninghoven-Frey K, Kliesch S, Neuhaus N, Stukenborg JB, Jahnukainen K. Z-scores for comparative analyses of spermatogonial numbers throughout human development. Fertil Steril. 2021;116:713–20.
28. Gille AS, Pondarre C, Dalle JH, Bernaudin F, Chalas C, Fahd M, Jean C, Lezeau H, Riou L, Drouineaud V, et al. Hydroxyurea does not affect the spermatogonial pool in prepubertal patients with sickle cell disease. Blood. 2021;137:856–9.
29. Feraille A, Liard A, Rives N, Bubenheim M, Barbotin AL, Giscard d'Estaing S, Mirallie S, Ancelle A, Roux C, Brugnon F, et al. Impact of low- or moderate-risk gonadotoxic chemotherapy prior to testicular tissue freezing on spermatogonia quantity in human (pre)pubertal testicular tissue. Hum Reprod. 2023;38:2105–18.
30. Medrano JV, Hervas D, Vilanova-Perez T, Navarro-Gomezlechon A, Goossens E, Pellicer A, Andres MM, Novella-Maestre E. Histologic analysis of testes from prepubertal patients treated with chemotherapy associates impaired germ cell counts with cumulative doses of cyclophosphamide, ifosfamide, cytarabine, and asparaginase. Reprod Sci. 2021;28:603–13.
31. Poganitsch-Korhonen M, Masliukaite I, Nurmio M, Lahteenmaki P, van Wely M, van Pelt AMM, Jahnukainen K, Stukenborg JB. Decreased spermatogonial quantity in prepubertal boys with leukaemia treated with alkylating agents. Leukemia. 2017;31:1460–3.
32. Allen CM, Lopes F, Mitchell RT, Spears N. How does chemotherapy treatment damage the prepubertal testis? Reproduction. 2018;156:R209–33.
33. Stukenborg JB, Jahnukainen K, Hutka M, Mitchell RT. Cancer treatment in childhood and testicular function: the importance of the somatic environment. Endocr Connect. 2018b;7:R69–87.
34. Wyns C, Kanbar M. In vitro spermatogenesis. In: Grynberg M, Patrizio P, editors. Female and male fertility preservation. Cham: Springer; 2022.
35. Green DM, Liu W, Kutteh WH, Ke RW, Shelton KC, Sklar CA, Chemaitilly W, Pui CH, Klosky JL, Spunt SL, et al. Cumulative alkylating agent exposure and semen parameters in adult survivors of childhood cancer: a report from the St Jude Lifetime Cohort Study. Lancet Oncol. 2014;15:1215–23.
36. Howell SJ, Shalet SM. Spermatogenesis after cancer treatment: damage and recovery. J Natl Cancer Inst Monogr. 2005:12–7. https://doi.org/10.1093/jncimonographs/lgi003.
37. Meistrich ML. Effects of chemotherapy and radiotherapy on spermatogenesis in humans. Fertil Steril. 2013;100:1180–6.
38. Mathiesen S, Andres-Jensen L, Nielsen MM, Sorensen K, Ifversen M, Jahnukainen K, Juul A, Muller K. Male gonadal function after pediatric hematopoietic stem cell transplantation: a systematic review. Transplant Cell Ther. 2022;28:503 e1–503 e15.

39. Lukusa AK, Vermylen C, Vanabelle B, Curaba M, Brichard B, Chantrain C, Dupont S, Ferrant A, Wyns C. Bone marrow transplantation or hydroxyurea for sickle cell anemia: long-term effects on semen variables and hormone profiles. Pediatr Hematol Oncol. 2009;26:186–94.
40. Joseph L, Jean C, Manceau S, Chalas C, Arnaud C, Kamdem A, Pondarre C, Habibi A, Bernaudin F, Allali S, et al. Effect of hydroxyurea exposure before puberty on sperm parameters in males with sickle cell disease. Blood. 2021;137:826–9.
41. Delgouffe E, Braye A, Goossens E. Testicular tissue banking for fertility preservation in young boys: which patients should be included? Front Endocrinol (Lausanne). 2022;13:854186.
42. Ntemou E, Delgouffe E, Goossens E. Immune checkpoint inhibitors and male fertility: should fertility preservation options be considered before treatment? Cancers (Basel). 2024;16
43. Adamczewska-Wawrzynowicz K, Wiacek A, Kozlowska A, Mikosza K, Szefler L, Dudlik W, Dey S, Varghese N, Derwich K. Modern treatment strategies in pediatric oncology and hematology. Discov Oncol. 2023;14:98.
44. Chang X, Zhou L, Chen X, Xu B, Cheng Y, Sun S, Fang M, Xiang Y. Impact of imatinib on the fertility of male patients with chronic myelogenous leukaemia in the chronic phase. Target Oncol. 2017;12:827–32.
45. Tauer JT, Ulmer A, Glauche I, Jung R, Suttorp M. Long-term imatinib treatment does not cause testicular toxicity in male adolescents with chronic myeloid leukemia and in a juvenile rat model. Klin Padiatr. 2014;226:169–74.
46. Butler E, Ludwig K, Pacenta HL, Klesse LJ, Watt TC, Laetsch TW. Recent progress in the treatment of cancer in children. CA Cancer J Clin. 2021;71:315–32.
47. Goossens E, Jahnukainen K, Mitchell RT, van Pelt A, Pennings G, Rives N, Poels J, Wyns C, Lane S, Rodriguez-Wallberg KA, et al. Fertility preservation in boys: recent developments and new insights. Hum Reprod Open. 2020;2020:hoaa016.
48. Wyns C, Collienne C, Shenfield F, Robert A, Laurent P, Roegiers L, Brichard B. Fertility preservation in the male pediatric population: factors influencing the decision of parents and children. Hum Reprod. 2015;30:2022–30.
49. Picton HM, Wyns C, Anderson RA, Goossens E, Jahnukainen K, Kliesch S, Mitchell RT, Pennings G, Rives N, Tournaye H, et al. A European perspective on testicular tissue cryopreservation for fertility preservation in prepubertal and adolescent boys. Hum Reprod. 2015;30:2463–75.
50. Brignardello E, Felicetti F, Castiglione A, Nervo A, Biasin E, Ciccone G, Fagioli F, Corrias A. Gonadal status in long-term male survivors of childhood cancer. J Cancer Res Clin Oncol. 2016;142:1127–32.
51. Romerius P, Stahl O, Moell C, Relander T, Cavallin-Stahl E, Wiebe T, Giwercman YL, Giwercman A. High risk of azoospermia in men treated for childhood cancer. Int J Androl. 2011;34:69–76.
52. Mathiesen S, Sorensen K, Nielsen MM, Suominen A, Ifversen M, Grell K, Lahteenmaki P, Frederiksen H, Juul A, Muller K, et al. Male gonadal function after allogeneic hematopoietic stem cell transplantation in childhood: a cross-sectional, population-based study. Biol Blood Marrow Transplant. 2020; https://doi.org/10.1016/j.bbmt.2020.05.009.
53. Curaba M, Poels J, van Langendonckt A, Donnez J, Wyns C. Can prepubertal human testicular tissue be cryopreserved by vitrification? Fertil Steril. 2011;95(2123):e9–12.
54. Poels J, Van Langendonckt A, Many MC, Wese FX, Wyns C. Vitrification preserves proliferation capacity in human spermatogonia. Hum Reprod. 2013;28:578–89.
55. Kvist K, Thorup J, Byskov AG, Hoyer PE, Mollgard K, Yding Andersen C. Cryopreservation of intact testicular tissue from boys with cryptorchidism. Hum Reprod. 2006;21:484–91.
56. Kanbar M, de Michele F, Wyns C. Cryostorage of testicular tissue and retransplantation of spermatogonial stem cells in the infertile male. Best Pract Res Clin Endocrinol Metab. 2019;33:103–15.
57. Benninghoven-Frey KM, Neuhaus N, Lahtinen AK, Krallmann C, Portela JMD, Jarisch A, Nordhoff V, Soave A, Ba Omar HAM, Sundin M, et al. Early testicular maturation is sensitive to depletion of spermatogonial pool in sickle cell disease. Haematologica. 2022;107:975–9.

58. Faes K, Goossens E. Short-term storage of human testicular tissue: effect of storage temperature and tissue size. Reprod Biomed Online. 2017;35:180–8.
59. Jahnukainen K, Ehmcke J, Hergenrother SD, Schlatt S. Effect of cold storage and cryopreservation of immature non-human primate testicular tissue on spermatogonial stem cell potential in xenografts. Hum Reprod. 2007;22:1060–7.
60. Hou M, Andersson M, Eksborg S, Soder O, Jahnukainen K. Xenotransplantation of testicular tissue into nude mice can be used for detecting leukemic cell contamination. Hum Reprod. 2007;22:1899–906.
61. Jahnukainen K, Hou M, Petersen C, Setchell B, Soder O. Intratesticular transplantation of testicular cells from leukemic rats causes transmission of leukemia. Cancer Res. 2001;61:706–10.
62. Kourta D, Kanbar M, Amorim CA, Wyns C. Cancer cell contamination and decontamination methods for ovaries and testes: special focus on prepubertal gonads with a view to safe fertility restoration. Hum Reprod. 2023; https://doi.org/10.1093/humrep/dead054.
63. Kourta D, Camboni A, Saussoy P, Kanbar M, Poels J, Wyns C. Evaluating testicular tissue for future autotransplantation: focus on cancer cell contamination and presence of spermatogonia in tissue cryobanked for boys diagnosed with a hematological malignancy. Hum Reprod. 2024;39:486–95.
64. Sadri-Ardekani H, Homburg CH, van Capel TM, van den Berg H, van der Veen F, van der Schoot CE, van Pelt AM, Repping S. Eliminating acute lymphoblastic leukemia cells from human testicular cell cultures: a pilot study. Fertil Steril. 2014;101:1072–8. e1
65. Ohta H, Wakayama T. Generation of normal progeny by intracytoplasmic sperm injection following grafting of testicular tissue from cloned mice that died postnatally. Biol Reprod. 2005;73:390–5.
66. Schlatt S, Kim SS, Gosden R. Spermatogenesis and steroidogenesis in mouse, hamster and monkey testicular tissue after cryopreservation and heterotopic grafting to castrated hosts. Reproduction. 2002;124:339–46.
67. Shinohara T, Inoue K, Ogonuki N, Kanatsu-Shinohara M, Miki H, Nakata K, Kurome M, Nagashima H, Toyokuni S, Kogishi K, et al. Birth of offspring following transplantation of cryopreserved immature testicular pieces and in-vitro microinsemination. Hum Reprod. 2002;17:3039–45.
68. Abrishami M, Anzar M, Yang Y, Honaramooz A. Cryopreservation of immature porcine testis tissue to maintain its developmental potential after xenografting into recipient mice. Theriogenology. 2010;73:86–96.
69. Honaramooz A, Megee SO, Dobrinski I. Germ cell transplantation in pigs. Biol Reprod. 2002;66:21 8.
70. Kaneko H, Kikuchi K, Nakai M, Somfai T, Noguchi J, Tanihara F, Ito J, Kashiwazaki N. Generation of live piglets for the first time using sperm retrieved from immature testicular tissue cryopreserved and grafted into nude mice. PLoS One. 2013;8:e70989.
71. Liu J, Cheng KM, Silversides FG. Production of live offspring from testicular tissue cryopreserved by vitrification procedures in Japanese quail (Coturnix japonica). Biol Reprod. 2013;88:124.
72. Fayomi AP, Peters K, Sukhwani M, Valli-Pulaski H, Shetty G, Meistrich ML, Houser L, Robertson N, Roberts V, Ramsey C, et al. Autologous grafting of cryopreserved prepubertal rhesus testis produces sperm and offspring. Science. 2019;363:1314–9.
73. Van Saen D, Goossens E, Bourgain C, Ferster A, Tournaye H. Meiotic activity in orthotopic xenografts derived from human postpubertal testicular tissue. Hum Reprod. 2011;26:282–93.
74. Van Saen D, Goossens E, Haentjens P, Baert Y, Tournaye H. Exogenous administration of recombinant human FSH does not improve germ cell survival in human prepubertal xenografts. Reprod Biomed Online. 2013;26:286–98.
75. Wyns C, Curaba M, Martinez-Madrid B, Van Langendonckt A, Francois-Xavier W, Donnez J. Spermatogonial survival after cryopreservation and short-term orthotopic imma-

ture human cryptorchid testicular tissue grafting to immunodeficient mice. Hum Reprod. 2007;22:1603–11.
76. Wyns C, Van Langendonckt A, Wese FX, Donnez J, Curaba M. Long-term spermatogonial survival in cryopreserved and xenografted immature human testicular tissue. Hum Reprod. 2008;23:2402–14.
77. Israely T, Nevo N, Harmelin A, Neeman M, Tsafriri A. Reducing ischaemic damage in rodent ovarian xenografts transplanted into granulation tissue. Hum Reprod. 2006;21:1368–79.
78. Poels J, Abou-Ghannam G, Herman S, Van Langendonckt A, Wese FX, Wyns C. In search of better spermatogonial preservation by supplementation of cryopreserved human immature testicular tissue xenografts with N-acetylcysteine and testosterone. Front Surg. 2014;1:47.
79. Del Vento F, Vermeulen M, Ucakar B, Poels J, des Rieux A, Wyns C. Significant benefits of nanoparticles containing a necrosis inhibitor on mice testicular tissue autografts outcomes. Int J Mol Sci. 2019;20
80. Del Vento F, Poels J, Vermeulen M, Ucakar B, Giudice MG, Kanbar M, Des Rieux A, Wyns C. Accelerated and improved vascular maturity after transplantation of testicular tissue in hydrogels supplemented with VEGF- and PDGF-loaded nanoparticles. Int J Mol Sci. 2021;22
81. Kanatsu-Shinohara M, Ogonuki N, Inoue K, Ogura A, Toyokuni S, Honjo T, Shinohara T. Allogeneic offspring produced by male germ line stem cell transplantation into infertile mouse testis. Biol Reprod. 2003;68:167–73.
82. Wu X, Goodyear SM, Abramowitz LK, Bartolomei MS, Tobias JW, Avarbock MR, Brinster RL. Fertile offspring derived from mouse spermatogonial stem cells cryopreserved for more than 14 years. Hum Reprod. 2012;27:1249–59.
83. Hermann BP, Sukhwani M, Winkler F, Pascarella JN, Peters KA, Sheng Y, Valli H, Rodriguez M, Ezzelarab M, Dargo G, et al. Spermatogonial stem cell transplantation into rhesus testes regenerates spermatogenesis producing functional sperm. Cell Stem Cell. 2012;11:715–26.
84. Dobrinski I, Avarbock MR, Brinster RL. Transplantation of germ cells from rabbits and dogs into mouse testes. Biol Reprod. 1999;61:1331–9.
85. Frederickx V, Michiels A, Goossens E, De Block G, Van Steirteghem AC, Tournaye H. Recovery, survival and functional evaluation by transplantation of frozen-thawed mouse germ cells. Hum Reprod. 2004;19:948–53.
86. Nagano M, Patrizio P, Brinster RL. Long-term survival of human spermatogonial stem cells in mouse testes. Fertil Steril. 2002;78:1225–33.
87. Schlatt S, Rosiepen G, Weinbauer GF, Rolf C, Brook PF, Nieschlag E. Germ cell transfer into rat, bovine, monkey and human testes. Hum Reprod. 1999;14:144–50.
88. Ning L, Goossens E, Geens M, Saen DV, Tournaye H. Spermatogonial stem cells as a source for regenerative medicine. Middle East Fertil Soc J. 2012;17:1–7.
89. Faes K, Tournaye H, Goethals L, Lahoutte T, Hoorens A, Goossens E. Testicular cell transplantation into the human testes. Fertil Steril. 2013; https://doi.org/10.1016/j.fertnstert.2013.06.016.
90. Komeya M, Kimura H, Nakamura H, Yokonishi T, Sato T, Kojima K, Hayashi K, Katagiri K, Yamanaka H, Sanjo H, et al. Long-term ex vivo maintenance of testis tissues producing fertile sperm in a microfluidic device. Sci Rep. 2016;6:21472.
91. Kanbar M, de Michele F, Poels J, Van Loo S, Giudice MG, Gilet T, Wyns C. Microfluidic and static organotypic culture systems to support ex vivo spermatogenesis from prepubertal porcine testicular tissue: a comparative study. Front Physiol. 2022a;13:884122.
92. Sato T, Katagiri K, Gohbara A, Inoue K, Ogonuki N, Ogura A, Kubota Y, Ogawa T. In vitro production of functional sperm in cultured neonatal mouse testes. Nature. 2011;471:504–7.
93. Matsumura T, Katagiri K, Yao T, Ishikawa-Yamauchi Y, Nagata S, Hashimoto K, Sato T, Kimura H, Shinohara T, Sanbo M, et al. Generation of rat offspring using spermatids produced through in vitro spermatogenesis. Sci Rep. 2023;13:12105.
94. Aden NL, Bleeke M, Kordes UR, Brunne B, Holstermann B, Biemann R, Ceglarek U, Soave A, Salzbrunn A, Schneider SW, et al. Germ cell maintenance and sustained testosterone and

precursor hormone production in human prepubertal testis organ culture with tissues from boys 7 years+ under conditions from adult testicular tissue. Cells. 2023;12

95. de Michele F, Poels J, Weerens L, Petit C, Evrard Z, Ambroise J, Gruson D, Wyns C. Preserved seminiferous tubule integrity with spermatogonial survival and induction of Sertoli and Leydig cell maturation after long-term organotypic culture of prepubertal human testicular tissue. Hum Reprod. 2017;32:32–45.
96. Medrano JV, Vilanova-Perez T, Fornes-Ferrer V, Navarro-Gomezlechon A, Martinez-Triguero ML, Garcia S, Gomez-Chacon J, Povo I, Pellicer A, Andres MM, et al. Influence of temperature, serum, and gonadotropin supplementation in short- and long-term organotypic culture of human immature testicular tissue. Fertil Steril. 2018;110:1045–57. e3
97. Portela JMD, de Winter-Korver CM, van Daalen SKM, Meißner A, de Melker AA, Repping S, van Pelt AMM. Assessment of fresh and cryopreserved testicular tissues from (pre) pubertal boys during organ culture as a strategy for in vitro spermatogenesis. Hum Reprod. 2019;34:2443–55.
98. Younis N, Caldeira-Brant AL, Chu T, Abdalla S, Orwig KE. Human immature testicular tissue organ culture: a step towards fertility preservation and restoration. Front Endocrinol (Lausanne). 2023;14:1242263.
99. de Michele F, Poels J, Vermeulen M, Ambroise J, Gruson D, Guiot Y, Wyns C. Haploid germ cells generated in organotypic culture of testicular tissue from prepubertal boys. Front Physiol. 2018;9:1413.
100. Vermeulen M, Del Vento F, Kanbar M, Pyr Dit Ruys S, Vertommen D, Poels J, Wyns C. Generation of organized porcine testicular organoids in solubilized hydrogels from decellularized extracellular matrix. Int J Mol Sci. 2019:20.
101. Robinson M, Bedford E, Witherspoon L, Willerth SM, Flannigan R. Using clinically derived human tissue to 3-dimensionally bioprint personalized testicular tubules for in vitro culturing: first report. F S Sci. 2022;3:130–9.
102. Richer G, Baert Y, Goossens E. In-vitro spermatogenesis through testis modelling: toward the generation of testicular organoids. Andrology. 2020;8:879–91.
103. Ishikura Y, Ohta H, Sato T, Murase Y, Yabuta Y, Kojima Y, Yamashiro C, Nakamura T, Yamamoto T, Ogawa T, et al. In vitro reconstitution of the whole male germ-cell development from mouse pluripotent stem cells. Cell Stem Cell. 2021;28:2167–79. e9
104. Kwaspen L, Kanbar M, Wyns C. Mapping the development of human spermatogenesis using transcriptomics-based data: a scoping review. Int J Mol Sci. 2024;25

Chapter 10
The Role of Varicocele Repair in Patients with Nonobstructive Azoospermia

Parviz K. Kavoussi, Imad Ziouziou, and Ates Kadioglu

Key Points

- Varicocele repair may allow for the return of sperm to the ejaculate in some men with nonobstructive azoospermia following varicocele repair.
- Varicocele repair may improve surgical sperm retrieval rate via microdissection, testicular sperm extraction, and assisted reproductive technology outcomes in some men who remain azoospermic following varicocele repair.
- The American Urological Association/American Society for Reproductive Medicine guidelines suggest an absence of definitive evidence supporting varicocele repair prior to assisted reproductive technology.
- The European Association of Urology suggests that some men with NOA who undergo varicocele repair will have a return of sperm to the ejaculate, and those who do not may have a higher surgical sperm retrieval rate and improved assisted reproductive technology outcomes.

Introduction

Approximately 15% of couples in the United States are infertile, failing to conceive after trying for pregnancy with unprotected intercourse for one year. Male factor is solely responsible in 20% of infertile couples and is a contributory factor in an

P. K. Kavoussi (✉)
Austin Fertility & Reproductive Medicine/Westlake IVF, Austin, TX, USA

I. Ziouziou
Department of Urology, University Hospital Souss Massa, Faculty of Medicine and Pharmacy, Ibn Zohr University, Agadir, Morocco

A. Kadioglu
Section of Andrology, Department of Urology, Istanbul Faculty of Medicine, Istanbul, Turkey

W. Zohdy et al. (eds.), *Non-Obstructive Azoospermia*,
https://doi.org/10.1007/978-3-031-99431-9_10

additional 40% of infertile couples, indicating that 60% of infertile couples have a male factor contributing [1]. One percent of men in the general population are azoospermic, and evaluations are found to have azoospermia [2, 3]. The definition of approximately 15% of men presenting for infertility azoospermia is a complete absence of sperm from the ejaculate, which is diagnosed by at least two semen analyses revealing no sperm in the ejaculate by high power light microscopy with the additional finding of no sperm in the centrifuged concentrated pellet after 15 min of centrifugation at a speed of at least 3000 × g or greater [4].

The three main categories of azoospermia include pre-testicular, testicular, and post-testicular causes. Pre-testicular causes include the different sources of hypogonadotropic hypogonadism. Testicular etiologies indicated primary testicular dysfunction with impaired spermatogenesis within the testicles. Post-testicular causes include obstructions of the reproductive tract at the level of the epididymides, vasa, or ejaculatory ducts. Most testicular causes of azoospermia cannot be corrected, with varicoceles being the exception. Varicoceles offer a cautious opportunity for men with nonobstructive azoospermia to have sperm appear in the ejaculate and achieve a pregnancy, either with timed intercourse or with assisted reproductive technology (ART), and obviate the need for surgical sperm retrieval.

This chapter reviews the effect of varicoceles on testicular function in men with azoospermia, the effect of varicocele repair on the semen of azoospermic men, and the effect of varicocele repair on sperm retrievals and ART outcomes when the male partner remains azoospermic following varicocele repair.

Varicocele and Nonobstructive Azoospermia

Varicoceles are defined as abnormally dilated scrotal veins draining into the pampiniform plexus, which are present in approximately 15% of men in the general population and occur in 40% of men presenting for infertility evaluations, resulting in varicoceles being the most common diagnosis made in infertile men [5]. As 1% of men in the general population are azoospermic and 15% of men presenting for infertility are azoospermic, overlap is inevitably found between the two [1, 5]. Varicoceles adversely impact spermatogenesis and testicular function, which may result in low sperm counts, and perhaps azoospermia in the most severe cases have many theories on the mechanisms of damage. The most prominent hypothesis described by the largest amount of data indicates that varicoceles primarily affect testicular function by elevating intratesticular temperatures by interrupting the counter-current heat exchange in the pampiniform plexus with opposing flows in a central arterial system [6–8]. Varicoceles have been demonstrated to induce cellular damage via sperm DNA fragmentation, apoptosis, increasing reactive oxygen species through oxidative stress, intracellular ionic and metabolic changes, and predisposition to sperm aneuploidy [9–16]. Men who have varicoceles have shown higher mean tubular apoptotic indices in comparison to controls without varicoceles [17].

The theory of the retrograde flow of adrenal and renal metabolites adversely inducing testicular cellular damage due to a varicocele was demonstrated in a murine model study [18]. Thermal abnormalities and class IIC meiotic abnormalities have been shown to be reversed after varicocele repair in the testes of men with nonobstructive azoospermia (NOA) 6 months after varicocele repair [19].

Despite some controversy and some conflicting studies, there may be a role of the repair of palpable varicoceles in men with NOA. Multiple publications have revealed the return of sperm to the semen in10–50% of men with NOA after varicocele repair. Return of sperm to the ejaculate has been shown to be more likely when testicular histology is favorable, such as hypospermatogenesis or late maturation arrest, rather than in men with Sertoli-cell-only or early maturation arrest [20–41]. In one small study, 3/25 men had the return of sperm 4 months after surgery, and this increased to 5/25 by the end of 1 year, suggesting it may take up to 1 year for some men to respond [37]. Although most men who have sperm return to the semen following varicocele repair, the post-varicocele repair sperm counts usually tend to remain low, and intracytoplasmic sperm injection (ICSI) is still necessary, there is a major benefit of avoiding a microdissection testicular sperm extraction (micro-TESE). Some men will relapse to azoospermia after having sperm return to the ejaculate following varicocele repair and there are no identifiable predictors for which men do so; therefore, cryopreservation of a semen sample is recommended soon after sperm returns to the ejaculate following varicocele repair in men who presented with NOA initially [29, 35, 42, 43]. Cryopreservation of sperm is recommended after return of sperm to the semen, regardless of whether the man underwent surgical varicocele repair or embolization, as cases have been reported of relapse to azoospermia as soon as 6 months after demonstrating sperm in the semen after both types of corrective procedures [25, 32, 44].

Seminal plasma micro-RNA (miR)-192a levels were demonstrated to be higher in azoospermic men who remained azoospermic following varicocele repair compared to those who had sperm return to the ejaculate. miR 192a induces GC-2 cell apoptosis through the activation of Caspase-3 protein and could be a predictor of response to varicocele repair in men with NOA and with a varicocele [45].

The presence of a Y chromosome microdeletion must be examined prior to consideration of varicocele repair in men with severe oligozoospermia or azoospermia, as the benefit is less likely if a Y chromosome microdeletion is present [46].

A publication of 33 men with varicoceles who were azoospermic revealed that 12 (34%) had return of sperm to the ejaculate within 2–14 months following varicocele repair [47]. Some small case series reported pregnancy rates in azoospermic men following varicocele repair when the men had no other treatments. A publication by Mehan revealed pregnancies in 2 out of 10 men who presented with azoospermia who were only treated with varicocele repair [48]. Another small series compared response rates to varicocele repair in men with azoospermia ($n = 24$) versus virtual azoospermia ($n = 14$). Sperm was identified in the semen of 5 (21%) of the azoospermic men after varicocele repair with a mean follow-up of 14 months, with 3 having testicular histology of maturation arrest at the spermatid stage, 1 demonstrating Sertoli-cell-only pattern with focal spermatogenesis, and 1 with hypospermatogenesis. All men in this study with pure Sertoli-cell-only or spermatocyte stage maturation arrest patterns remained azoospermic after varicocele repair. Of the virtually azoospermic men, 12 (85%) had improvement in semen parameters and 4 (28%) achieved a total motile count of greater than five million. After varicocele repair, 3 of the virtually azoospermic men (21%) were able to conceive with timed intercourse due to a significant improvement in semen parameters [49]. One publication included 32 men with azoospermia who underwent percutaneous embolization and 18 (56%) had sperm return to the semen with a mean sperm concentration of $3.81 \pm 1.69 \times 10^6$/ml following embolization [50].

Controversy exists regarding the outcomes of sperm returning to the semen after varicocele repair in men with NOA due to variable results in studies [51].

Varicocele and Sperm Retrieval

Having sperm return to the semen following varicocele repair with a baseline status of NOA does not necessarily ensure sufficient sperm for use with assisted reproductive technology (ART). One study of 32 men with NOA who underwent varicocele repair revealed that 7 (22%) had sperm in the ejaculate following varicocele repair; however, only 3 (9.6%) had adequate motile sperm in the semen for use with in vitro fertilization/intracytoplasmic sperm injection (IVF/ICSI) [51]. Therefore, there will be many NOA, who will still require microTESE following varicocele repair, in cases where they remain azoospermic or because the sperm in the semen are not adequate for ICSI. Data exists suggesting that varicocele repair in NOA men can improve sperm retrieval rates at the time of microTESE and improve IVF/ICSI outcomes. One publication reported a surgical sperm retrieval rate of 60.8% in men who remained azoospermic following varicocele repair versus a sperm retrieval rate of 38.5% in men who left varicoceles untreated. There were significantly higher clinical pregnancy rates and live birth rates with IVF/ICSI in the group that had undergone varicocele repair and then successful sperm retrieval via microTESE, than the men who did not undergo repair, 74.2% versus 52.3% and 64.5% versus 41.5%, respectively [52]. Another study compared couples who underwent IVF/ICSI when men underwent varicocele repair versus men who did not have varicoceles repaired prior to microTESE sperm retrieval. The sperm retrieval rate with microTESE was significantly higher in the varicocele repair group, 53% versus 30%, respectively. However, they reported no difference in fertilization rate, rate of high-quality embryo formation, or mean number of transferred embryos. The clinical pregnancy rate was significantly higher in the varicocele repair group in comparison to the group who had varicoceles left intact, at 31% versus 22%, respectively [53]. Other studies have reported similar findings of improved sperm retrieval rates, fertilization rates, pregnancy rates, and live birth rates with microTESE/IVF/ICSI following varicocele repair when compared to varicoceles that are left intact [36, 38, 40, 41, 54–56]. One study reported an improvement in the severity of testicular histology after varicocele repair in men with NOA. At the time of varicocele repair, testicular biopsy was performed for diagnostic histology and repeated at the time of microTESE in men who failed to have sperm return to the ejaculate after varicocele repair. Fourteen men revealed Sertoli-cell-only patterns from the biopsies at the time of varicocele repair and had improvement in the severity of histology to focal spermatogenesis in 2 of them and late maturation arrest in 3 of them from the biopsies at the time of microTESE [57]. This study was limited by the possibility of baseline heterogeneity in testicular histology.

There is controversy in the data in the medical literature. A publication of a small cohort of 31 men reported that varicocele repair resulted in adequate sperm in the semen in only three of these men (9.6%) that was adequate for use with ART, and varicocele repair did not impact surgical sperm retrieval rates. A major limitation of this study was the sample size [51].

Sperm Retrieval/Testicular Biopsy at the Time of Varicocele Repair

Histologic pattern has been strongly associated with the success rates of varicocele repair in NOA men with varicoceles [34]. Multiple studies have reported the usefulness of testicular histology to predict sperm returning to the semen following varicocele repair as well as success in ICSI outcomes with sperm retrieved via microTESE [22, 25, 29, 58, 59].

NOA men with primary infertility and a clinical varicocele should be evaluated extensively by physical, hormonal, and genetic assessments (Y-chromosome microdeletions and karyotyping). For men who are candidates following this evaluation, the option of a testicular biopsy first may be offered. If the biopsy reveals hypospermatogenesis or late maturation arrest at the spermatid stage, then varicocele repair can be recommended. Since patients with Sertoli-cell-only [22, 25, 29, 58, 59] or early maturation arrest [22, 29] have very low chances of the appearance of spermatozoa in the ejaculate following varicocele repair, they should be counseled cautiously despite data suggesting some men with Sertoli-cell-only pattern may improve their histopathology with varicocele repair [57].

Men with NOA who have varicocele symptoms such as orchialgia or those whose testis size and consistency and hormonal profile are not consistent with Sertoli-cell-only pattern histopathology may undergo varicocele repair and testicular biopsy simultaneously, both of which can be performed through a single subinguinal incision. The biopsy is used to assist with prognosis.

A meta-analysis demonstrated that the overall return of sperm to the semen following varicocele repair was 30% [34], suggesting that the majority of patients with NOA and a palpable varicocele will ultimately need microTESE for surgical sperm retrieval for use with ART. This prompted the recommendation for testicular sperm retrieval as well as a diagnostic testicular biopsy and cryopreservation of testicular tissue to be performed in one setting to obviate the need for multiple surgical procedures at asynchronous settings.

Sperm Retrieval at the Time of Varicocele Repair Versus Sperm Retrieval 6 months After Varicocele Repair (Pros and Cons)

The rationale for repairing clinical varicoceles in NOA patients is to improve the sperm retrieval rate and the ART outcomes [38]. If the sperm extraction is performed simultaneously with varicocele repair, this beneficial effect will be obviously missed. This simultaneous approach could be suggested for couples with a female partner older than 35 years or with diminished ovarian reserve. However, couples should be informed about the low quality of evidence in favor of varicocele repair in the NOA setting and also the risk of surgical complications that could be increased.

Delayed sperm extraction seems to be the best approach even though there is a lack of comparative studies between simultaneous and delayed strategies.

Varicocele repair has no specific contraindication in NOA patients. Microsurgical subinguinal varicocele repair is a minimally invasive procedure with low complication rates in experienced hands; patients should be advised about complications.

Counseling the Couple on Odds of Pregnancy Following Varicocele Repair in NOA Men

A meta-analysis approximated the overall return of spermatozoa in the semen following varicocele repair at 34% when all patterns of testicular histopathology (hypospermatogenesis, maturation arrest, and Sertoli-cell-only) were included. Excluding men with Sertoli-cell-only improved the overall rate of sperm returning to the ejaculate following varicocele repair to 54% [34]. The recovery of spermatogenesis after varicocele surgery in NOA cases obviates the need for surgical sperm retrieval for ART in a proportion of patients, which is very beneficial for the patient. Live birth rates with ejaculated sperm after varicocele repair have been reported in three studies [21, 54, 60]. Elzanaty et al. published a meta-analysis indicating that 13.6% of couples achieved pregnancy with timed intercourse after having sperm return to the semen after varicocele repair [34].

Publications have demonstrated improvement in clinical pregnancy rates and live birth rates in ART cycles using testicular surgically retrieved sperm following varicocele repair. Inci et al. revealed that clinical pregnancy rates of 31.4% vs 22.4% and live birth rates of 25.7% vs 22.2% were not statistically different in the varicocele-repaired versus varicocele-intact patients, respectively [53]. Conversely, both clinical pregnancy rates (74.4% vs 52.3%; $P = 0.03$) and live birth rates (64.5% vs 41.5%; $P = 0.02$) were significantly higher in the varicocele-repaired group in the publication by Haydardedeoglu et al. [52]. Several studies have reported significant improvement in sperm retrieval rates in cases following varicocele repair prior to surgical sperm retrieval. Inci et al. demonstrated a surgical sperm retrieval rate of 53% in varicocele-repaired compared with 30% in varicocele-intact patients (OR: 2.63; 95% CI: 1.05–6.60; $P = 0.036$) [53].

Professional Guideline Statements on Varicoceles in Men with NOA

The American Urological Association/American Society for Reproductive Medicine (AUA/ASRM) guideline statement regarding men with NOA and a varicocele states, "The couple should be informed of the absence of definitive evidence supporting varicocele repair prior to assisted reproductive technology" [61]. The European Association of Urology (EUA) guidelines state regarding NOA men with varicoceles that varicocele repair may allow for the return of sperm to the ejaculate in 20.8–55% of these men. They also state that varicocele repair results in improved surgical sperm retrieval rate in cases where men remain azoospermic following varicocele repair. The EUA statement does caution that this data is from observational studies and recommends discussing the risks and benefits of varicocele repair with the man with a clinically palpable varicocele and NOA [62]. Yan et al. published a study suggesting that guidelines should be revised to recommend varicocele repair in men with NOA based on the current level of data available in the medical literature [63].

Expert Opinion on Varicocele Repair in Men with NOA

The data on varicocele repair in men with NOA is conflicting and limited. NOA men should only have varicocele repair considered when there is a large, clinically palpable varicocele. A man without a palpable varicocele on physical examination should not have an ultrasound obtained for the purpose of trying to identify a varicocele. Shared decision-making between the clinician and the patient should include a discussion of the risks, benefits, and alternatives. If sperm appears in the semen following varicocele repair, cryopreservation should be recommended, as there are reported cases of relapse to azoospermia [29]. An additional option to consider is percutaneous needle biopsy for histopathological analysis and, if sperm are present, for cryopreservation. The histopathology may guide the option of varicocele repair in cases with more favorable histological patterns. In cases where varicocele repair is performed without a preoperative biopsy, a biopsy may be considered at the time of varicocele repair to establish a histopathologic diagnosis, and if sperm are present, they can be cryopreserved at that time. Controversy still remains about varicocele repair in men with NOA, highlighted by the survey by Shah et al., revealing that 15% of respondents reported they never recommend varicocele repair in men with NOA, and 35% reported advising varicocele repair in less than 10% of their patients with NOA. At present, shared decision-making between the physician and patient is recommended due to the lack of well-controlled studies in this patient population [64].

Conclusions

Considering that 1% of men presenting for primary infertility evaluations will be found to be azoospermic and 40% will have clinical varicoceles on physical examination, the overlap of clinical varicoceles and azoospermia is not uncommonly seen in reproductive practices. Counseling on options for these men and couples based on the level of data available is important. After a complete reproductive assessment has ruled out other causes of azoospermia, it is appropriate to discuss varicocele repair as a potential next step. This intervention may improve spermatogenesis sufficiently to allow for the presence of sperm in the semen, and in cases where sperm do not return to the ejaculate, it may optimize surgical sperm retrieval and improve pregnancy outcomes. Consideration of the female partners' age and ovarian reserve status is critical in the shared decision-making process for the ultimate goal of live birth (Fig. 10.1).

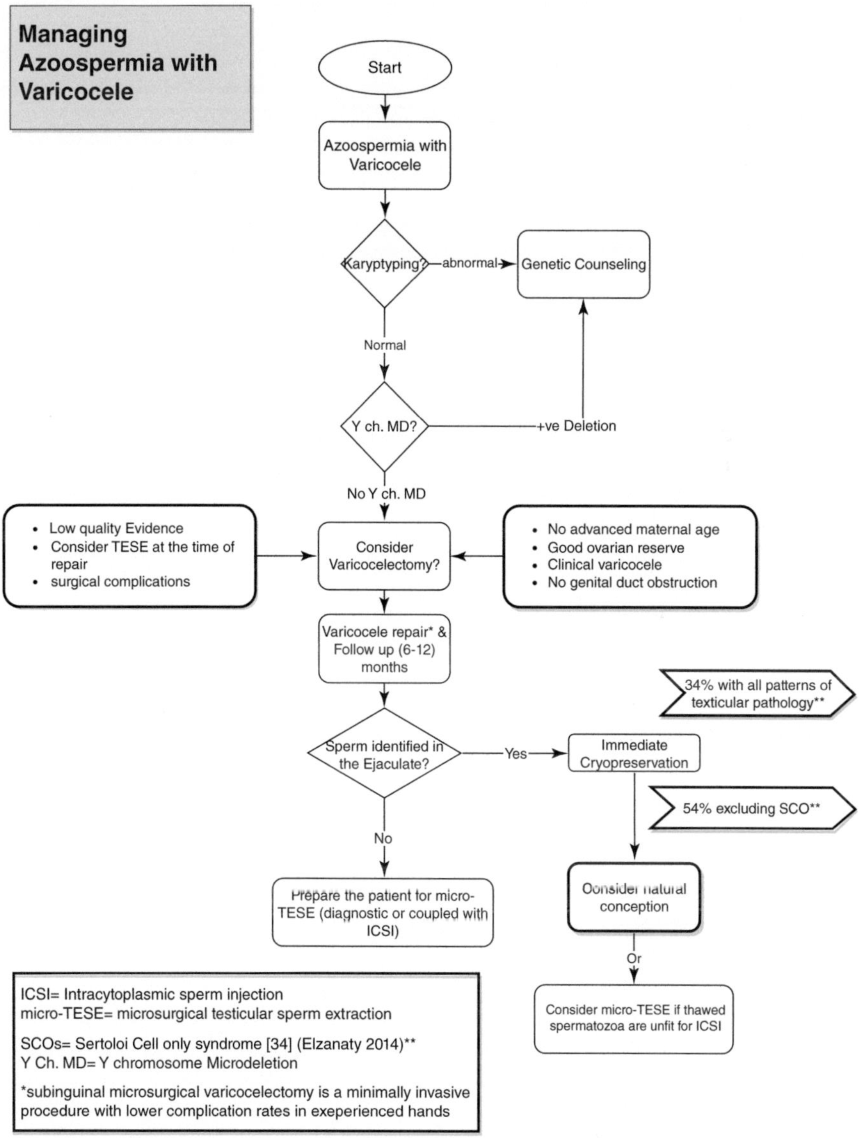

Fig. 10.1 Suggested decision-making algorithm for men with nonobstructive azoospermia and a palpable varicocele

References

1. Thonneau P, et al. Incidence and main causes of infertility in a resident population (1,850,000) of three French regions (1988-1989). Hum Reprod. 1991;6(6):811–6.
2. Willott GM. Frequency of azoospermia. Forensic Sci Int. 1982;20(1):9–10.
3. Jarow JP, Espeland MA, Lipshultz LI. Evaluation of the azoospermic patient. J Urol. 1989;142(1):62–5.
4. WHO. WHO laboratory manual for the examination of human semen and semen-cervical mucus interaction. New York: Cambridge University Press; 2010.
5. Nagler HM, Luntz RK, Martinis FG. Varicocele. Infertility in the male. St. Louis: Mosby Year Book; 1997. p. 336–59.
6. Zorgniotti AW, Macleod J. Studies in temperature, human semen quality, and varicocele. Fertil Steril. 1973;24(11):854–63.
7. Goldstein M, Eid JF. Elevation of intratesticular and scrotal skin surface temperature in men with varicocele. J Urol. 1989;142(3):743–5.
8. Masson P, Brannigan RE. The varicocele. Urol Clin North Am. 2014;41(1):129–44.
9. Smith R, et al. Increased sperm DNA damage in patients with varicocele: relationship with seminal oxidative stress. Hum Reprod. 2006;21(4):986–93.
10. Bertolla RP, et al. Sperm nuclear DNA fragmentation in adolescents with varicocele. Fertil Steril. 2006;85(3):625–8.
11. Enciso M, et al. Infertile men with varicocele show a high relative proportion of sperm cells with intense nuclear damage level, evidenced by the sperm chromatin dispersion test. J Androl. 2006;27(1):106–11.
12. Agarwal A, Makker K, Sharma R. Clinical relevance of oxidative stress in male factor infertility: an update. Am J Reprod Immunol. 2008;59(1):2–11.
13. Blumer CG, et al. Sperm nuclear DNA fragmentation and mitochondrial activity in men with varicocele. Fertil Steril. 2008;90(5):1716–22.
14. Pasqualotto FF, et al. Semen quality and oxidative stress scores in fertile and infertile patients with varicocele. Fertil Steril. 2008;89(3):602–7.
15. Wu GJ, et al. Apoptosis-related phenotype of ejaculated spermatozoa in patients with varicocele. Fertil Steril. 2009;91(3):831–7.
16. El-Domyati MM, et al. The expression and distribution of deoxyribonucleic acid repair and apoptosis markers in testicular germ cells of infertile varicocele patients resembles that of old fertile men. Fertil Steril. 2010;93(3):795–801.
17. Hassan A, el-Nashar EM, Mostafa T. Programmed cell death in varicocele-bearing testes. Andrologia. 2009;41(1):39–45.
18. Camoglio FS, et al. Varicocele and retrograde adrenal metabolites flow. An experimental study on rats. Urol Int. 2004;73(4):337–42.
19. North MO, et al. Reversible meiotic abnormalities in azoospermic men with bilateral varicocele after microsurgical correction. Cell Mol Biol (Noisy-le-Grand). 2004;50(3):281–9.
20. Matthews GJ, Matthews ED, Goldstein M. Induction of spermatogenesis and achievement of pregnancy after microsurgical varicocelectomy in men with azoospermia and severe oligoasthenospermia. Fertil Steril. 1998;70(1):71–5.
21. Kim ED, et al. Varicocele repair improves semen parameters in azoospermic men with spermatogenic failure. J Urol. 1999;162(3 Pt 1):737–40.
22. Cakan M, Altug U. Induction of spermatogenesis by inguinal varicocele repair in azoospermic men. Arch Androl. 2004;50(3):145–50.
23. Karayi MK, Maraj BH. Re: effect of varicocelectomy on patients with unobstructive azoospermia and severe oligospermia. BJU Int. 2008;101(9):1181. author reply 1181
24. Ishikawa T, et al. Effect of varicocelectomy on patients with unobstructive azoospermia and severe oligospermia. BJU Int. 2008;101(2):216–8.
25. Lee JS, Park HJ, Seo JT. What is the indication of varicocelectomy in men with nonobstructive azoospermia? Urology. 2007;69(2):352–5.

26. Saleh R, et al. Histopathologic patterns of testicular biopsies in infertile azoospermic men with varicocele. Fertil Steril. 2010;94(6):2482–5. 2485 e1-2
27. Weedin JW, Khera M, Lipshultz LI. Varicocele repair in patients with nonobstructive azoospermia: a meta-analysis. J Urol. 2010;183(6):2309–15.
28. Youssef T, et al. Varicocelectomy in men with nonobstructive azoospermia: is it beneficial? Int J Surg. 2009;7(4):356–60.
29. Abdel-Meguid TA. Predictors of sperm recovery and azoospermia relapse in men with nonobstructive azoospermia after varicocele repair. J Urol. 2012;187(1):222–6.
30. Esteves SC, Miyaoka R, Agarwal A. Surgical treatment of male infertility in the era of intracytoplasmic sperm injection – new insights. Clinics (Sao Paulo). 2011;66(8):1463–78.
31. Saleh R, Agarwal A, Farouk H. A rational approach to the management of varicocele-associated nonobstructive azoospermia. Fertil Steril. 2011;95(2):489–90.
32. Elzanaty S. Non-obstructive azoospermia and clinical varicocele: therapeutic options. Int Urol Nephrol. 2013;45(3):669–74.
33. Inci K, Gunay LM. The role of varicocele treatment in the management of non-obstructive azoospermia. Clinics (Sao Paulo). 2013;68(Suppl 1):89–98.
34. Elzanaty S. Varicocele repair in non-obstructive azoospermic men: diagnostic value of testicular biopsy – a meta-analysis. Scand J Urol. 2014;48(6):494–8.
35. Aboutaleb HA, et al. Testicular biopsy histopathology as an indicator of successful restoration of spermatogenesis after varicocelectomy in non-obstructive azoospermia. World J Mens Health. 2014;32(1):43–9.
36. Esteves SC, et al. Outcome of varicocele repair in men with nonobstructive azoospermia: systematic review and meta-analysis. Asian J Androl. 2016;18(2):246–53.
37. Alves LS, Oliveira FB. Should azoospermic patients with varicocele disease undergo surgery to recover fertility? Rev Assoc Med Bras (1992). 2017;63(4):332–5.
38. Sajadi H, et al. Varicocelectomy May Improve Results for Sperm Retrieval and Pregnancy Rate in Non-Obstructive Azoospermic Men. Int J Fertil Steril. 2019;12(4):303–5.
39. Tian RH, et al. Efficacy and safety study of microsurgical varicocelectomy in the treatment of non-obstructive azoospermia with varicocele. Zhonghua Yi Xue Za Zhi. 2018;98(46):3737–40.
40. Jensen S, Ko EY. Varicocele treatment in non-obstructive azoospermia: a systematic review. Arab J Urol. 2021;19(3):221–6.
41. Kaltsas A, et al. Varicoceles in men with non-obstructive azoospermia: the dilemma to operate or not. Front Reprod Health. 2022;4:811487.
42. Schlegel PN, Goldstein M. Alternate indications for varicocele repair: non-obstructive azoospermia, pain, androgen deficiency and progressive testicular dysfunction. Fertil Steril. 2011;96(6):1288–93.
43. Shiraishi K, Oka S, Matsuyama H. Predictive factors for sperm recovery after varicocelectomy in men with nonobstructive azoospermia. J Urol. 2017;197(2):485–90.
44. Pasqualotto FF, et al. Induction of spermatogenesis in azoospermic men after varicocelectomy repair: an update. Fertil Steril. 2006;85(3):635–9.
45. Zhi EL, et al. Seminal plasma miR-192a: a biomarker predicting successful resolution of nonobstructive azoospermia following varicocele repair. Asian J Androl. 2018;
46. Dada R, et al. Azoospermia factor deletions in varicocele cases with severe oligozoospermia. Indian J Med Sci. 2007;61(9):505–10.
47. Czaplicki M, Bablok L, Janczewski Z. Varicocelectomy in patients with azoospermia. Arch Androl. 1979;3(1):51–5.
48. Mehan DJ. Results of ligation of internal spermatic vein in the treatment of infertility in azoospermic patients. Fertil Steril. 1976;27(1):110–4.
49. Kadioglu A, et al. Microsurgical inguinal varicocele repair in azoospermic men. Urology. 2001;57(2):328–33.
50. Gat Y, et al. Induction of spermatogenesis in azoospermic men after internal spermatic vein embolization for the treatment of varicocele. Hum Reprod. 2005;20(4):1013–7.

51. Schlegel PN, Kaufmann J. Role of varicocelectomy in men with nonobstructive azoospermia. Fertil Steril. 2004;81(6):1585–8.
52. Haydardedeoglu B, et al. The effect of prior varicocelectomy in patients with nonobstructive azoospermia on intracytoplasmic sperm injection outcomes: a retrospective pilot study. Urology. 2010;75(1):83–6.
53. Inci K, et al. Sperm retrieval and intracytoplasmic sperm injection in men with nonobstructive azoospermia, and treated and untreated varicocele. J Urol. 2009;182(4):1500–5.
54. Kirac M, Deniz N, Biri H. The effect of microsurgical varicocelectomy on semen parameters in men with non-obstructive azoospermia. Curr Urol. 2013;6(3):136–40.
55. Zampieri N, et al. Relationship between testicular sperm extraction and varicocelectomy in patients with varicocele and nonobstructive azoospermia. Urology. 2013;82(1):74–7.
56. Kirby EW, et al. Undergoing varicocele repair before assisted reproduction improves pregnancy rate and live birth rate in azoospermic and oligospermic men with a varicocele: a systematic review and meta-analysis. Fertil Steril. 2016;106(6):1338–43.
57. Ustuner M, et al. Varicocele repair improves testicular histology in men with nonobstructive azoospermia. Biomed Res Int. 2015;2015:709452.
58. Cocuzza M, et al. Use of subinguinal incision for microsurgical testicular biopsy during varicocelectomy in men with nonobstructive azoospermia. Fertil Steril. 2009;91(3):925–8.
59. Esteves SC, Glina S. Recovery of spermatogenesis after microsurgical subinguinal varicocele repair in azoospermic men based on testicular histology. Int Braz J Urol. 2005;31(6):541–8.
60. Poulakis V, et al. Induction of spermatogenesis in men with azoospermia or severe oligoteratoasthenospermia after antegrade internal spermatic vein sclerotherapy for the treatment of varicocele. Asian J Androl. 2006;8(5):613–9.
61. Schlegel PN, et al. Diagnosis and treatment of infertility in men: AUA/ASRM guideline part II. Fertil Steril. 2021;115(1):62–9.
62. Salonia ABC, Boeri L, Capogrosso P, Carvalho J, Cilesiz NC, et al. EAU Working Group on Male Sexual and Reproductive Health. European Association of Urology guidelines on sexual and reproductive health-2021 update: male inferility. Eur Urol. 2021;80:603–20.
63. Yan S, et al. Should the current guidelines for the treatment of varicoceles in infertile men be re-evaluated? Hum Fertil (Camb). 2021;24(2):78–92.
64. Shah R, et al. Consensus and diversity in the management of varicocele for male infertility: results of a global practice survey and comparison with guidelines and recommendations. World J Mens Health. 2023;41(1):164–97.

Chapter 11
Surgical Approaches for Sperm Retrieval

Wael Zohdy, Nazim Gherabi, and Ponco Birowo

Testicular Anatomy

The testes represent the male sex glands that serve endocrine and exocrine functions. They are located in the scrotal sac and separated by a septum. Each testis is smooth, soft, and measures approximately 5 × 3 cm. The testicles are suspended by the spermatic cord and attached to the scrotum by the scrotal ligament (a remnant of the gubernaculum). In general, the left testis is positioned slightly lower than the right testis [1].

Two layers of the peritoneum surround the testis and the epididymis. These layers are known as the tunica vaginalis. During the second and third embryonic months, the tunica vaginalis extends into the scrotum [2]. The inner (visceral) layer of the tunica vaginalis is close to the epididymis, testes, and vas deferens. The sinus of the epididymis is a tiny space located between the body of the epididymis and the testis. The tough and durable layer represents the fibrous covering of the testes and is deep to the tunica vaginalis [3].

The epididymis is a highly convoluted and tightly compressed tubule. Its length is estimated to be around 20 feet. The epididymis is situated on the posterior aspect of the testis and consists of three parts: the head (caput), which receives sperm and testicular fluid from the efferent ducts; the body (corpus), and the tail (cauda). Because of its length, the epididymis can store a significant number of maturing sperm cells [3].

W. Zohdy (✉)
Department of Andrology, Cairo University, Cairo, Egypt

N. Gherabi
University of Algiers Benyoucef Benkhedda, Algiers, DZ, Algeria

P. Birowo
Faculty of Medicine, Department of Urology, Universitas Indonesia-Cipto Mangunkusumo Hospital, Jakarta, Indonesia

W. Zohdy et al. (eds.), *Non-Obstructive Azoospermia*,
https://doi.org/10.1007/978-3-031-99431-9_11

The testes start their descent into the inguinal canal during the third trimester and then to their final scrotal destination. Consequently, the inguinal canal contains the processus vaginalis, which is a structure that develops from the peritoneum. Failure of its closure may result in communicating hydrocele and inguinal hernia.

During the third trimester of pregnancy, the testes, which are located in the abdomen, start their descent into the inguinal canal and then to their final destination in the scrotum. During this journey, they pass through the peritoneum, the abdominal wall, and the inguinal canal. During development, the inguinal canal contains the processus vaginalis, which is a structure that develops from the peritoneum. It allows the testes to descend and then eventually undergoes apoptosis and becomes the tunica vaginalis, which surrounds part of the testis. Failure of the closure of the processus vaginalis may lead to complications such as communicating hydrocele and inguinal hernia [4].

The testicular artery represents the main blood supply of the testis. The cremasteric and the vas deferens arteries supplement its blood flow [5]. Moreover, the upper polar, mediastinum testis, and posterolateral segments are rich vascular areas. The intratesticular arterial supply is mainly provided by two sets of arteries—branches of the testicular arteries. The first set consists of the predominant superficial arteries that course through the tunica albuginea and penetrate the parenchyma from the anterior testicular border. The second set comprises centrifugal transmediastinal blood vessels crossing the mediastinum testis and heading to the periphery (toward the anterior border) [6]. Achermann and their colleague explained in their review that these anatomical observations are crucial during mTESE because the tunica albuginea is widely incised to ensure adequate exploration of the testicular parenchyma and find active spermatogenic foci that are deeply located in the testicular lobes and consequently securing the testicular blood flow and minimizing segmental devascularization [7].

Surgical Sperm Retrieval

In Obstructive Azoospermia

Earlier, reconstructive surgery was the only way to treat men with obstructive azoospermia [8]. Reconstructive surgery is not possible in certain conditions, such as congenital bilateral absence of the vas deferens (CBAVD), failed prior reconstruction [9, 10], or multiple genital duct obstructions as seen in genitourinary tuberculosis [11]. Sperm retrieval in men with obstructive azoospermia is easier and always successful. The harvested sperm could be used for in vitro fertilization by using a micro-pipette to aspirate the sperm from a punctured epididymal ductule [12]. Men with CBAVD could have their sperm retrieved through microsurgical epididymal sperm aspiration (MESA) [13] or by simply aspirating sperm from the exposed epididymis with a 26-G needle without any microsurgical dissection (OFNA) [14].

In 1994, Shrivastav and colleagues suggested percutaneous epididymal sperm aspiration (PESA) [15]. The testis could also be an excellent source for sperm cells when ICSI is planned [16, 17, 18, 19].

In Nonobstructive Azoospermia

Conventional Testicular Sperm Extraction (C-TESE)

This technique is performed through a scrotal approach where the testis is exposed and a smaller incision(s) are performed in the tunica albuginea to excise the protruding tissues. This approach is simple, doesn't require microsurgical skills, and harvests a significant amount of tissue for processing and sperm extraction [20]. However, this technique is open as compared to the closed aspiration approach. Moreover, the indiscriminate incisions in the tunica albuginea may injure subtunical vessels and the end arteries and may result in impaired gonadal function [21, 22, 23, 24]. Another study by Dadkhah and coworkers ($n = 741$ patients) used the multibiopsy approach and found that sperm retrieval rates ranged from 44% for a single biopsy to 58% for four biopsies [25].

Testicular Sperm Aspiration and Fine Needle Aspiration (TESA & FNA) Including Imaging-Guided Retrieval

TESA is performed using an 18–23-G butterfly needle jabbed around the testicular parenchyma. The assistant ensures a suction with a 20-ml syringe. The aspirated fluid is examined for spermatozoa [26]. However, the blind nature of the procedure means there is a risk of puncturing a tunical vessel and causing a hematocele. Therefore, Belenky and colleagues refined this approach by deploying color Doppler ultrasonography to avoid intratesticular vascular injury and subsequently reduce hematoma formation [27]. Testicular sperm aspiration is relatively simple, rapid, and cost-effective and doesn't need microsurgical skills or expensive equipment [9, 10]. Multiple needle-pass percutaneous testicular sperm aspiration has been suggested as first-line treatment in azoospermic men with a reasonable sperm retrieval rate (SRR) of 30% and a 3% complication rate [28]. Nevertheless, multiple passages of the needle through the testicular parenchyma may result in substantial damage to the seminiferous tubules with a relatively scanty cellular material [29, 9, 10]. Although some investigators reported comparable results between TESA and TESE [30], others reported that TESA has often failed to retrieve spermatozoa in men with NOA in whom sperm could be found when the testicular biopsy was examined [9, 10]. Smaller gauge needles have been described. Lewin et al. used a 23-gauge butterfly needle connected to a 20-ml syringe with an aspiration handle. Using this approach, they performed an average of 15 punctures and aspirations per testis, a technique referred to as testicular fine needle aspiration (TEFNA). The authors suggested that this technique could be considered the first choice whenever sperm recovery is attempted in men with nonobstructive azoospermia [31]. Jarvis and colleagues evaluated the ability of fine-needle aspiration (FNA) mapping to find spermatozoa and to guide sperm extraction after failed microdissection testicular sperm extraction (m-TESE). The authors reported that in a significant proportion of failed m-TESE procedures, sperm were detected by FNA mapping and could be reliably retrieved through an FNA map-guided approach. They also claimed that sperm were more likely to be found in the testis periphery rather than centrally with FNA mapping [32]. Contrast-enhanced ultrasound (CEUS) has been reported to recognize major perfusion areas by cognitive fusion and the quantitative CEUS features. The authors concluded that CEUS-guided TESA with cognitive fusion cannot yield improved sperm recovery outcomes of TESA in men with NOA, possibly because of an imprecise correlation between biopsy sites and the main perfusion area analyzed by CEUS; however, they observed that quantitative CEUS features can be useful predictors of TESA success [33].

Microdissection Testicular Sperm Extraction (m-TESE)

Soon after the description of multibiopsy TESE, m-TESE was developed by Schlegel [34] and then by Amer et al. [35], which allowed improved localization of testicular sperm with the aid of intraoperative microscopy (Fig. 11.1). m-TESE was developed from observing that seminiferous tubules with active spermatogenesis seem bigger and opaque under magnification than those with inactive production (Fig. 11.2). In terms of procedure, the testicle is exposed in a fashion like that of a standard. However, a much larger longitudinal or equatorial incision is made through the tunica albuginea over the full length or width of the testicle, and the testicular parenchyma is wholly extruded through this incision. The exposed seminiferous tubules are studied by operative microscopy and are selectively biopsied for sperm [36, 37].

Several modifications have been developed to maximize surgical sperm retrieval. Investigators explored the combination of trifocal TESE with mTESE in low-chance retrieval NOA (Fig. 11.2). In trifocal TESE, the tunica albuginea of the testis is

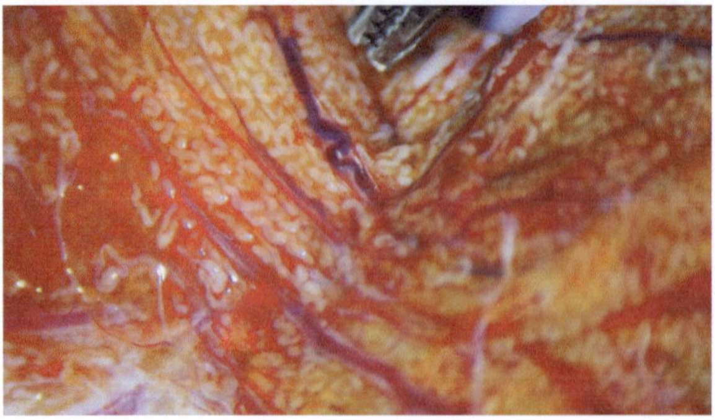

Fig. 11.1 Testicular tissue under optical magnification. The image shows that intraparenchymal blood vessels are well visualized, and injuries could be avoided

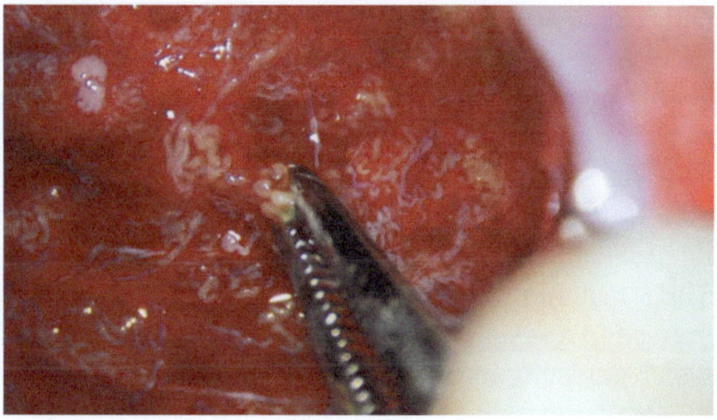

Fig. 11.2 Well-defined dilated tubules under optical magnification within surrounding tissue of atretic (collapsed) tubules

exposed, and three incisions are placed at the upper pole, midline, and lower pole of the testis. The authors claimed that the combined trifocal and m-TESE approach is safe and may increase the sperm retrieval rate significantly [38, 39].

As shown in Fig. 11.2, in m-TESE, a magnification of 20–25× is achieved using an operative optic microscope to identify the more dilated, opaque, and whitish seminiferous tubules, which are often located near blood vessels. In trifocal TESE, three incisions are placed at the upper, middle, and lower poles of the testis [38].

Another innovative approach was reported by Ichioka et al. [40], who proposed maximizing the surface area coverage by performing a longitudinal incision on the tunica albuginea and following transverse slicing incisions of testicular parenchyma. The authors claim that the new technique increased the sperm retrieval rate from 29% to 45%. Furthermore, they reported that transverse resections of parenchyma run parallel to the courses of intratesticular arteries and will not interfere with testicular blood flow. Although the authors noted that postoperative pain was comparable to the ordinary m-TESE, they did not include information on gonadal functions after surgery.

The objective measurement of the seminiferous tubule diameter during m-TESE was suggested by Amer et al. The technique minimizes the harvested tissues, resulting in a single-tubule biopsy to retrieve sufficient spermatozoa. The authors observed that m-TESE is often successful when the seminiferous tubules measure 300 microns or more [41]. Unfortunately, objective assessment may not be helpful in many cases. Therefore, other investigators focused their research on the relationship between seminiferous tubule caliber patterns and surgical sperm retrieval [42]. They suggested that spermatozoa may be retrieved even from slightly dilated tubules in about half of the cases. The pattern of tubules retrieved, together with histology, may represent an additional outcome measure of m-TESE [42].

Franco et al. [43] described a stepwise m-TESE approach in 64 poor-prognosis NOA men undergoing sperm retrieval for ICSI. The technique consisted of three steps: (1) single conventional TESE biopsy; (2) micro-TESE on the same testis; and (3) contralateral multiple TESE. The SRR was 28.1% (18/64). Sperm was obtained in both the initial single conventional TESE and in the following m-TESE. The positive or negative sperm retrieval was further confirmed by a contralateral multiple TESE. The stepwise m-TESE approach was considered to reduce the cost, time, and effort associated with the surgery. Recently, Li et al. [44, 45] conducted a retrospective study on 20 NOA men with a history of orchidopexy for whom a modified stepwise mini-incision m-TESE was employed. The technique consisted of three steps: (1) mini-incision m-TESE; (2) standard m-TESE of the ipsilateral testis; (3) contralateral m-TESE. The overall sperm retrieval rate (SRR) was 80% (16/20). In 50% of patients (10/20), mini-incision m-TESE alone was required because of the rapid identification of spermatozoa harvested from the superficial testicular tissue. The remaining ten patients underwent a standard m-TESE, and four patients progressed to a bilateral m-TESE. The modified stepwise mini-incision micro-TESE, which gradually increases surgical invasiveness, may represent an optimal approach for sperm retrieval for patients affected by NOA with a history of orchidopexy. The modified stepwise m-TESE approach was considered to reduce the time and effort associated with the surgical treatment [44, 45].

Evolution of m-TESE

The use of robotic assistance for m-TESE offers real-time synchronous imaging of the testicular tissue and evaluation by the embryologist while the surgeon is operating [46]. The approach is helpful in identifying areas or tubules that may be more likely to harbor spermatozoa. As future sperm imaging detection techniques evolve, such as Raman spectroscopy [47] and multiphoton microscopy [48], integration of this technology will be easier with the robotic platform. Intuitive Surgical, Inc. (Sunnyvale, CA, USA) offers a four-arm da Vinci-type Si robotic system with high-definition digital visual magnification (up to 310–315). The left and right arms are loaded with Black Diamond microforceps [49]. The fourth arm offers the microsurgeon an additional tool, such as Micro Potts Scissors [50]. Robotic assistance for microsurgical procedures has potential practical benefits, including reduction of tremors, high-quality, 3-dimensional visualization, improved surgeon comfort, reduced morbidity associated with microsurgery, and decreased need for skilled surgical assistance [51, 52, 53]. This surgical technique could facilitate real-time simultaneous imaging of the testicular tissue and evaluation by the embryologist while the surgeon is operating. This helps identify areas or tubules that may be more likely to bear sperm, resulting in improved operative workflow and efficiency [51].

Clinical Decisions in SSR

Clinical Factors and Utilities That Favor the Choice or the Approach and Cost Implications

The decision regarding the optimum method for sperm retrieval in azoospermic men depends on several factors:

1. The cause of azoospermia.
2. The gonadal function.

3. Previous surgical sperm retrieval technique and outcome.
4. Testicular location (cryptorchidism).
5. The available resources (skills of the surgeon, equipment).
6. Anesthesia.
7. Patient's decision.
8. The potential risks and complications.
9. The cost of the procedure and the insurance coverage.

Table 11.1 discusses the above factors and matches them to a suggested approach. We need to brainstorm regarding the contents of this table.

From the above review, m-TESE seems to be the cornerstone in surgical sperm retrieval, and Fig. 11.3 shows the various approaches used in m-TESE based on the clinical situation and available resources.

The decision to perform diagnostic TESE or to proceed with TESE/ICSI requires extensive counselling and enables a patient-centered approach.

TESE and Sperm Freezing Versus TESE-ICSI (Decision Algorithm)

An essential consideration in the management of NOA is the timing of sperm retrieval. Surgical sperm retrieval can be performed during an IVF cycle to coincide with oocyte retrieval with the intent of using fresh sperm for ICSI. Alternatively, sperm retrieval can be performed before ovarian stimulation with the plan for cryopreservation if sperm are identified for use in future ICSI cycles [54].

Table 11.1 Factors affecting the surgical sperm retrieval approach

Decision criteria	PESA	MESA	TESA	FNA	cTESE	mTESE	Others
Cause of azoospermia	OA	OA	OA/ NOA	OA/ NOA	NOA	NOA	
Gonadal function	NS	NS	NS/DS	NS/ DS	NS/DS	NS/D	Trifocal or 3D simulations
Prev. failed attempt	No	No	NA	NA	Maybe	Yes	Trifocal or 3D simulations
Cryptorchidism	No	No	No	No	Maybe	Maybe	Modified stepwise mini-incision m-TESE
Skills/resources	+	+++	+	+	++	+++	
Anesthesia	L/ None	L/S	L/S	L/S	L/S/G	S/G	
Patients' decision	++	++	++	++	++	++	
Risk	–	+	++	+	++	++	
Cost/time	+	+++	+	+	++	+++	

NS= Normal Spermatogenesis, L=local, S=Spinal, G=General, OA= Obstructive azoospermia, NOA=Non-obstructive azoospermia, PESA= percutaneous epididymal sperm preparation, MESA= Microsurgical epididymal sperm aspiration, FNA= Fine needle aspiration, TESE= Testicular sperm Extraction, cTESE= Conventional TESE, mTESE= Microsurgical TESE

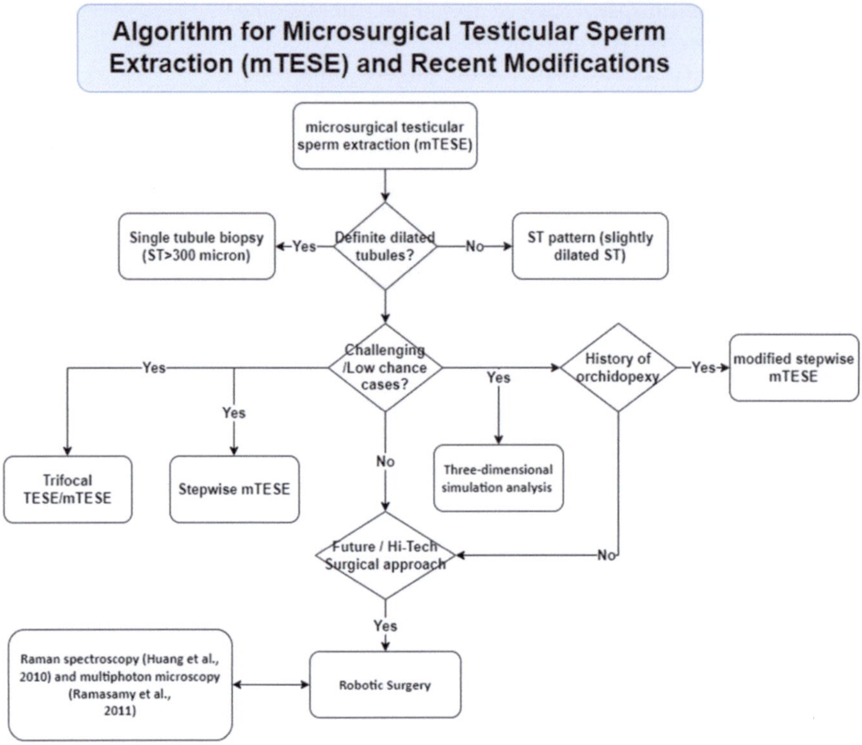

Fig. 11.3 m-TESE in men with NOA. Various approaches and a literature-based algorithm in managing challenging cases of gonadal failure

There are theoretical advantages to each strategy. The use of freshly extracted sperm allows sperm to avoid the stress of cryopreservation. Freezing the extracted sperm for later use separates the timing of the ICSI from sperm extraction so that if sperm is not found, the female partner can potentially avoid unnecessary ovarian stimulation. In addition, both couple members will be undergoing gamete retrieval on separate days, allowing each to help the other rather than involving a third party for transportation/assistance. Moreover, due to the inherent workflows of coordinating an operating room, scheduling a sperm extraction for a precise day or time can be challenging when the exact timing is known only a few days prior. Establishing the efficacy of frozen sperm can also allow men to undergo a single sperm extraction rather than a separate procedure for each cycle [55].

We believe that the decision algorithm in ICSI with synchronous or asynchronous surgical sperm retrieval should follow a patient-centered approach. Interestingly, neither the timing of sperm retrieval (on the day of or the day before oocyte retrieval) nor the use of frozen-thawed testicular sperm affects ICSI outcomes when motile spermatozoa are obtained in azoospermic men. Moreover, the etiology of azoospermia does not influence the result with different timing of the m-TESE procedure for ICSI [56, 57]. However, we are presenting the clinical decision table (Table 11.2) to discuss the cost-effectiveness and risk of sperm loss in advanced cases of NOA and propose alternate pathways that enable a couple-centered approach and improve patients' counseling.

Table 11.2 Major clinical decisions in azoospermic men undergoing ICSI

Male status	Female status	Clinical decision	Advantage/risk	Caution
Obstructive azoospermia	Young with good ovarian reserve	TESE/ICSI and freezing of surplus spermatozoa	Cost-effective	None
Obstructive azoospermia	Advanced maternal age or poor ovarian reserve	TESE second (delays surgical sperm retrieval untill mature oocytes are harvested first), ICSI is performed and surpulus spermatozoa are frozen)	Cost-effective	None
NOA/easy TESE[a]	Young with good ovarian reserve	TESE/ICSI and freezing of surplus spermatozoa	Cost-effective	Low risk of pointless ovarian stimulation[b]
NOA/easy TESE[a]	Advanced maternal age or poor ovarian reserve	TESE 2nd (start with egg collection before TESE and freezing of surplus spermatozoa	Cost-effective	Low risk of pointless ovarian stimulation[b]
NOA/ Difficult TESE[c]	Young with good ovarian reserve	TESE/ICSI and freezing of surplus spermatozoa	Maximize ICSI outcome and avoid the risk of sperm loss during freezing	High risk of pointless ovarian stimulation[b] Oocyte number may exceed sperm number[d]
NOA/difficult TESE[c]	Advanced maternal age or poor ovarian reserve	TESE 2nd (start with egg collection before TESE and freezing of surplus spermatozoa	Maximize ICSI outcome and avoid the risk of sperm loss during freezing	Low risk of having oocytes exceeding the sperm harvested
NOA any status	Not willing to start COS before ensuring sperm availability	ICSI frozen/thawed testicular sperm ± standby TESE during egg collection day[e]	Couple-centered approach	Sperm loss during freezing/ thawing[e]

COS Controlled ovarian stimulation, *NOA* Nonobstructive azoospermia, *TESE* Testicular sperm extraction

[a]NOA/easy TESE: favorable pathology (e.g., hypospermatogenesis), previous successful TESE

[b]Offer oocyte vitrification

[c]Difficult TESE: small size testes, Klinefelter's, KS or XXY, unfavorable pathology (Sertoli cell only or complete maturation arrest), and previous negative or difficult TESE or harvest of few spermatozoa

[d]Offer oocyte vitrification for the remaining un-injected oocytes

[e]In patients with few sperm cells frozen: prepare the male partner of TESE during the egg collection day

Comparison of SRR Techniques in Terms of Pregnancy and LBRs

Fresh vs. Frozen Sperm

ICSI outcomes for patients with NOA were evaluated in a meta-analysis involving 38 studies (14 used fresh sperm, 8 frozen sperm, and 16 used both cryopreserved and fresh sperm). A cumulative pregnancy rate (PR) of 29% per ICSI cycle was revealed as a cumulative LBR of 24% per ICSI cycle. Patients' age, testicular volume, and hormonal parameters did not influence the pregnancy outcome. Fresh testicular spermatozoa yielded a significantly higher pregnancy rate (35%) than cryopreserved sperm (20%). However, when the cumulative LBR per ICSI cycle was analyzed, LBR was 30% for fresh compared to 20% for cryopreserved sperm (not significant) [58]. On the other hand, another meta-analysis gathered data from 11 studies reporting on 275 fresh and 299 frozen cycles in men with NOA revealed no difference between fresh and frozen sperm concerning clinical pregnancy rate (95% CI 0.75–1.33) or fertilization rate (95% CI 0.92–1.02) [55]. Three additional studies, including 401 cycles, could not demonstrate a difference in outcomes between fresh versus frozen sperm in patients with NOA [56, 57, 59, 60]. New existing evidence suggests that testicular sperm in men with cryptozoospermia offers higher embryo quality and implantation rates as compared to ejaculated sperm. Almekaty and colleagues reported outcomes on 141 ICSI cycles and 23 frozen embryo transfers. Clinical pregnancy rates were observed in 62 and LBRs in 37. The longitudinal LBR, crude, and expected cumulative delivery rates after five cycles were 15.5%, 48.7%, and 71.1%, respectively. Reassuringly, there was no significant difference in pregnancy rate ($P = 0.37$) or LBR ($P = 0.68$) using fresh or frozen sperm or embryos ($P = 0.74$). Female age was the only significant predictor of LBR ($P = 0.04$). The authors documented that the longitudinal LBR for a couple embarking on m-TESE is only 15.5%, although the cumulative delivery rates are promising [61].

Sperm Origin and Functional Outcomes for Offspring

With continued success in sperm extraction and the achievement of live birth via IVF/ICSI, there has been an increasing focus on determining which sperm characteristics will lead to the best pregnancy and functional outcomes for offspring. A study in Denmark approached the questions of gamete source location from a developmental standpoint and compared functional outcomes of children born via IVF/ICSI using epididymal versus ejaculated sperm. Children born from epididymal sperm had equivalent motor skills, language skills, and rates of malformation compared with children born with ejaculated sperm [62]. This finding is in contrast with a 2012 report on the higher risk of congenital disabilities compared with children born naturally or even via conventional IVF [63]. Such findings could be explained by bypassing the intrinsic sperm selection processes through the ICSI procedure. In response to this concern, Akerman et al. focused their research on technologies for sperm selection, including the role of DNA fragmentation and sperm selection with microfluidics and nanotechnology [64].

Surgical Sperm Retrieval in Specific Situations

- M-TESE in men with KS and in men with other chromosomal anomalies.
- M-TESE in men with undescended testicles.
- ONCO-TESE and TESE in the context of malignant disease (pending).

Surgical Retrieval in Specific Situations

TESE in Men with KS and in Men with Other Chromosomal Anomalies

Although the surgical sperm retrieval may be lower in patients with Klinefelter syndrome (KS) compared to non-KS counterparts [65], this is still a debated issue, with studies reporting opposite results [66, 67]. It must be pointed out that SSR in KS may be significantly affected by factors like age and serum testosterone level. Hence, the heterogeneity of study populations makes synthesizing studies' results difficult [66].

While the role of adjuvant medical and surgical treatments in improving sperm retrievals in men with NOA was supported by some authors [65], this is still a controversial matter, with studies reporting opposite results [66]. Whereas there is quite a consensus that men with hypogonadism should have their testosterone optimized before attempting surgery, the literature is unable to provide definitive results about the role of hormonal treatment in eugonadal men [66, 68]. Moreover, limited evidence from cohort studies suggests that NOA men with treated varicoceles are more likely to have an SSR than their untreated counterparts [65, 69, 70, 71].

Majzoub and colleagues evaluated the surgical sperm retrieval rate in patients with KS and to investigate the approach associated with the highest SSR. The surgical sperm retrieval was significantly higher in the m-TESE group when compared with the cTESE group (30% versus 0%, respectively). In the m-TESE group, hormonal stimulation was given to 16 patients, while four patients received no treatment. Sperm retrieval was only successful in hormonally treated patients (6/16). The authors explored the type of hormone stimulation and found that sperm retrieval was higher in men receiving aromatase inhibitors (27.8%). They concluded that hormonal stimulation, particularly aromatase enzyme inhibitors, improves m-TESE outcomes [72]. In respect to ICSI outcomes, 88 KS patients were investigated by Vicdan, who reported that the fertilization and clinical pregnancy rates were comparable at 52.7% and 51.6% with fresh and 48.3% and 60% with cryopreserved-thawed testicular spermatozoa groups, respectively. Twenty-two clinical pregnancies were obtained, including 14 singletons, 5 twins, 2 triplets, and 1 quadruplet and ended with the delivery of 13 singletons and 6 twins [73]. Other investigators had reported similar results [74, 75]. Corona et al., in their meta-analysis of 37 articles including 1248 men with KS, suggested that performing TESE/micro-TESE in subjects with KS results in a retrieval rate close to 50%, and then pregnancy rate and live birth rates close to 50%, with the results being independent of any clinical or biochemical parameters tested [76].

TESE in Men with Undescended Testicles

Several factors can predict, to some extent, the TESE outcome in men with cryptorchidism. Chen et al. [77] revealed that four factors, including laterality of cryptorchidism, location of cryptorchidism, age of orchidopexy, and testicular volume, could together preoperatively evaluate the success rate of mTESE for patients with NOA and cryptorchidism. However, Ozan et al. [78], Barbotin et al. [79], and Li et al. [44, 45] reported no significant difference in SRR between cases with a history of bilateral and unilateral cryptorchidism. Osaka et al. [80] reported that testicular volume is a predictor for successful sperm recovery. They noted that the mean testicular volume in men with positive and negative TESE was 11.7 and 7.3 ml, respectively. Marcelli and colleagues reported that FSH level was not a predictor for the presence of sperm on testicular biopsies in non-obstructive azoospermia. Even when combined with testicular volume, the prediction of sperm presence was not improved [81].

Wiser et al. [82] did not find the age of orchidopexy as a predictor of SRR. The authors classified 42 patients into two groups based on orchidopexy done at the age of 10. The authors reported SRRs of 61.9% and 57.1% for those who had the orchidopexy done before and after the age of 10, respectively [82].

Likewise, Osaka et al. [80], in a cohort of 36 men with an SRR of 55.6%, reported that there were no significant differences between TESE-positive and TESE-negative groups regarding age at mTESE, age at orchidopexy, the interval from orchidopexy to TESE, or serum testosterone levels.

Regarding testicular location, Sangster et al. [83] reported an SRR of 33% in inguinal testes compared to 0% in abdominal testes. AlGosaibi et al. [84] observed a lower SRR of 10% in inguinal testes and 0% in abdominal testes. In contrast, Chen et al. [77] reported a higher SRR of 44.8% in inguinal testes versus 27% in abdominal testes. However, other investigators have reported no consistent clinical predictive factors for successful testicular sperm extraction in NOA patients with a history of cryptorchidism [85].

References

1. Tsili AC, Sofikitis N, Stiliara E, Argyropoulou MI. MRI of testicular malignancies. Abdom Radiol (NY). 2019;44(3):1070–82.
2. Oyen RH. Scrotal ultrasound. Eur Radiol. 2002;12:19–34.
3. Tiwana MS, Leslie SW. Anatomy, abdomen and pelvis: testes. 2023. In: StatPearls [Internet]. Treasure Island (FL): StatPearls; 2024. PMID: 29261881.
4. Dagur G, Gandhi J, Suh Y, Weissbart S, Sheynkin YR, Smith NL, Joshi G, Khan SA. Classifying hydroceles of the pelvis and groin: an overview of etiology, secondary complications, evaluation, and management. Curr Urol. 2017 Apr;10(1):1–14.
5. Mostafa T, Labib I, El-Khayat Y, El-Rahman El-Shahat A, Gadallah A. Human testicular arterial supply: gross anatomy, corrosion cast, and radiologic study. Fertil Steril. 2008;90:2226–30.
6. Pais D, Fontoura P, Esperança-Pina JA. The transmediastinal arteries of the human testis: an anatomical study. Surg Radiol Anat. 2004;26:379–83.
7. Achermann APP, Pereira TA, Esteves SC. Microdissection testicular sperm extraction (micro-TESE) in men with infertility due to nonobstructive azoospermia: summary of current literature. Int Urol Nephrol. 2021;53(11):2193–210.
8. Nagy Z, Liu J, Cecile J, Silber S, Devroey P, Van Steirteghem A. Using ejaculated, fresh, and frozen-thawed epididymal and testicular spermatozoa gives rise to comparable results after intracytoplasmic sperm injection. Fertil Steril. 1995;63:808–15.
9. Shah R. Surgical sperm retrieval: techniques and their indications. Indian J Urol. 2011a;27(1):102–9.
10. Hussein TM, Zakaria NH, Zahran AM. Clinical, laboratory and genetic assessment of patients with congenital bilateral absent vas deferens. Andrologia. 2011;43(1):16–22.
11. Kumar R. Reproductive tract tuberculosis and male infertility. Indian J Urol. 2008;24(3):392–5.
12. Temple-Smith PD, Southwick GJ, Yates CA, Trounson AO, de Kretser DM. Human pregnancy by in vitro fertilization (IVF) using sperm aspirated from the epididymis. J In Vitro Fert Embryo Transf. 1985;2:119–22.
13. Patrizio P, Silber S, Ord T, Balmaceda JP, Asch RH. Two births after microsurgical sperm aspiration in congenital absence of vas deferens. Lancet. 1988;2:1364.
14. Shah RS. Recent advances in infertility management. In: Goenka ML, Goenka D, editors. Operative sperm retrieval for ART. Guwahati: Goenka; 2001. p. 179–83.
15. Shrivastav P, Nadkarni P, Wensvoort S, Craft I. Percutaneous epididymal sperm aspiration for obstructive azoospermia. Hum Reprod. 1994;9:2058–61.
16. Craft I, Bennett V, Nicholson N. Fertilising ability of testicular spermatozoa. Lancet. 1993;342:864.
17. Devroey P, Liu J, Nagy Z, Tournaye H, Silber SJ, Van Steirteghem AC. Normal fertilization of human oocytes after testicular sperm extraction and intracytoplasmic sperm injection. Fertil Steril. 1994;62:639–41.
18. Mansour RT, Aboulghar MA, Serour GI, Fahmi I, Ramzy AM, Amin Y. Intracytoplasmic sperm injection using microsurgically retrieved epididymal and testicular sperm. Fertil Steril. 1996;65(3):566–72.
19. Schoysman R, Vanderzwalmen P, Nijs M, Segal L, Segal-Bertin G, Geerts L, et al. Pregnancy after fertilisation with human testicular spermatozoa. Lancet. 1993;342:1237.
20. Devroey P, Liu J, Nagy Z, Goossens A, Tournaye H, Camus M, et al. Pregnancies after testicular sperm extraction and intracytoplasmic sperm injection in non-obstructive azoospermia. Hum Reprod. 1995;10:1457–60.
21. Eliveld J, van Wely M, Meißner A, Repping S, van der Veen F, van Pelt AMM. The risk of TESE-induced hypogonadism: a systematic review and meta-analysis. Hum Reprod Update. 2018;24(4):442–54.
22. Eliveld J, van der Bles I, van Wely M, Meißner A, Soufan AT, Heijboer AC, Repping S, van der Veen F, van Pelt AMM. The risk of hypogonadism after testicular sperm extraction in men with various types of azoospermia: a prospective cohort study. Reprod Biomed Online. 2023;46(6):973–81. https://doi.org/10.1016/j.rbmo.2023.02.003. Epub 2023 Feb 10

23. Manning M, Junemann KP, Alken P. Decrease in testosterone blood concentrations after testicular sperm extraction for intracytoplasmic sperm injection in azoospermic men (letter). Lancet. 1998;352:37.
24. Schlegel PN, Su LM. Physiological consequences of testicular sperm extraction. Hum Reprod. 1997;12:1688–92.
25. Dadkhah F, Hosseini SJ, Gilani MAS, Farrahi F, Amini E, Kazeminejad B. Optimal number of biopsies and impact of testicular histology on the outcome of testicular sperm extraction. Urol J. 2013;10(1):795–801.
26. Turek PJ, Givens CR, Schriock ED, Meng MV, Pedersen RA, Conaghan J. Testis sperm extraction and intracytoplasmic sperm injection guided by prior fine-needle aspiration mapping in patients with non-obstructive azoospermia. Fertil Steril. 1999;71:552–7.
27. Belenky A, Avrech O, Bachar G, Zuckerman Z, Ben Rafael Z, Fisch B, et al. Ultrasound-guided testicular sperm aspiration in azoospermic patients: a new sperm retrieval method for intracytoplasmic sperm injection. J Clin Ultrasound. 2001;29:33.
28. Jensen CF, Ohl DA, Hiner MR, Fode M, Shah T, Smith GD, Sonksen J. Multiple needle-pass percutaneous testicular sperm aspiration as first-line treatment inazoospermic men. Andrology. 2016;4(2):257–62.
29. Friedler S, Raziel A, Strassburger D, Soffer Y, Komarovsky D, Ron-El R. Testicular sperm retrieval by percutaneous fine needle aspiration compared with testicular sperm extraction by open biopsy in men with NOA. Hum Reprod. 1997;12:1488–93.
30. Nowroozi MR, Ahmadi H, Ayati M, Jamshidian H, Sirous A. Testicular fine-needle aspiration versus testicular open biopsy: Comparable sperm retrieval rate in selected patients. Indian J Urol. 2012;28(1):37–42.
31. Lewin A, Reubinoff B, Porat-Katz A, Weiss D, Eisenberg V, Arbel R, Bar-el H, Safran A. Testicular fine needle aspiration: the alternative method for sperm retrieval in non-obstructive azoospermia. Hum Reprod. 1999;14(7):1785–90.
32. Katz MJ, Huland DM, Ramasamy R. Multiphoton microscopy: applications in urology and andrology. Transl Androl Urol. 2014;3(1):77–83.
33. Xue H, Wang SY, Cui LG, Hong K. Can contrast-enhanced ultrasound increase or predict the success rate of testicular sperm aspiration in patients with azoospermia? AJR Am J Roentgenol. 2019;212(5):1054–9.
34. Schlegel PN. Testicular sperm extraction: microdissection improves sperm yield with minimal tissue excision. Hum Reprod. 1999;14:131–5.
35. Amer M, Ateyah A, Hany R, Zohdy W. Prospective comparative study between microsurgical and conventional testicular sperm extraction in non-obstructive azoospermia: follow-up by serial ultrasound examinations. Hum Reprod. 2000;15(3):653–6.
36. Cirigliano L, Falcone M, Gül M, Preto M, Ceruti C, Plamadeala N, Gontero P. Onco-TESE (testicular sperm extraction): insights from a tertiary center and comprehensive literature analysis. Medicina. 2023;59(7):1226.
37. Joshi R, Singh A, Sudharsan SB, Ganpule A, Sabnis RB, Desai MR. Abstracts-USICON 2019. Indian J Urol. 2019;35(Suppl 1):S1–S49.
38. Falcone M, Boeri L, Timpano M, Cirigliano L, Preto M, Russo GI, Peretti F, Ferro I, Plamadeala N, Gontero P. Combined trifocal and microsurgical testicular sperm extraction enhances sperm retrieval rate in low-chance retrieval non-obstructive azoospermia. J Clin Med. 2022;11(14):4058.
39. Marconi M, Keudel A, Diemer T, Bergmann M, Steger K, Schuppe HC, Weidner W. Combined trifocal and microsurgical testicular sperm extraction is the best technique for testicular sperm retrieval in “low-chance” nonobstructive azoospermia. Eur Urol. 2012 Oct;62(4):713–9.
40. Ichioka K, Matsui Y, Terada N, Negoro H, Goto T, Ogawa O. Three-dimensional simulation analysis of microdissection testicular sperm extraction for patients with non-obstructive azoospermia. Andrology. 2020;8(5):1214–21.
41. Amer M, Zohdy W, Abd El Naser T, Hosny H, Arafa M, Fakhry E. Single tubule biopsy: a new objective microsurgical advancement for testicular sperm retrieval in patients with nonobstructive azoospermia. Fertil Steril. 2008;89(3):592–6.

42. Caroppo E, Colpi EM, Gazzano G, Vaccalluzzo L, Piatti E, D'Amato G, Colpi GM. The seminiferous tubule caliber pattern as evaluated at high magnification during microdissection testicular sperm extraction predicts sperm retrieval in patients with non-obstructive azoospermia. Andrology. 2019;7(1):8–14.
43. Franco G, Scarselli F, Casciani V, De Nunzio C, Dente D, Leonardo C, Greco PF, Greco A, Minasi MG, Greco E. A novel stepwise micro-TESE approach in non-obstructive azoospermia. BMC Urol. 2016;16(1):1–8.
44. Li P, Yao CC, Zhi EL, Xu Y, Wan Z, Jiang YC, Huang YH, Gong YH, Chen HX, Tian RH, Yang C. Modified stepwise mini-incision microdissection testicular sperm extraction: a useful technique for patients with a history of orchidopexy affected by non-obstructive azoospermia. J Zhejiang Univ Sci B. 2020a;21(1):87–92.
45. Li S, Zhao Y, Nie M, Ma W, Wang X, Ji W. Clinical characteristics and spermatogenesis in patients with congenital hypogonadotropic hypogonadism caused by FGFR1 mutations. Int J Endocrinol. 2020;2020:8873532.
46. Schlegel PN. Non-obstructive azoospermia: a revolutionary surgical approach and results. Semin Reprod Med. 2009;27:165–70.
47. Huang WE, Li M, Jarvis RM, et al. Shining light on the microbial world the application of Raman microspectroscopy. Adv Appl Microbil. 2010;70:153–86.
48. Ramasamy R, Sterling J, Fisher ES, et al. Identification of spermatogenesis with multiphoton microscopy: an evaluation in a 2011;186:2487–92.
49. Parekattil SJ, Gudeloglu A. Robotic assisted andrological surgery. Asian J Androl. 2013;15(1):67–74.
50. Etafy M, Gudeloglu A, Brahmbhatt JV, Parekattil SJ. Review of the role of robotic surgery in male infertility. Arab J Urol. 2018;16(1):148–56.
51. Darves-Bornoz A, Panken E, Brannigan RE, Halpern JA. Robotic surgery for male infertility. In: Robotic urology: the next frontier, an issue of urologic clinics., E-Book, vol. 5; 2020. p. 127.
52. Gudeloglu A, Brahmbhatt JV, Parekattil SJ. Robotic microsurgery in male infertility and urology – taking robotics to the next level. Transl Androl Urol. 2014;3(1):102–12.
53. Howarth AL, Hallbeck S, Mahabir RC, et al. Workrelated musculoskeletal discomfort and injury in microsurgeons. J Reconstr Microsurg. 2019;35(5):322–8.
54. Fainberg J, Hayden RP, Schlegel PN. Fertility management of Klinefelter syndrome. Expert Rev Endocrinol Metab. 2019;14(6):369–80.
55. Ohlander S, Hotaling J, Kirshenbaum E, Niederberger C, Eisenberg ML. Impact of fresh versus cryopreserved testicular sperm upon intracytoplasmic sperm injection pregnancy outcomes in men with azoospermia due to spermatogenic dysfunction: a metaanalysis. Fertil Steril. 2014;101:344–9.
56. Karacan M, Alwaeely F, Erkan S, Cebi Z, Berberoglugil M, Batukan M, et al. Outcome of intracytoplasmic sperm injection cycles with fresh testicular spermatozoa obtained on the day of or the day before oocyte collection and with cryopreserved testicular sperm in patients with azoospermia. Fertil Steril. 2013a;100:975–80.
57. Karacan M, Alwaeely F, Erkan S, Çebi Z, Berberoğlugil M, Batukan M. Outcome of intracytoplasmic sperm injection cycles with fresh testicular spermatozoa obtained on the day of or the day before oocyte collection and with cryopreserved testicular sperm in patients with azoospermia. Fertil Steril. 2013b;100(4):975–80.
58. Corona G, Minhas S, Giwercman A, Bettocchi C, Dinkelman-Smit M, Dohle G, Fusco F, Kadioglou A, Kliesch S, Kopa Z, Krausz C. Sperm recovery and ICSI outcomes in men with non-obstructive azoospermia: a systematic review and meta-analysis. Hum Reprod Update. 2019;25(6):733–57.
59. Park YS, Lee SH, Lim CK, Cho JW, Yang KM, Seo JT. Effect of testicular spermatozoa on embryo quality and pregnancy in patients with non-obstructive azoospermia. Syst Biol Reprod Med. 2015;61:300–6.
60. Tavukcuoglu S, Al-Azawi T, Al-Hasani S, Khaki AA, Khaki A, Tasdemir S. Using fresh and frozen testicular sperm samples in couples undergoing ICSI MicroTESE treatment. J Reprod Infertil. 2013;14:79–84.

61. Almekaty K, Abomelha S, Thum Y, Nicopoullos J, Bracewell-Milnes T, Yap T, Minhas S. Reporting on longitudinal live birth rates and cumulative delivery rates are more realistic outcome measures than sperm retrieval rates in couples undergoing mTESE-ICSI. Hum Fertil (Camb). 2019;22(2):139–44.
62. Woldringh GH, Horvers M, Janssen AJ, Reuser JJ, de Groot SA, Steiner K, D'Hauwers KW, Wetzels AM, Kremer JA. Follow-up of children born after ICSI with epididymal spermatozoa. Hum Reprod. 2011;26(7):1759–67.
63. Davies MJ, Moore VM, Willson KJ, Van Essen P, Priest K, Scott H, Haan EA, Chan A. Reproductive technologies and the risk of birth defects. N Engl J Med. 2012;366(19):1803–13.
64. Akerman JP, Hayon S, Coward RM. Sperm extraction in obstructive azoospermia: what's next? Urol Clin. 2020;47(2):147–55.
65. Arshad MA, Majzoub A, Esteves SC. Predictors of surgical sperm retrieval in non-obstructive azoospermia: summary of current literature. Int Urol Nephrol. 2020;52(11):2015–38.
66. Colpi GM, Caroppo E. Re: predictors of surgical sperm retrieval in non-obstructive azoospermia: summary of current literature. Int Urol Nephrol. 2020;11:1–3.
67. Dohle GR, Elzanaty S, van Casteren NJ. Testicular biopsy: clinical practice and interpretation. Asian J Androl. 2012;14(1):88–93.
68. Kato Y, Shiraishi K, Matsuyama H. Expression of testicular androgen receptor in non-obstructive azoospermia and its change after hormonal therapy. Andrology. 2014;2(734):740.
69. Esteves SC, Miyaoka R, Roque M, Agarwal A. Outcome of varicocele repair in men with nonobstructive azoospermia: systematic review and meta-analysis. Asian J Androl. 2016;18(2):246–53.
70. Haydardedeoglu B, Turunc T, Kilicdag EB, Gul U, Bagis T. The effect of prior varicocelectomy in patients with nonobstructive azoospermia on intracytoplasmic sperm injection outcomes: a retrospective pilot study. Urology. 2010;75(1):83–6.
71. Inci K, Hascicek M, Kara O, Dikmen AV, Gurgan T, Ergen A. Sperm retrieval and intracytoplasmic sperm injection in men with nonobstructive azoospermia, and treated and untreated varicocele. J Urol. 2009;182(4):1500–5.
72. Majzoub A, Arafa M, Al Said S, Agarwal A, Seif A, Al Naimi A, El Bardisi H. Outcome of testicular sperm extraction in nonmosaic Klinefelter syndrome patients: what is the best approach? Andrologia. 2016;48(2):171–6.
73. Vicdan K, Akarsu C, Sözen E, Buluç B, Vicdan A, Yılmaz Y, Biberoğlu K. Outcome of intracytoplasmic sperm injection using fresh and cryopreserved-thawed testıcular spermatozoa in 83 azoospermic men with Klinefelter syndrome. J Obstet Gynaecol Res. 2016;42(11):1558–66.
74. Greco E, Scarselli F, Minasi MG, Casciani V, Zavaglia D, Dente D, Tesarik J, Franco G. Birth of 16 healthy children after ICSI in cases of nonmosaic Klinefelter syndrome. Hum Reprod. 2013;28(5):1155–60.
75. Madureira C, Cunha M, Sousa M, Neto AP, Pinho MJ, Viana P, Gonçalves A, Silva J, Teixeira da Silva J, Oliveira C, Ferraz L, Dória S, Carvalho F, Barros A. Treatment by testicular sperm extraction and intracytoplasmic sperm injection of 65 azoospermic patients with non-mosaic Klinefelter syndrome with birth of 17 healthy children. Andrology. 2014;2(4):623–31.
76. Corona G, Pizzocaro A, Lanfranco F, Garolla A, Pelliccione F, Vignozzi L, Ferlin A, Foresta C, Jannini EA, Maggi M, Lenzi A, Pasquali D, Francavilla S, Klinefelter Italian Group (KING). Sperm recovery and ICSI outcomes in Klinefelter syndrome: a systematic review and meta-analysis. Hum Reprod Update. 2017;23(3):265–75.
77. Chen XL, Wei YA, Ren XH, Zhang X, Li GY, Lu ZW, et al. Predictive factors for successful sperm retrieval by microdissection testicular sperm extraction in men with nonobstructive azoospermia and a history of cryptorchidism. Asian J Androl. 2022;24(5):503–8.
78. Ozan T, Karakeci A, Kaplancan T, Pirincci N, Firdolas F, Orhan I. Are predictive factors in sperm retrieval and pregnancy rates present in nonobstructive azoospermia patients by microdissection testicular sperm extraction on testicle with a history of orchidopexy operation? Andrologia. 2019;51(11):e13430.

79. Barbotin AL, Dauvergne A, Dumont A, Ramdane N, Mitchell V, Rigot JM, Robin G. Bilateral versus unilateral cryptorchidism in nonobstructive azoospermia: testicular sperm extraction outcomes. Asian J Androl. 2019;21(5):445–51.
80. Osaka A, Iwahata T, Kobori Y, Shimomura Y, Yoshikawa N, Onota S, Okada H. Testicular volume in non-obstructive azoospermia with a history of bilateral cryptorchidism may predict successful sperm retrieval by testicular sperm extraction. Reprod Med Biol. 2020;19(4):372–7.
81. Marcelli F, Mahe P, Soulez B, Herbaut JC, Hermand E, Rigot JM. Testicular sperm extraction in 50 men with nonobstructive azoospermia associated with cryptorchidism: Clinical parameters predictive of successful sperm extraction. Andrologie. 2005;15:19–23.
82. Wiser A, Raviv G, Weissenberg R, Elizur SE, Levron J, Machtinger R, Madgar I. Does age at orchidopexy impact on the results of testicular sperm extraction? Reprod Biomed Online. 2009;19(6):778–83.
83. Sangster P, Alnajjar HM, Ahmed K, Christodoulidou M, Williamson E, Kelly JD, Muneer A. Microdissection TESE (mTESE) following adult orchidopexy for undescended intra-abdominal and inguinal testicles–surgical techniques and outcomes from a single-centre cohort. Andrology. 2020;8(1):166–70.
84. AlGosaibi A, AlMulhim A, AlThekafi S, AlHatha N. Chances of sperm retrieval during testicular sperm extraction in adult cryptorchid testes. Urol Nephrol Open Access J. 2017;4(2):54–6.
85. Vernaeve V, Krikilion A, Verheyen G, Van Steirteghem A, Devroey P, Tournaye H. Outcome of testicular sperm recovery and ICSI in patients with non- obstructive azoospermia with a history of orchidopexy. Hum Reprod. 2004;19(10):2307–12.

Chapter 12
Predictors of Sperm Retrieval for Nonobstructive Azoospermia

Balagobi Balasingam, Baris Altay, and Ramadan Saleh

Introduction

Infertility is one of the trending problems in the population and is becoming a growing subspecialty in medicine. Infertility affects 1 in 6 couples, with 20% of infertility cases solely attributed to male factor, while an additional 30–40% are influenced by male contribution. Azoospermia accounts for 1% of the male population and about 10–15% of all men with infertility. Azoospermia is defined as the complete absence of sperm in two separate centrifuged semen specimens. It should not be mistaken for aspermia, which refers to the total lack of ejaculate [1].

Azoospermia is classified as nonobstructive azoospermia (NOA) and obstructive azoospermia (OA). NOA occurs as a result of impairment of spermatogenesis and is usually categorized by anatomical positions of the cause into pretesticular or testicular types. Pretesticular NOA (hypogonadotropic hypogonadism) is due to hormone abnormalities in which a structurally normal testis is not stimulated properly. This is also known as secondary hypogonadism, where defects in the hypothalamus or pituitary gland result in low testosterone levels due to insufficient stimulation of the Leydig cells. Pretesticular causes of NOA may be congenital, as seen in cases of

B. Balasingam (✉)
Faculty of Medicine, Department of Surgery, University of Jaffna, Jaffna, Sri Lanka

B. Altay
Department of Urology, Ege University School of Medicine, İzmir, Turkey

R. Saleh
Faculty of Medicine, Department of Dermatology, Venereology and Andrology, Sohag University, Sohag, Egypt

Ajyal IVF Center, Ajyal Hospital, Sohag, Egypt

W. Zohdy et al. (eds.), *Non-Obstructive Azoospermia*,
https://doi.org/10.1007/978-3-031-99431-9_12

Kallmann syndrome, Prader–Willi syndrome, and Laurence–Moon syndrome, or acquired, such as tumors, radiation, or trauma to the pituitary or hypothalamus. Additionally, hypogonadotropic hypogonadism may be caused by spermatogenesis suppression by excessive or prolonged use of exogenous steroids or androgens. On the other hand, testicular failure or primary hypogonadism refers to intrinsic defects in the testis leading to impaired spermatogenesis [2].

Primary testicular failure may be due to underlying genetic defects, as in cases of Klinefelter syndrome or Y chromosome microdeletions. Testicular causes of NOA also include cryptorchidism, infection, ischemia, and gonadotoxic exposures [3]. Further details of diagnosis and management of NOA are discussed elsewhere in this book and are not in the scope of this chapter.

Historically, azoospermic men were considered sterile but, with modern advancements in assisted reproductive techniques (ART), particularly intracytoplasmic sperm injection (ICSI), these men are now able to biologically father their own children. The mainstay of treating infertile men with azoospermia is testicular sperm extraction (TESE). Currently, it is combined with ICSI to improve the success rate of fertilization. Testicular sperm aspiration, conventional testicular sperm extraction, and more optimal techniques like microdissection testicular sperm extraction (micro-TESE) have been used for sperm retrieval [2].

In this chapter, we aim to highlight the significance of predictive models in the clinical management of NOA. Additionally, we describe various predictive models developed to improve the success rates of sperm retrieval in those patients. Furthermore, we comprehensively discuss the factors influencing sperm retrieval success in infertile men with NOA.

Importance of Predictive Models in NOA

Challenges in Sperm Retrieval for NOA

Sperm retrieval techniques such as TESE and micro-TESE have revolutionized the field of male infertility by enabling the retrieval of sperm directly from the testes in men with NOA. However, these procedures are not always successful. A systematic review and meta-analysis found an overall SSR rate of 47% in patients with NOA [4]. Additionally, the likelihood of finding sperm can vary significantly among those patients based on individual circumstances. Indeed, this presents a challenge for clinicians in accurately predicting the success rates of sperm retrieval procedures and advising patients on the most appropriate treatment options. Without reliable predictive tools, patients with NOA may undergo invasive procedures with limited chances of success, leading to emotional distress, financial burden, and potential delays in pursuing alternative fertility options such as sperm donation or adoption [3].

Advantages of Predictive Models

Generally, predictive models provide clinicians with objective data to guide patient counselling and treatment decision-making [5]. In the context of NOA, predictive models can offer a valuable solution to overcome the challenges associated with sperm retrieval. By integrating various clinical and histopathological factors, these models can provide a quantitative estimate of the likelihood of finding sperm during the sperm retrieval procedure. The advantages of using predictive models in the management of patients with NOA are described in the following subsections.

Informed Decision-Making

By assessing the probability of successful sperm retrieval, clinicians can discuss the realistic chances of achieving biological fatherhood and help patients make informed choices about the most appropriate course of action.

Patient Selection

Predictive models aid in identifying patients who are more likely to benefit from sperm retrieval procedures. By considering factors such as hormonal profiles, testicular volume, genetic markers, and histopathological findings, these models can stratify patients into different risk categories, allowing clinicians to select those with higher chances of success for the procedure [4]. This targeted approach improves the efficiency of sperm retrieval procedures, reduces unnecessary interventions, and minimizes patient frustration.

Surgical Planning

Knowing the likelihood of finding sperm in advance allows surgeons to plan the surgical approach accordingly. For example, in cases where the chances of sperm retrieval are low, surgeons may opt for micro-TESE instead of conventional TESE due to its higher precision and better visualization of testicular tissue. This tailored surgical planning optimizes the chances of successful sperm retrieval and minimizes surgical complications [6, 7].

Outcome Prediction

Predictive models provide an estimation of the success rates of sperm retrieval procedures, allowing clinicians to discuss the expected outcomes with patients [8]. This information enables couples to manage their expectations, emotionally prepare for potential outcomes, and explore alternative fertility options if necessary.

Research and Development

Predictive models serve as valuable tools for researchers and clinicians to identify new factors and refine existing models. By analyzing the outcomes and predictors, researchers can uncover novel associations, validate the performance of the models, and develop more accurate and robust models in the future [9].

Clinical Significance of Predictive Models

Optimizing the use of predictive models can enhance SSR in patients with NOA and therefore can significantly improve reproductive outcomes of these patients. These models not only enhance patient counselling and treatment decision-making but also improve the overall success rates and cost-effectiveness of sperm retrieval procedures. Attempts to improve their potential to accurately predict the chances of successful SSR, predictive models may help optimize the allocation of healthcare resources and reduce the physical and emotional burden on patients. Additionally, predictive models can help schedule TESE procedures based on the likelihood of successful sperm retrieval. Therefore, busy IVF centers can better manage their staff, ensuring that experienced personnel are available for high-probability cases. Indeed, integrating predictive models will allow IVF centers to allocate resources more effectively and provide a higher standard of care. Furthermore, these models contribute to ongoing research efforts in male infertility by identifying new predictors and improving our understanding of the underlying mechanisms of NOA [4].

In summary, predictive models offer numerous advantages in the context of sperm retrieval for NOA. By providing evidence-based estimates of the likelihood of finding sperm, these models facilitate informed decision-making, improve patient selection, enhance surgical planning, predict outcomes, and contribute to ongoing research. The development and validation of accurate predictive models hold great promise for improving the management and outcomes of men with NOA, ultimately helping them achieve their goal of fatherhood.

Factors Influencing Sperm Retrieval Success

The sperm retrieval rate in patients with NOA differs widely based on several factors, including patient-related factors, techniques used and experience of the performing surgeon, and the experience of the IVF team in handling and processing of harvested testicular tissue. Various studies have been done to formulate predictive models in various settings.

Patient-Related Factors

Age

The impact of age on sperm production has been described in various studies. Spermatogenesis declines with advancing age. Studies have found that there is a significant association between age in sperm retrieval success.

In patients with Klinefelter's syndrome, the success rates of testicular sperm extraction differ between age groups. Specifically, the percentage of successful spermatozoa recovery significantly decreases in those aged 35 years and older compared to those under 35, with the difference being statistically significant [10]. Bernie et al. showed no relationship between male age and micro-TESE results, the overall sperm recovery rate (SRR) was highest in men aged ≥40 years, and there was no upper age limit for men for the success of micro-TESE. There are no studies stating a specific cutoff for age, but some studies have incorporated age in their predictive model [11].

Hormone Levels

Hormones play an important role in spermatogenesis. Testosterone, FSH, and Inhibin B are the most important and studied ones.

Follicle-stimulating hormone is essential for stimulating sperm production within the testicles. In NOA, elevated FSH levels are often observed due to the lack of sperm production. Higher FSH levels usually indicate a poorer prognosis for sperm retrieval. To the contrary, a study by Cissen et al. [12] found low serum FSH levels to be predictive of positive sperm retrieval with TESE.

Inhibin is a glycoprotein secreted by the testicles, which has an inhibitory effect on spermatogenesis. Its levels are found to be low in males with testicular dysfunction, and some studies have advocated its use as a predictive marker for sperm retrieval. However, some studies refute this claim due to its poor sensitivity. These contradictory findings have made the role of inhibin B as a predictive marker controversial. While it may have limited predictive value when used alongside other preoperative markers, we do not use it as a routine evaluation tool in men with NOA prior to sperm retrieval [13].

The predictive value of serum testosterone levels for successful sperm retrieval in men with NOA has been investigated, but findings are inconsistent. Some studies suggest that testosterone levels alone do not significantly correlate with sperm retrieval outcomes. For instance, a study found no significant association between serum testosterone levels and successful micro-TESE outcomes in NOA patients [14].

Conversely, other research indicates that the ratio of testosterone to luteinizing hormone (LH) may have predictive value. A recent study by Kim and Koo reported that a lower testosterone/LH ratio was associated with unsuccessful sperm retrieval, suggesting that this ratio could serve as a potential predictor for sperm retrieval outcomes in NOA patients [15].

Additionally, the AMH to testosterone ratio has been explored as a predictive marker. Research published in Scientific Reports found that a higher AMH-to-testosterone ratio was predictive of positive sperm retrieval in men with idiopathic NOA [16].

In conclusion, while serum testosterone levels alone may not be reliable predictors of sperm retrieval success in NOA, ratios involving testosterone and other hormones like LH and AMH could provide more insight. However, these findings are not universally accepted, and further research is needed to establish definitive predictive markers.

Genetic Factors

The American Urological Association guidelines recommend karyotype and Y-chromosome microdeletion testing for men presenting with NOA or severe oligospermia. Microdeletions in the AZFa and AZFb regions are associated with a worse prognosis, as no man has been reported to have retrievable sperm in these cases. Isolated AZFa deletions are rare but result in a Sertoli cell-only histologic pattern with no sperm, while AZFb deletions are often observed with focal maturation arrest.

Therefore, micro-TESE is not recommended for patients with complete AZFa or AZFb microdeletions. However, patients with deletions in the AZFc region, the most common microdeletion seen, may have rare sperm in the ejaculate or can often achieve successful sperm retrieval with micro-TESE. A study by Stahl et al. demonstrated a 71.4% sperm retrieval rate in men with AZFc deletions, while no sperm was retrieved in those with AZFa, AZFb, AZFb+c, or complete Yq deletions [17].

A study by Cissen et al. [12] indicated that detection of an AZFc deletion has good prognosis for the chances of success with TESE.

Klinefelter syndrome (KS) is the most common genetic abnormality seen in men with infertility. Overall, the SRR ranges from 22.5% to 51.5% in patients with KS [18–21]. A study found that KS patients who responded to preoperative therapy with clomiphene citrate, aromatase inhibitors, HCG, or a combination of these hormonal interventions with increased serum testosterone levels to ≥250 ng/dL had a higher SRR than men who did not respond [6]. Several studies have evaluated factors that influence SRR in Klinefelter patients, including age, testicular volume, or hormone levels, with mixed results.

Cryptorchidism

Cryptorchidism is the most common genital problem encountered in pediatrics. Cryptorchidism literally means hidden or obscure testis and generally refers to an undescended or maldescended testis. Untreated cryptorchidism clearly has deleterious effects on the testis over time. A predictive model using an artificial neural network found the diagnosis of cryptorchidism to be a significant predictor of sperm retrieval. Cryptorchid men tend to have slightly higher sperm retrieval rates (74%)

relative to all other men with NOA (58%) [23]. The age at which the intervention is performed has also been considered a predictor in various studies [23]. The retrieval success rate is higher in males who have undergone orchidopexy before the age of 10 years.

Testicular Volume

Since seminiferous tubules contribute to approximately 80% of testis volume, testicular volume has been classically correlated with spermatogenesis. A meta-analysis evaluating 117 studies found that testis volume significantly predicted sperm retrieval rate. Volume higher than 12.5 mL predicted a retrieval rate of >60%, with a 73% specificity and 74% sensitivity [24]. Even though lower testicular volume has lower predictive value, attempts must be taken to retrieve sperm after proper patient counselling.

Body Mass Index (BMI)

Patients with NOA and an elevated BMI have a high sperm DNA fragmentation index, high FSH levels, low testosterone levels, and low spontaneous pregnancy. However, studies found no relationship between BMI and sperm retrieval rate. The sperm retrieval rate remained almost equal in patients with high, normal, and low BMI [25]. Research indicates that higher BMI is associated with altered hormone levels, such as reduced serum testosterone and elevated gonadotropins, which can adversely affect spermatogenesis. However, these hormonal changes do not directly correlate with TESE outcomes.

Histopathology

Various studies [26, 27] have proved histopathology as a good predictor of sperm retrieval success rate. Retrieval success is highest (85%) in cases with hypospermatogenesis, while Sertoli-cell-only syndrome shows the lowest success rate (22.5%). Maturation arrest falls in between these extremes; within this category, late and focal maturation arrest is associated with higher retrieval rates compared to early and diffuse maturation arrest. Although histology can be used as a predictive tool, its limitation lies in the fact that tissue samples can only be obtained after surgery. Nevertheless, it remains valuable for counseling patients regarding the likelihood of success in future sperm retrieval attempts. The level of spermatogenesis in each testicular biopsy sample is measured based on the Johnsen score system [28]. Patients with idiopathic NOA who have Johnsen scores of 1–2 will be identified as having Sertoli-cell-only syndrome (SCOS), those with Johnsen scores of 3–7 will be identified as having maturation arrest (MA), and those with Johnsen scores of 8–9 will be identified as having hypospermatogenesis (HS).

Varicocele

Varicocele in men often leads to poor sperm quality and azoospermia in some cases. It occurs due to venous pooling in the testicular vein, which compromises the maintenance of effective temperature for spermatogenesis. Studies have found that the repair of a varicocele in men with NOA may play a predictive role in the success of micro-TESE [29]. A systematic review evaluated the benefits of repairing clinical varicoceles in infertile men with NOA. The primary outcomes assessed were sperm retrieval rates (SRR) and pregnancy rates following assisted reproductive technology (ART) using retrieved testicular sperm. The study aimed to summarize evidence on the effectiveness of varicocele repair in this patient population [30].

Research has explored predictive factors for successful varicocele repair in men with infertility. Kaltsas and coworkers [31] suggest that certain clinical parameters may help predict favorable outcomes post-repair, although specific indicators require further validation [31].

A study assessed the effect of varicocele repair on testicular histology in men with NOA. Results indicated that varicocele repair could lead to histological improvements, potentially enhancing the chances of sperm retrieval [32]. Czaplicki et al. reported the reappearance of spermatozoa in the ejaculate in 12 out of 33 men with NOA (34%) who underwent varicocele repair [32]. It is not clear how many patients could have had sperm in the ejaculate with no treatment (or may have had cryptozoospermia prior to therapy), as there was no control group followed over time [33]. Tung et al. [34] also reported no success on 8 patients with azoospermia who underwent varicocelectomy. These studies collectively suggest that varicocele repair in men with NOA may improve TESE success rates and subsequent ART outcomes. However, individual results can vary, and further research is needed to establish definitive predictive factors and standardized treatment protocols.

History of Acquired Etiological Factors

Acquired etiological factors such as mumps, testicular ischemia, and chemotherapy can affect spermatogenesis. Mumps orchitis, damaging seminiferous tubules and impacting Leydig cells, is crucial for testosterone production [35]. Chemotherapy's direct toxicity on germ cells and hormonal disruption in the reproductive system can lead to temporary or permanent declines in sperm count and quality [36].

Chemical Biomarkers

Studies are underway in using biomarkers as predictors for successful sperm retrieval. A study found that the seminal plasma level of ESX1 has a sensitivity of 84% and a specificity of 28% [37]. Research has also been done to use seminal plasma protamine 1 as a predictor. It was found to have a sensitivity of 89% and a specificity of 90%. There is also further research in using germ cell-specific mRNA [38].

Radiological Predictors

Predictors of retrieval in the realm of medical imaging have evolved significantly with the advent of advanced technologies such as contrast enhanced ultrasound (CEUS), magnetic resonance imaging (MRI) spectroscopy, apparent diffusion coefficient (ADC), and fractional anisotropy (FA). These cutting-edge techniques have revolutionized the way healthcare professionals diagnose and predict outcomes in various medical conditions. Let's delve a little deeper into the efficiency of each of these advanced imaging techniques:

Doppler Ultrasound

Doppler ultrasound and traditional ultrasound scans are valuable tools in the assessment of male reproductive anatomy and can play a role in sperm retrieval procedures. In sperm retrieval procedures, such as TESE or percutaneous epididymal sperm aspiration (PESA), evaluating testicular blood flow using Doppler can help identify areas with optimal vascularity for sampling. Adequate blood flow is essential for spermatogenesis, and regions with good blood supply may have a higher likelihood of containing viable sperm. Thus, real-time ultrasound imaging during procedures like TESE can enhance the precision of sperm retrieval, increasing the chances of obtaining viable sperm for assisted reproductive techniques [39].

Contrast Ultrasound

Contrast ultrasound is highly efficient in assessing blood flow and perfusion in real time. It is noninvasive and does not involve ionizing radiation, making it a safe option for patients. Contrast ultrasound provides dynamic imaging, allowing healthcare professionals to monitor blood flow continuously. Its efficiency lies in its ability to enhance the visualization of vascular structures; this can help assess testicular blood flow by providing enhanced imaging of the testicular vasculature and provides insights into the vascular status of the testes. Poor blood flow to the testes may indicate conditions such as testicular ischemia, vascular abnormalities, or inflammation that could contribute to azoospermia [40].

Magnetic Resonance Imaging (MRI) Spectroscopy

MRI spectroscopy is a noninvasive imaging technique that measures the chemical composition of tissues, including testicles. It is highly efficient in providing detailed information about cellular metabolism and biochemical changes within organs. By analyzing specific metabolites, MRI spectroscopy helps in the diagnosis and monitoring of various conditions and potentially aids in the characterization of conditions contributing to impaired spermatogenesis in NOA [41].

MRI spectroscopy is occasionally used in male subfertility research settings to explore metabolic and molecular aspects of testicular function and dysfunction. Studies employing MRI spectroscopy may seek to understand the biochemical changes occurring in the testicular microenvironment in cases of infertility [42].

Apparent Diffusion Coefficient

Apparent diffusion coefficient (ADC) is a quantitative parameter derived from diffusion-weighted magnetic resonance imaging (DWI-MRI). It measures the random motion of water molecules within tissues, including the testis. High ADC values indicate increased water diffusion, often seen in benign lesions, while low ADC values suggest restricted diffusion, characteristic of malignant tumors or areas of cellular density. ADC is highly efficient in distinguishing between different tissue types. Its efficiency lies in its ability to provide valuable information about tissue microstructure and cellularity [43].

In NOA, where there is often impaired spermatogenesis, changes in the cellular and structural composition of the testicular tissue can be assessed through ADC values. In the testes, variations in ADC may help differentiate between normal and abnormal testicular tissue, potentially providing information on the severity and nature of the underlying pathology contributing to NOA [43].

Fractional Anisotropy

Fractional anisotropy (FA) is a measure derived from diffusion tensor imaging (DTI) and indicates the directionality and coherence of water diffusion within tissues. While DTI and FA are more commonly associated with imaging neural tissues like the brain, there has been some exploration of their use in the evaluation of testicular tissues, including in cases of male infertility, such as NOA. In the context of NOA, alterations in testicular microstructure, such as changes in the arrangement of seminiferous tubules or fibrosis, may be reflected in FA values.

Shear Wave Elastography

Shear wave elastography (SWE) is a medical imaging technique that measures tissue stiffness or elasticity. It is commonly used in the field of liver assessment, but its application in other areas, including reproductive medicine, is an emerging area of research. By assessing the elasticity of testicular tissue, SWE could potentially help identify areas of the testes with better sperm production or distinguish between areas of normal and abnormal tissue.

In their 2021 study, Abdelaal and colleagues examined shear wave elastography (SWE) as a predictor for sperm retrieval in NOA patients undergoing TESE. They found significant differences in SWE values between patients with successful and unsuccessful sperm retrieval. SWE demonstrated a 94.7% negative predictive value and a 50.0% positive predictive value for sperm retrieval in NOA patients, with 75.0% sensitivity and 85.71% specificity ($P = 0.0001$). The mean stiffness index measured by SWE also correlated significantly with histopathological types, particularly in severe hypospermatogenesis cases [44]. These findings indicate that SWE, being noninvasive and easily applicable, holds promise as a reliable sonographic modality for predicting sperm retrieval outcomes in NOA patients.

Technique of Surgical Sperm Retrieval

There are studies done comparing microdissection testicular sperm extraction, conventional testicular sperm extraction, and testicular sperm aspiration for NOA. In a direct comparison, the performance of microdissection TESE was 1.5 (95% CI, 1.4–1.6) times more likely to result in successful sperm retrieval than conventional TESE [45]. Similarly, in a direct comparison, conventional TESE was 2.0 times (95% CI, 1.8–2.2) more likely to result in successful sperm retrieval compared to testicular sperm aspiration [46].

Likewise, a risk-predictive model of sperm retrieval failure with fine needle aspiration in males states that FSH level, testicular volume, and age were significantly associated with higher success rates. The model's sensitivity was 67.7% and its specificity was 86.3% [46].

Experience of the Surgeon

The experience of a surgeon plays a significant role in sperm retrieval procedures for individuals with NOA. Sperm retrieval techniques such as TESE, microdissection TESE, or PESA are commonly employed to retrieve sperm directly from the testicles or epididymis in such cases. The success of these procedures relies on the surgeon's expertise and experience in identifying and extracting viable sperm [47].

An experienced surgeon in the field of male infertility is well-versed in the intricacies of sperm retrieval techniques. They possess a thorough understanding of the anatomy of the male reproductive system and can accurately locate potential areas within the testicles or epididymis where viable sperm may be present.

The surgeon's experience enables them to perform the procedure efficiently, minimizing potential complications and maximizing the chances of successful sperm retrieval. They are adept at handling delicate tissues, using specialized instruments, and employing meticulous surgical techniques, which significantly improve the overall outcome of the procedure.

A systematic review examined the impact of surgeons' experience on sperm retrieval techniques for nonobstructive azoospermia [27]. The review concluded that surgeons' expertise played a crucial role in achieving successful sperm retrieval and minimizing complications. Experienced surgeons had higher retrieval rates, lower complication rates, and improved pregnancy outcomes.

The experience of a surgeon in sperm retrieval procedures for NOA is crucial. Their expertise, technical skills, and ability to adapt to individual cases significantly impact the success rates of sperm retrieval, ultimately providing hope for couples seeking to overcome male infertility and achieve their reproductive goals [48].

Experience of the Embryologist

The expertise of an embryologist is paramount in ART procedures, playing a pivotal role in the delicate process of fertilization and early embryo development. Embryologists are highly trained professionals responsible for handling gametes (sperm and eggs) and creating a suitable environment for fertilization and embryo culture. Their experience and proficiency significantly influence the success of procedures like in vitro fertilization (IVF) and ICSI, offering hope to couples struggling with infertility [49].

Embryologists are extensively trained in the intricacies of gamete manipulation and embryo culture. Their deep understanding of reproductive biology, cell physiology, and embryonic development equips them to handle gametes with precision and care. Expert embryologists can assess the quality of sperm and eggs, identifying the most viable ones for fertilization. They employ advanced laboratory techniques to optimize the conditions for fertilization, ensuring the best possible chance of successful embryo formation.

The experience of an embryologist is particularly crucial during procedures like ICSI, where a single sperm is injected directly into an egg to achieve fertilization. The embryologist's skill in performing this intricate procedure can significantly impact fertilization rates. They must have a keen eye and steady hands to handle the delicate manipulation required for ICSI, maximizing the chances of successful fertilization.

Furthermore, embryologists play a key role in embryo culture and selection. They monitor the developing embryos closely, assessing their growth and morphology to select the healthiest ones for transfer into the uterus. Experienced embryologists can accurately identify embryos with the highest potential for implantation, increasing the likelihood of a successful pregnancy.

In the realm of ART, embryologists often collaborate with other medical professionals, including reproductive endocrinologists and fertility nurses. Their expertise ensures seamless coordination and communication within the healthcare team, fostering a supportive environment for patients undergoing fertility treatments.

Numerous studies and clinical reports have underscored the significant impact of embryologists' experience on the outcomes of ART procedures. Research published in reputable journals such as the Journal of Assisted Reproduction and Genetics has highlighted the correlation between embryologists' skills and the success rates of IVF and ICSI. Experienced embryologists demonstrate higher fertilization rates, better embryo quality, and increased pregnancy rates compared to their less-experienced counterparts [49].

Existing Predictive Models

Predicting the success of sperm retrieval in NOA is a complex task and involves considering various factors related to the patient's medical history, clinical examination, and diagnostic tests. While there is ongoing research in this area, it's essential to note that predicting success with absolute certainty can be challenging due to the heterogeneity of NOA cases. Several individual factors are commonly considered in predictive models for successful sperm retrieval in NOA, which are discussed above. While these factors are considered in predicting success, it's important to emphasize that predicting outcomes in individual cases can be challenging. Some predictive models have been proposed, incorporating multiple parameters, but the success of sperm retrieval can still vary.

Several studies have attempted to develop combined predictive models for the success of sperm retrieval in NOA. These models often integrate various clinical, hormonal, genetic, and histological parameters to provide a more comprehensive prediction. Keep in mind that the field is continually evolving, and newer models may emerge in the future [50, 51].

Limitations of the Current SSR Techniques

While SSR techniques have proven effective in many cases of NOA, they do have some limitations. Here are some of these limitations:

1. Limited Success Rates: Success rates for sperm retrieval can vary widely depending on the technique used and the underlying cause of azoospermia. NOA cases, where sperm production is impaired, may have lower success rates compared to OA.

2. Inability to Guarantee Pregnancy: Even if sperm are successfully retrieved, there is no guarantee of a successful pregnancy. The quality and viability of the retrieved sperm, as well as the fertility of the female partner, play crucial roles in achieving a pregnancy.
3. Risk of Complications: Surgical procedures, including TESE and micro-TESE, carry inherent risks such as bleeding, infection, and damage to surrounding structures. These risks need to be carefully considered, especially in patients with comorbidities.
4. Limited Information on Sperm Quality: Surgical techniques focus on obtaining sperm from the testes, but they do not provide information about the sperm's functional or genetic quality. Advanced sperm analysis and genetic testing may be necessary to assess sperm quality and guide further treatment.
5. Possible Multiple Procedures: In some cases, multiple sperm retrieval procedures may be required to find viable sperm. Each surgical intervention carries its own set of risks and requires time for recovery.
6. Cost and Resource Intensive: SSR techniques can be costly, and they may not be readily available in all medical centers. The financial and logistical aspects of these procedures can be limiting factors for some patients.
7. Psychological Impact: The process of undergoing multiple surgical procedures, along with the uncertainty of success, can have a psychological impact on individuals and couples. It is important to consider the emotional well-being of patients.
8. Ethical Considerations: The use of SSR techniques raises ethical considerations, especially in cases where the retrieved sperm will be used for assisted reproductive technologies. Ethical discussions may involve considerations of the potential risks and benefits, as well as the disposition of unused sperm.
9. Despite these limitations, SSR techniques remain valuable options for many couples facing male infertility. Advances in technology and ongoing research aim to improve success rates, minimize risks, and provide a better understanding of the underlying causes of male infertility. As with any medical procedure, individualized assessment and consultation with a reproductive specialist are crucial to determining the most appropriate course of action for each patient.

Future Research and Development

Future research is to advance the prediction models of SSR in infertile men with NOA by exploring genomic markers, seminal fluid biomarkers, advanced imaging, artificial intelligence, functional sperm assessments, in vitro testicular culture, and patient-specific factors. Future precision approaches aim to tailor interventions based on genetic and molecular characteristics, optimize sperm retrieval conditions, and assess long-term outcomes. Staying informed about these evolving areas is crucial for researchers, clinicians, and patients as they contribute to the dynamic field of male infertility, fostering more accurate and individualized diagnosis and treatment strategies.

Summary

Infertility is a growing concern, affecting 1 in 6 couples, with male factors accounting for approximately 50% of infertility cases, including azoospermia. Advances in SSR techniques like micro-TESE have revolutionized male infertility treatment. Multiple factors affect the outcome of SRR, including the underlying etiology of NOA, the available facilities, and the skills of the surgeon and expertise of the embryologist. Predicting the success rates of SSR in NOA patients is crucial. Ongoing research explores combined prediction models, genomic markers, imaging, AI, and personalized medicine. Future precision interventions aim to tailor treatments based on genetic factors, optimizing conditions for SSR and ensuring better outcomes in the dynamic field of male infertility.

References

1. Sudhakar DVS, Shah R, Gajbhiye RK. Genetics of male infertility – present and future: a narrative review. J Hum Reprod Sci. 2021;14(3):217–27. https://doi.org/10.4103/jhrs.jhrs_115_21. Epub 2021 Sep 28. PMID: 34759610; PMCID: PMC8527069
2. Tharakan T, Luo R, Jayasena CN, Minhas S. Non-obstructive azoospermia: current and future perspectives. Fac Rev. 2021;10:7. https://doi.org/10.12703/r/10-7. PMID: 33659925; PMCID: PMC7894261
3. Cocuzza M, Alvarenga C, Pagani R. The epidemiology and etiology of azoospermia. Clinics (Sao Paulo). 2013;68 Suppl 1(Suppl 1):15-26.
4. Corona G, Minhas S, Giwercman A, Bettocchi C, Dinkelman-Smit M, Dohle G, et al. Sperm recovery and ICSI outcomes in men with non-obstructive azoospermia: a systematic review and meta-analysis. Hum Reprod Update. 2019;25(6):733–757.
5. Markham S. Patient perspective on predictive models in healthcare: translation into practice, ethical implications and limitations? BMJ Health Care Inform. 2025;32(1):e101153.
6. Shah R, Gupta C. Advances in sperm retrieval techniques in azoospermic men: a systematic review. Arab J Urol. 2017;16(1):125–31. https://doi.org/10.1016/j.aju.2017.11.010. PMID: 29713543; PMCID: PMC5922005
7. Deng CY, Liu DF, Zhao LM, Lin HC, Mao JM, Zhang Z, Yang YZ, Zhang HT, Hong K, Xu HY, Jiang H. Development of a predictive model for increasing sperm retrieval success by microdissection testicular sperm extraction in patients with nonobstructive azoospermia. Asian J Androl. 2023;25(5):598–603. https://doi.org/10.4103/aja2022111. Epub ahead of print. PMID: 36814170; PMCID: PMC10521962
8. Jamalirad H, Jajroudi M, Khajehpour B, Sadighi Gilani MA, Eslami S, Sabbaghian M, et al. AI predictive models and advancements in microdissection testicular sperm extraction for non-obstructive azoospermia: a systematic scoping review. Hum Reprod Open. 2024;2025(1):hoae070.
9. Ng MY, Youssef A, Pillai M, Shah V, Hernandez-Boussard T. Scaling equitable artificial intelligence in healthcare with machine learning operations. BMJ Health Care Inform. 2024;31(1):e101101.
10. Okada H, Goda K, Yamamoto Y, Sofikitis N, Miyagawa I, Mio Y, et al. Age as a limiting factor for successful sperm retrieval in patients with nonmosaic Klinefelter's syndrome. Fertil Steril. 2005;84(6):1662–4.

11. Achermann APP, Pereira TA, Esteves SC. Microdissection testicular sperm extraction (micro-TESE) in men with infertility due to nonobstructive azoospermia: summary of current literature. Int Urol Nephrol. 2021;53(11):2193–210.
12. Cissen M, Meijerink AM, D'Hauwers KW, Meissner A, van der Weide N, Mochtar MH, et al. Prediction model for obtaining spermatozoa with testicular sperm extraction in men with non-obstructive azoospermia. Hum Reprod. 2016;31(9):1934–41.
13. Meachem SJ, Nieschlag E, Simoni M. Inhibin B in male reproduction: pathophysiology and clinical relevance. Eur J Endocrinol. 2001;145(5):561–71. https://doi.org/10.1530/eje.0.1450561. PMID: 11720872
14. Althakafi SA, Mustafa OM, Seyam RM, Al-Hathal N, Kattan S. Serum testosterone levels and other determinants of sperm retrieval in microdissection testicular sperm extraction. Transl Androl Urol. 2017;6(2):282–287.
15. Kim TJ, Koo KC. Testosterone to Luteinizing Hormone Ratio as a Potential Predictor of Sperm Retrieval in Non-bstructive Azoospermia Patients. Yonsei Med J. 2023;64(7):433–439.
16. Alfano M, Ventimiglia E, Locatelli I, Capogrosso P, Cazzaniga W, Pederzoli F, et al. Anti-Mullerian hormone-to-testosterone ratio is predictive of positive sperm retrieval in men with idiopathic non-obstructive Azoospermia. Sci Rep. 2017;7(1):17638.
17. Stahl PJ, Masson P, Mielnik A, Marean MB, Schlegel PN, Paduch DA. A decade of experience emphasizes that testing for Y microdeletions is essential in American men with azoospermia and severe oligozoospermia. Fertil Steril. 2010;94(5):1753–6. PMID: 19896650
18. Rohayem J, Fricke R, Czeloth K, Mallidis C, Wistuba J, et al. Age and markers of Leydig cell function, but not of Sertoli cell function predict the success of sperm retrieval in adolescents and adults with Klinefelter's syndrome. Andrology. 2015;3(5):868–75
19. Schiff JD, Palermo GD, Veeck LL, Goldstein M, Rosenwaks Z, Schlegel PN. Success of testicular sperm injection and intracytoplasmic sperm injection in men with Klinefelter syndrome. J Clin Endocrinol Metab. 2005;90(11):6263–7.
20. Greco E, Scarselli F, Minasi MG, Casciani V, Zavaglia D, Dente D, et al. TESEICSI in patients with non-mosaic Klinefelter syndrome: a comparative study. Reprod Biomed Online. 2010;21(6):756–60.
21. Okada H, Goda K, Yamamoto Y, et al. Age as a limiting factor for successful sperm retrieval in patients with nonmosaic Klinefelter's syndrome. Fertil Steril. 2005;84(6):1662–4.
22. Ramasamy R, Padilla WO, Osterberg EC, Srivastava A, Reifsnyder JE, Niederberger C, et al. A comparison of models for predicting sperm retrieval before microdissection testicular sperm extraction in men with nonobstructive azoospermia. J Urol. 2013;189(2):638–42.
23. Çayan S, Orhan İ, Altay B, Aşcı R, Akbay E, Ayas B, et al. Fertility outcomes and predictors for successful sperm retrieval and pregnancy in 327 azoospermic men with a history of cryptorchidism who underwent microdissection testicular sperm extraction. Andrology. 2021;9(1):253–9.
24. Corona G, Minhas S, Giwercman A, Bettocchi C, Dinkelman-Smit M, Dohle G, et al. Sperm recovery and ICSI outcomes in men with non-obstructive azoospermia: a systematic review and meta-analysis. Hum Reprod Update. 2019;25(6):733–757. https://doi.org/10.1093/humupd/dmz028.
25. Qi L, Liu YP, Zhang NN, Su YC. Predictors of testicular sperm retrieval in patients with non-obstructive azoospermia: a review. J Int Med Res. 2021;49(4):3000605211002703. https://doi.org/10.1177/03000605211002703. PMID: 33794677
26. Gnessi L, Scarselli F, Minasi MG, Mariani S, Lubrano C, Basciani S, et al. Testicular histopathology, semen analysis and FSH, predictive value of sperm retrieval: supportive counseling in case of reoperation after testicular sperm extraction (TESE). BMC Urol. 2018;18(1):63.
27. Caroppo E, Colpi EM, Gazzano G, Vaccalluzzo L, Scroppo FI, D'Amato G, Colpi GM. Testicular histology may predict the successful sperm retrieval in patients with non-obstructive azoospermia undergoing conventional TESE: a diagnostic accuracy study. J Assist Reprod Genet. 2017;34(1):149–54. https://doi.org/10.1007/s10815-016-0812-3. Epub 2016 Sep 21. PMID: 27655389; PMCID: PMC5330973

28. Cito G, Coccia ME, Dabizzi S, et al. Relevance of testicular histopathology on prediction of sperm retrieval rates in case of non-obstructive and obstructive azoospermia. Urologia. 2018;85:60–7. https://doi.org/10.1177/0391560318758940.
29. Inci K, Gunay LM. The role of varicocele treatment in the management of non-obstructive azoospermia. Clinics (Sao Paulo). 2013;68(Suppl 1):89–98. https://doi.org/10.6061/clinics/2013(sup01)10. PMID: 23503958
30. Dudley T, Hotaling J, et al. Azoospermia: etiology, diagnosis and management. Asian J Androl. 2016;18(3):333–42.
31. Kaltsas A, Markou E, Zachariou A, Dimitriadis F, Mamoulakis C, Andreadakis S, et al. Varicoceles in men with non-obstructive azoospermia: the dilemma to operate or not. Front Reprod Health. 2022;4:811487
32. Czaplicki M, Bablok L, Janczewski Z. Varicocelectomy in Patients with Azoospermia. Archives of Andrology. 1979;3:51–5.
33. Schlegel PN, Goldstein M. Alternate indications for varicocele repair: non-obstructive azoospermia, pain, androgen deficiency and progressive testicular dysfunction. Fertil Steril. 2011;96(6):1288–93.
34. Tung MC, Huang WJ, Chen KK. Modified subinguinal varicocelectomy for painful varicocele and varicocele-associated infertility. J Chin Med Assoc 2004;67:296–300.
35. Wu H, Jiang X, Gao Y, Liu W, Wang F, Gong M, Chen R, Yu X, Zhang W, Gao B, Song C, Han D. Mumps virus infection disrupts blood-testis barrier through the induction of TNF-α in Sertoli cells. FASEB J. 2019;33(11):12528–40. https://doi.org/10.1096/fj.201901089R. Epub 2019 Aug 26. PMID: 31450968; PMCID: PMC6902681
36. Qu N, Itoh M, Sakabe K. Effects of chemotherapy and radiotherapy on spermatogenesis: the role of testicular immunology. Int J Mol Sci. 2019;20(4):957. https://doi.org/10.3390/ijms20040957. PMID: 30813253; PMCID: PMC6413003
37. Li J, Yang F, Dong L, Chang D, Yu X. Seminal plasma biomarkers for predicting successful sperm retrieval in patients with nonobstructive azoospermia: a narrative review of human studies. Basic Clin Androl. 2023;33(1):9.
38. Barceló M, Mata A, Bassas L, Larriba S. Exosomal microRNAs in seminal plasma are markers of the origin of azoospermia and can predict the presence of sperm in testicular tissue. Hum Reprod. 2018;33(6):1087–98. https://doi.org/10.1093/humrep/dey072. PMID: 29635626; PMCID: PMC5972609
39. Souza CA, Cunha-Filho JS, Fagundes P, Freitas FM, Passos EP. Sperm recovery prediction in azoospermic patients using Doppler ultrasonography. Int Urol Nephrol. 2005;37(3):535–40. https://doi.org/10.1007/s11255-005-0918-5. PMID. 16307338
40. Zhang S, Du J, Tian R, Xie S, Li F, Li Z. Assessment of the use of contrast enhanced ultrasound in guiding microdissection testicular sperm extraction in nonobstructive azoospermia. BMC Urol. 2018;18(1):48. https://doi.org/10.1186/s12894-018-0367-y. PMID: 29792185; PMCID: PMC5966902
41. Çelik Ö, Hatırnaz Ş, Erşahin A, Başbuğ A, Yetkin Yıldırım G, Özener V, Gürpınar N, Çelik S, Çelik N, Küçük T, Ünlü C. Testis spectroscopy may predict sperm retrieval rate in men with non-obstructive azoospermia undergoing micro-TESE: a pilot study. J Turk Ger Gynecol Assoc. 2020;21(2):70–8. https://doi.org/10.4274/jtgga.galenos.2019.2018.0154. Epub 2019 Oct 23. PMID: 31640305; PMCID: PMC7294832
42. Hesham Said A, Ragab A, Zohdy W, Ibrahim AS, Abd El Basset AS. Diffusion-weighted magnetic resonance imaging and magnetic resonance spectroscopy for non-invasive characterization of azoospermia: a prospective comparative single-center study. Andrology. 2023;11(6):1096–106. https://doi.org/10.1111/andr.13392. Epub 2023 Feb 6. PMID: 36690593
43. Ntorkou A, Tsili AC, Goussia A, Astrakas LG, Maliakas V, Sofikitis N, Argyropoulou MI. Testicular apparent diffusion coefficient and magnetization transfer ratio: can these MRI parameters be used to predict successful sperm retrieval in nonobstructive azoospermia? AJR Am J Roentgenol. 2019;213(3):610–8. https://doi.org/10.2214/AJR.18.20816. Epub 2019 May 7. PMID: 31063417

44. Abdelaal AMA, El-Azizi HM, GamalEl Din SF, Abdulsalam Mohammad Azzazi O, Shokr Mohamed M. Evaluation of the potential role of shear wave elastography as a promising predictor of sperm retrieval in non-obstructive azoospermic patients: a prospective study. Andrology. 2021;9(5):1481–9.
45. Bernie AM, Mata DA, Ramasamy R, Schlegel PN. Comparison of microdissection testicular sperm extraction, conventional testicular sperm extraction, and testicular sperm aspiration for nonobstructive azoospermia: a systematic review and meta-analysis. Fertil Steril. 2015;104(5):1099–1103.e3.
46. Ma Y, Li F, Wang L, Zhao W, Li D, Xian Y, et al. A risk prediction model of sperm retrieval failure with fine needle aspiration in males with non-obstructive azoospermia. Hum Reprod Oxf Engl. 2019;34(2):200–8.
47. Tiseo BC, Hayden RP, Tanrikut C. Surgical management of nonobstructive azoospermia. Asian J Urol. 2015;2(2):85–91. https://doi.org/10.1016/j.ajur.2015.04.020. Epub 2015 Apr 16. PMID: 29264125; PMCID: PMC5730741
48. Esteves SC, Miyaoka R, Orosz JE, Agarwal A. An update on sperm retrieval techniques for azoospermic males. Clinics (Sao Paulo). 2013;68(Suppl 1):99–110. https://doi.org/10.6061/clinics/2013(sup01)11. PMID: 23503959; PMCID: PMC3583154
49. Shapiro H, Brown TJ, Pat Chronis-Brown G, Hamilton S, Bentley DC, Kandel R, Gotlieb AI. Education of the clinical embryology laboratory professional: development of a novel program delivered in a laboratory medicine department. F S Rep. 2023;4(3):262–9. https://doi.org/10.1016/j.xfre.2023.03.001.
50. Chen X, Ma Y, Zou S, Wang S, Qiu J, Xiao Q, Zhou L, Ping P. Comparison and outcomes of nonobstructive azoospermia patients with different etiology undergoing MicroTESE and ICSI treatments. Transl Androl Urol. 2019;8(4):366–73. https://doi.org/10.21037/tau.2019.04.08. PMID: 31555560; PMCID: PMC6732089
51. Donoso P, Tournaye H, Devroey P. Which is the best sperm retrieval technique for non-obstructive azoospermia? A systematic review. Hum Reprod Update. 2007;13(6):539–49.

Chapter 13
Overview of the Technical Aspects in the Lab

Israel Maldonado Rosas, Vijay Mangoli, and Krishna Chaitanya Mantravadi

Retrieval of Testicular Sperm: Techniques and Recommendations

Introduction of Techniques Used for the Retrieval of Testicular Sperm in NOA Patients

For the recovery of testicular sperm, the most used methods include testicular sperm aspiration (TESA), random open biopsy sperm extraction (TESE), and microdissection-TESE (m-TESE) [1, 2, 3]. The m-TESE procedure using microscopic magnification is considered the best method for sperm recovery rates with little tissue loss and has been advocated as the gold standard. Interestingly, high rates of sperm recovery and live births are ensured in NOA patients when an m-TESE is performed after a conventional TESE has failed to retrieve sperm [4]. After testicular sperm extraction, sperm quality and selection play an essential role in the success of in vitro fertilization (IVF). The retrieval of testicular sperm of patients with NOA continues to be a challenge since sometimes very few sperm may be present [2].

I. M. Rosas (✉)
IVF Laboratory, Citmer Reproductive Medicine, Mexico City, Mexico
e-mail: imaldonado@citmer.mx

V. Mangoli
Fertility Clinic & IVF Centre, Mumbai, India

K. C. Mantravadi
Department of Embryology, Oasis Fertility, Chennai, India
e-mail: krishna@oasisindia.in

W. Zohdy et al. (eds.), *Non-Obstructive Azoospermia*,
https://doi.org/10.1007/978-3-031-99431-9_13

Description of the sperm Retrieval Techniques from NOA Patients (mTESE and Others)

Advancements in surgical sperm retrieval (SSR) techniques have helped men with NOA to father their own genetic child. TESA (testicular sperm aspiration) is a fine needle aspiration method done under minimal sedation or local anesthesia. It is a quick procedure and is practiced widely. Blind approach and risk of hematoma are the potential downsides of this process [5]. TESE (testicular sperm extraction) is an open procedure involving testis dissection and tissue extraction [6]. With the invention of micro-TESE, a blind open extraction is not recommended. Use of the microscope to directly visualize the testicular parenchyma allows the identification of dilated seminiferous tubules that have a higher chance of sperm retrieval. However, this procedure is time-consuming and expensive and needs an experienced urologist and embryologist [7].

Tissue Separation and Enzymatic Digestion (When and How)

The optimal method to separate extracted testicular tissue must be considered according to the tissue's characteristics, the laboratory's capacity, and personal experiences [2]. Different methods are used in the laboratory, and one of the most commonly used is the disintegration of testicular tissue by mechanical treatment by shredding the tissue with fine needles or mechanical mincing of the tissue [2, 8]. Another way to release germ cells trapped in the seminiferous tubules or the tissue after the biopsy is through enzymatic digestion, which allows the loosening of the cellular contacts between the wall of the seminiferous tubules and the sperm, allowing their release. In this sense, the use of collagenase, mainly type IV, has been evaluated with good results, which does not affect the viability of the gamete [2, 9]. The use of enzymes is recommended, especially when it is perceived that there will be a low number of sperm cells in the testicular tissue. The segment below provides an in-depth understanding of various processing techniques.

Sperm Processing and Selection

Classic Techniques to Obtain Sperm from Seminiferous Tubules

Methods for Sperm Recovery

From tissue recovery to sperm separation, it is crucial to maintain the physiologically optimum conditions to retain the membrane structure integrity, viability, and reproductive ability of the sperm present in the tubules. Immediately after taking out the tubules from the testicles, they should be placed in a buffered medium with a balanced salt composition, fulfilling these requirements of the sperm [10]. Even during the surgical procedure, continuous hydration of the open tissue is recommended to prevent tubules from becoming dehydrated, which may adversely affect the osmolarity, thus affecting the fertilizing characteristics of the sperm.

Once the tubules are handed over to the laboratory, they must be handled cautiously to maximize the probability of getting intact sperm for fertilization. Methods for obtaining sperm entrapped in the seminiferous tubules include shredding and mechanical mincing, with or without enzymatic digestion, tailored to different lab preferences.

Oates et al. [11] proposed mechanical homogenization of the testicular tissue using a glass slide pestle. This homogenate is then aspirated through a 16 G hypodermic needle to release sperm, whereas Tucker et al. suggested using 21 G hypodermic needles for tissue dissection [12]. The tubules are then separated with the help of a needle attached to a tuberculin syringe (Fig. 13.1)

Advantages

Relatively simple technique.
Minimizes physiological fluctuations of pH, temperature, and osmolarity.
Effective in obtaining most of the inner content, including sperm.
Less possibility of damage to the sperm.

Limitations

Unsuitable for torn-off or amorphous tubules.
Sperm comes along with other debris and cells, which are to be separated.
Sperm may remain embedded in interstitial, Sertoli, or epithelial cells; hence, there is still a need to separate them.

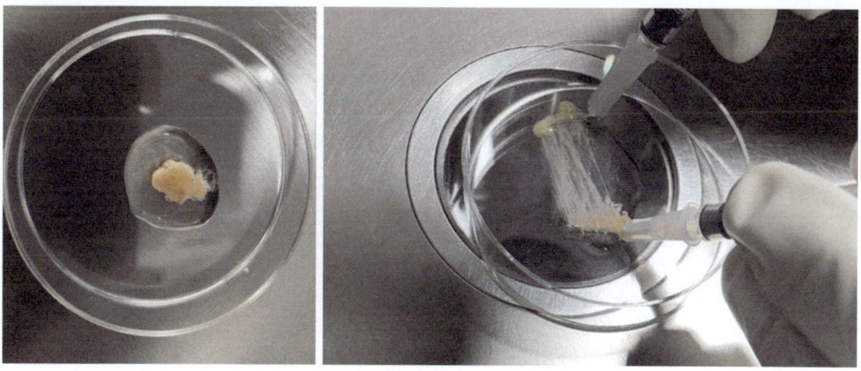

Fig. 13.1 Teasing of seminiferous tubules using two needles

Technical Challenges in Laboratory Processing

Laboratory process to prepare surgically retrieved testicular sperm from NOA patients is a tedious process and takes a longer time. Improper processing methods may result in a final pellet with plenty of red blood cells, round cells, and tissue debris. These cellular debris make the sperm selection process tricky and difficult. These cellular debris at times will also result in the blockage of the micromanipulation pipettes used for the ICSI technique.

In certain instances, the medium drop becomes too turbid to find and separate intact sperm.

The sperm retrieved from NOA patients may be nonmotile, but viable. It needs to be checked either by a Hypo Osmotic Swelling Test (HOST) or using methylxanthine derivatives like pentoxifylline [13].

If the extraction results in accompanying excess blood, the contamination with RBCs in the tissue is taken care of using Erythrocyte Lysing Buffer, which makes the teased suspension clearer, making finding the sperm easier [14].

Jow et al. proposed a different sperm preparation method for obtaining sperm from testicular tissues. Fresh tissue is placed on a sterile slide, and culture media is added. A coverslip is placed on the tissue, and the specimen is compressed to release embedded sperm [15]. The crushed tubule material may need to be incubated for up to 24 h and extensively examined to search for any injectable sperm with twitching motility [16].

Enzymatic Testicular Tissue Treatment

Salzbrunn et al. described a method of enzymatic extraction using collagenase and a trypsin inhibitor, the enzymatic use of collagenase optimizes testicular gamete preparation by gentle dissolving tissue, yielding higher numbers of mature spermatids or spermatozoa. Compared to traditional shredding, this approach reduces debris, simplifies microscopic visualization, and facilitates accurate sperm isolation, providing ideal conditions for sperm aspiration and subsequent microinjection during ICSI procedures [17].

Sperm Microinjection Techniques

If, during initial observation, poor motility is seen, sperm can be retrieved using a direct pick-up method. The dissected suspension is divided into multiple droplets and diluted appropriately to disperse debris. These droplets with poor motility sperm are deposited at the center of a larger culture medium of 6–8 μl. These sperm can be picked up either immediately while observing under the inverted microscope using an ICSI injection pipette or after 30–45 min when sperm migrate to the periphery [18].

Prospects About Sperm Selection

The testicular tissue samples are assessed in the operating room by an experienced andrologist. Visualization of at least one spermatozoon per slide at 200× magnification is defined as a successful retrieval. Once sperm are observed, the procedure can be concluded. When several spermatozoa are present, their motility is the main criterion considered. The preparation of testicular sperm in the laboratory level requires special handling. The success of an ICSI procedure in patients with NOA is closely related to the recovery of viable spermatozoa from the TESE, which is why sperm selection of sufficient quality and quantity is very important [2, 19]. The selection of sperm for ICSI is mainly based on morphology and motility. However, testicular spermatozoa may be immotile since motility is acquired during epididymal transit [20]. On the other hand, some compounds such as pentoxifylline [21] can induce motility, which may not be a critical criterion when it comes to characterizing the best sperm [2]. On the other hand, morphological criteria also become essential, especially for those who have access to magnification - based classification using more strict morphology criterion [2]. We will discuss some of these methodologies and see their advantages.

Mechanical Touch Technique (MTT)

Marques de Oliveira et al. [22] introduced the mechanical touch technique (MTT) to identify viable immotile spermatozoa. This method involves applying a lateral force to the flagella using an ICSI micropipette, where flexible tails indicate viability while rigid ones signify non-viability. In their sole clinical trial, they found no discernible differences in ICSI outcomes, including deliveries, between motile sperm and those immotile but selected via MTT in both fresh and frozen samples.

Hypoosmotic Swelling Test (HOST)

The hypoosmotic swelling test (HOST), introduced by Jayendran et al., for ejaculated sperm, is a useful test of sperm function [23]. It helps assess the functional integrity of sperm cell membranes. This test involves exposing sperm to a hypoosmotic solution, containing sodium citrate and fructose, which induces swelling in structurally intact sperm cells. The hypoosmotic swelling test (HOST) is a method for assessing sperm membrane integrity by observing swelling in response to a hypoosmotic solution. Mix the sperm cells with 1 mL of hypoosmotic solution and incubate the mixture at 37 °C for 30 min. After incubation, examine the sample under a microscope at 400× magnification for signs of swelling in the sperm tails, which indicate intact membrane function. The viable sperm can then be microinjected into mature oocytes. The osmolarity of normal saline is about 287 mOsmol/kg. A hypoosmotic solution can be prepared by adjusting distilled water to an osmolality of 50 mOsmol/kg or by using a readily available HOS solution. Five microliters of liquified semen solution containing sperm is mixed with 50 μl of HOS solution and incubated at 37°C for 5–30 min. For NOA samples, testicular extracts obtained through the TESE procedure are diluted with the appropriate culture medium and incubated at 37°C. A 10-μl drop is taken in a Petri dish containing a 20-μl modified HOS solution having a composition of 50% culture medium and 50% Milli Q water [24]. They reported tail curling of viable sperm in 1–2 s. The curling occurs due to the influx of water into the sperm through functional cell membranes [23]. The hypoosmotic swelling test (HOST) plays a significant role in testicular sperm extraction (TESE), a procedure crucial for retrieving sperm directly from the testes of men with severe infertility issues [24].

The significance of HOST in TESE lies in its ability to identify the most viable and functionally intact sperm cells among the immotile sperm retrieved from the testicular tissue. Sperm cells exhibiting swelling in the hypoosmotic solution are more likely to possess better membrane integrity and functionality [25].

The above method of HOST is usually performed for diagnostic purposes. However, HOST is also used to pick viable spermatozoa that do not demonstrate active motility or twitching during the process of ICSI. In this situation, the tail of the immotile sperm is carefully touched using micromanipulation, and once we notice a coil of the distal end of the tail, we immediately move the sperm to a buffer drop and wash the sperm and later use it for injecting the oocyte [2].

Chemical Inducers of Motility

Chemical inducers of motility, like pentoxifylline, can be used effectively [13]. A 3 mM solution of pentoxifylline (Sigma Aldrich, St Louis, MO P-1784) is prepared by adding 0.5 g of the powder to 2.5 ml of distilled water. Subsequently, 2–3 μl of this is added to the dissected suspension drops, which are aliquoted into multiple 6–8 μl culture medium droplets. The motility of the sperm is enhanced for a short duration, sufficient for them to migrate toward the periphery. These sperm are picked up using an injecting pipette and used for fertilization.

Importance of Sperm Characteristics and Their Impact on ICSI Results in Men with NOA

Sperm characteristics improve fertilization rates and embryonic development. The most recognized parameters of sperm quality are morphology and motility. However, motility is minimal for testicular sperm since this is acquired during the passage of sperm through the epididymis. Additionally, with the use of pentoxifylline and other strategies, sperm can be evaluated and chosen according to their motility. That is why Aboukhshaba et al. [19] carried out an investigation where they evaluated sperm characteristics of a group of NOA patients after mTESE and examined the impact of abnormal testicular sperm characteristics on fertilization and clinical pregnancy rates. These investigators concluded that the use of immotile or morphologically abnormal spermatozoa obtained surgically from men with NOA does not prevent fertilization or clinical pregnancy in women undergoing ICSI. Despite these results, it is necessary to consider that there is limited data on the health of the offspring resulting from the sperm from testicular tissue [19]. To ensure healthy offspring and increased pregnancy rates, it is essential to find the best parameters or characteristics of quality sperm. Emerging technologies in gamete selection for ART procedures, including advanced microscopy and functional sperm evaluations beyond conventional semen analysis, offer a promising outlook for optimizing male infertility treatments and deepening our understanding of its molecular and biological underpinnings, enabling timely diagnosis and successful interventions [26].

Intracytoplasmic Morphologically Selected Sperm Injection (IMSI)

Intracytoplasmic morphologically selected sperm injection (IMSI) represents a refined form of intracytoplasmic sperm injection (ICSI) that involves a meticulous selection process for sperm. IMSI enhances the sperm selection process by utilizing high-magnification microscopy, allowing embryologists to scrutinize sperm morphology at a level of detail that was not previously feasible with conventional microscopy. In testicular sperm extraction (TESE), IMSI becomes particularly significant due to its emphasis on selecting the better-quality sperm for injection into the egg [27].

The significance of IMSI (intracytoplasmic morphologically selected sperm injection) in TESE (testicular sperm extraction) primarily lies in its capacity to enhance sperm selection. IMSI enables a thorough morphological assessment of sperm, allowing for the identification of structurally superior sperm cells from others. This targeted approach may increase the likelihood of selecting sperm with fewer structural abnormalities, potentially leading to improved embryo development [27]. However, no significant differences have been found between ICSI and IMSI regarding pregnancy outcomes, chemical pregnancies, first-trimester miscarriages, or adverse results related to embryonic chromosomal abnormalities [28].

The role of IMSI remains contentious, and it is not routinely recommended for sperm selection in ART (assisted reproductive technology) procedures, particularly when only a limited number of viable sperm are available after mTESE. IMSI aims to enhance fertilization rates during the ICSI procedure. Selected sperm with normal structures are expected to have a higher potential to successfully fertilize the egg and improve embryo quality. However, when ejaculated sperm have been used, more evidence is still needed to confirm whether the use of IMSI significantly improves clinical outcomes [29–33]. Another concern is that IMSI process can take considerably longer, especially with low sperm motility or morphology [34, 35].

Automated Sperm Selection (Robotic System to Select Sperm with Low Sperm DNA Fragmentation)

Sperm DNA fragmentation significantly reduces the fertilization rate and embryonic development in ART treatments, in addition to increasing the rate of spontaneous abortions and producing genetic disorders in the offspring [36]. Many research groups are focused on generating tools that allow the selection of the best sperm from the point of view of morphology and DNA integrity. Zhang and collaborators developed a quantitative criterion based on the fact that DNA integrity is associated with normal morphology and motility and developed an algorithm that allows these parameters to be evaluated (according to normality criteria established by the WHO) in single living cells and selected sperm with lower DNA fragmentation for use in ICSI procedures. This development enabled the creation of a noninvasive sperm selection software program designed to minimize the risk of injecting sperm with damaged DNA [37]. However, it is important to note that this automated sperm selection method has yet to be tested on sperm obtained from testicular biopsies.

Computer Software-Assisted Real-Time Search for Single Sperm After Testicular Biopsy

Another emerging tool in sperm selection for ICSI is artificial intelligence (AI). Identifying viable sperm in surgically retrieved testicular samples for ICSI is a time-consuming process and the application of AI to aid the process of sperm searching will enhance the outcomes of assisted reproduction cycles. Goss et al. [38] conducted a trial using AI-powered image analysis and demonstrated that an AI-assisted sperm selection tool for testicular samples significantly reduces the time required to identify viable sperm and enhances reproductive outcomes. Other algorithms where deep neural netwoks were applied allowed the analysis of images of the testicular tissue, and through a CASA system, an authomated identification algorithm [39].

Machine Learning Algorithm-Based Testicular Sperm Selection

Machine learning is an automated method of data analysis that, through algorithms, allows computers to identify patterns in massive data and make predictions [40]. This methodology is increasingly used in healthcare to improve diagnosis and treatments. In assisted reproduction, this tool has been used for the selection of good-quality embryos and to improve the sperm finding for ART after mTESE [39, 41]. This offers excellent opportunities for machine learning to contribute to male fertility treatments. Bachelot and collaborators have developed a machine learning algorithm based on clinical and laboratory parameters to predict successful sperm retrieval in men with NOA undergoing microsurgical TESE with promising performance [42]. Despite this advance, the authors recommend additionally conducting a formal prospective multicenter validation study before any clinical application. Other algorithms where deep neural networks were applied allowed the analysis of images of the testicular tissue, and through the CASA system, an automated identification algorithm was applied [39]. Accurately predicting the success of sperm recovery in TESE procedures has become a growing need to contribute to improving the success of ART treatments in patients with NOA. These and other investigations are a valuable contribution to improving the success of ART in patients with NOA. However, the search continues for machine learning tools that can accurately predict the success of sperm retrieval in TESE.

Post-Retrieval TissueHandling

Tissue Handling Conditions

TESE or mTESE procedures can be scheduled either on the same day as oocyte retrieval, or on the day before. In either case, fragments of testicular tissue are placed in sperm medium, where seminiferous tubules are identified and blood clots removed. Following washing, tubules are mechanically minced with tuberculin syringes to disperse cells and release spermatozoa. The resulting suspension is examined under inverted microscope to confirm sperm presence. The surgeon is promptly informed if sufficient sperm for ICSI are available, If sperm are limited, seminiferous tubules can be further processed through additional mechanical shredding or enzymatic digestion to optimize recovery [20]. Incubating testicular tissue samples in a medium supplemented with recombinant follicle-stimulating hormone (FSH) for 24 h may enhance sperm motility and, consequently, improve fertilization rates during ICSI [16]. While there is no consensus, studies suggest that performing testicular sperm retrieval the day before and following in vitro sperm culture may potentially enhance sperm motility and overall pregnancy outcomes [44]. However, it has also been observed that prolonged sperm incubation at 37 °C may increase sperm DNA fragmentation. Therefore, it is recommended that recovered spermatozoa be utilized as soon as possible [45].

Role of FSH and Technical Aspects in Short-Term In Vitro Sperm Culture

The studies by Hosseini and Khalili [46], Wu et al. [47], and Balaban et al. [16] provide valuable insights into short-term in vitro culture conditions for spermatozoa in three different studies, particularly focusing on the role of follicle-stimulating hormone (FSH) and the technical conditions of incubation. Wu et al. and Hosseini and Khalili did not use recombinant FSH (rFSH) in their culture media, whereas Balaban et al. [16] included rFSH, which may enhance sperm viability.

Additionally, the enhancement of sperm motility in nonobstructive azoospermia (NOA) patients has been linked to specific in vitro incubation conditions. Moreover, incubating sperm for 24 h at 37 °C significantly increased motility, peaking at 72 h, with thawed samples performing similarly to fresh ones. Lee et al. [44] observed that a 24-h in vitro culture improved pregnancy outcomes in TESE-ICSI cycles, regardless of whether sperm samples were obtained on the day of or the day before ovarian puncture.

Sperm Freezing Recommendations for NOA Patients

Sperm cryopreservation plays a critical role in assisted reproduction. The following subsections outline the main considerations, including back up strategies , elimination of time constraints, success rates and the potential to reduce stress and costs in clinical practice.

Backup for Assisted Reproductive Techniques
Cryopreservation ensures a backup of sperm samples obtained through TESE. These samples can be stored for extended periods without compromising their viability. Various devices have been tested for cryopreserving few sperm, with different success rates and technical challenges. One cryopreservation technique which preserves rare sperm directly within the original microdroplet may enhance recovery, and this technique shows promise for broader assisted reproduction applications [48].

Elimination of Time Constraints
Cryopreservation eliminates time constraints associated with using fresh sperm. It allows for the sperm to be stored until needed, providing flexibility in the timing of assisted reproductive procedures such as IVF or ICSI [49].

Comparable Success Rates
Cryopreserved sperm obtained from TESE can yield comparable success rates in fertilization and pregnancy outcomes to fresh sperm when used in assisted reproductive techniques [50], with similar neonatal outcomes in men with OA. This ensures that individuals undergoing TESE have options for reproductive success regardless of when they decide to pursue fertility treatments [49].

Reduced Stress and Cost
Having cryopreserved sperm available from a TESE procedure offers individuals the opportunity to preserve their fertility, provides flexibility in reproductive planning, and ensures the availability of viable sperm for future use in ART, thereby offering hope for parenthood in challenging fertility circumstances [47, 49].

Sperm cryopreservation of rare testicular sperm samples through techniques like slow cooling and vitrification has been a subject of interest in ART. Comparing these methods is crucial due to their impact on sperm viability and potential success rates of fertility treatments [51].

Cryopreservation of testicular sperm may play a role in reducing the surgical sperm retrieval-induced hypogonadism [51].

Slow Freezing Versus Vitrification

Slow Cooling
This traditional cryopreservation method involves gradually reducing the temperature of sperm samples. It allows for a controlled decrease in temperature, minimizing potential damage to the cells from ice crystal formation. However, slow cooling may still pose risks of ice crystal formation within the cells, potentially impacting sperm viability [52].

Vitrification
In contrast, vitrification is a rapid freezing technique that involves transforming the sperm into a glass-like state without forming ice crystals. This swift process prevents ice crystal formation, which can harm cell integrity. Vitrification is known for its speed and efficacy in preserving cellular structures, including rare sperm, with minimal damage. While slow cooling has been a traditional method for sperm cryopreservation, vitrification has emerged as a promising alternative, especially for preserving rare sperm obtained through TESE. Vitrification's ability to prevent ice crystal formation and maintain cell integrity has shown advantages in preserving the viability and functionality of rare sperm, potentially leading to better outcomes in assisted reproductive treatments. However, ongoing research is essential to evaluate further and compare the efficacy of both methods in preserving rare sperm for successful fertility treatments [53].

Zhou et al. [54] showed that vitrification achieves better results for several sperm protection parameters than slow freezing; vitrification achieves a higher recovery rate ($P < 0.05$), motility ($P < 0.05$), morphology ($P < 0.05$), and curve line velocity ($P < 0.05$) than slow freezing. Furthermore, DNA fragmentation was decreased ($P < 0.05$), and better acrosome protection ($P < 0.05$) was exhibited in the spermatozoa after vitrification.

Freeze-drying or lyophilization of sperm is another method of sperm cryopreservation, which did not become a routinely applied technique due to the majority of the cryopreserved sperm becoming non-motile post-procedure. However, it was claimed that such sperm can be utilized for ICSI after confirming their viability [55].

Single-Sperm Cryopreservation Advances

Researchers have reported various methods for cryopreserving a few or single sperm obtained through TESE, including the empty zona method [56], microdroplet method [57], Volvox globator spheres method [58], agarose microspheres method [59], and sperm vitrification.

Of these, sperm vitrification with various modifications is effective in cryopreserving rare sperm. Desai et al. employed Cryoloop using an open system and reported 73% retention of motility, though reduced to just twitching movement; further investigations of sperm function tests revealed that the sperm could undergo sperm head decondensation, thus being capable of successful fertilization. They reported cryopreservation of five testicular sperm on the cryoprotectant layer in the loop. Three sperm were recovered post-warming, and two sperm could fertilize the oocytes [60].

Mangoli et al. [61] reported the effective use of closed system VitriMate® to cryopreserve sperm, achieving recovery and viability rates of 78.6% and 84.5%, respectively. In this study, both raw and processed samples (without cryoprotectant) were loaded onto the carrier and inserted into a pre-cooled lower sleeve of a specialized device that creates temperatures near that of liquid nitrogen, allowing sperm vitrification without direct contact with liquid nitrogen.

Berkovitz et al. [62] used a different device in which a few sperm overlayed with mineral oil were vitrified in a close system and reported a recovery rate of 96%, motility retention rate of 37%, fertilization rate of 59%, and pregnancy rate of 55%.

Proper Cryoprotectant

Cryoprotectants are chemicals specifically formulated to shield sperm cells from the detrimental effects of freezing temperatures. They mitigate freezing injury by reducing ice crystal formation within the cells, minimizing cellular damage, and preserving the structural integrity and viability of sperm during freezing and thawing [63].

Various cryoprotectants, including glycerol, ethylene glycol, dimethyl sulfoxide (DMSO), and propanediol, are used in sperm preservation. Each type has specific properties and concentrations that impact the effectiveness of preserving sperm cells [63].

Reduced Harmful Effects of Cryopreservation

The emerging trend of cryopreserving sperm without additional cryoprotective agents represents an innovative approach in assisted reproductive technologies. This strategy aims to simplify the cryopreservation process and potentially improve post-thaw sperm viability without relying on external cryoprotectants [64, 65].

Conclusion

Assisted reproduction outcomes in patients with nonobstructive azoospermia (NOA) face several challenges due to the limited availability and quality of viable sperm [66]. NOA is characterized by a severe reduction or absence of sperm in the ejaculate, necessitating the retrieval of sperm directly from the testes through procedures like testicular sperm extraction (TESE) or microdissection-TESE (m-TESE) [3]. However, the success rate of sperm retrieval in NOA patients can vary depending on factors such as testicular histology, testicular volume, and hormonal levels [3]. This limited availability of viable sperm poses a significant challenge in achieving successful assisted reproduction outcomes.

Furthermore, the quality of the retrieved sperm can also impact the success of these procedures. Sperm obtained from the testes of NOA patients may exhibit reduced motility, abnormal morphology, or DNA fragmentation [67]. These factors can negatively affect the fertilization potential and subsequent embryo development. Various techniques have been developed to address this challenge and improve the selection of high-quality sperm for fertilization. These include sperm selection based on morphology, DNA integrity, or advanced imaging technologies [68, 69]. By utilizing these methods, embryologists can identify the most viable and functionally intact sperm cells, increasing the chances of successful fertilization and embryo development.

In addition to the challenges associated with sperm quality and availability, the overall health and fertility of the female partner also play a crucial role in the success of assisted reproduction outcomes in NOA patients. Factors such as the female partner's age, ovarian reserve, and any other female infertility factors can impact the chances of successful fertilization, embryo development, and pregnancy [66].

To overcome these challenges, ongoing advancements in sperm retrieval techniques, sperm selection methods, and laboratory technologies are being made [69]. Researchers are continuously exploring new approaches to improve the success rates of assisted reproduction in NOA patients. However, it is important to note that each NOA patient is unique, and a personalized approach is necessary to optimize the chances of success based on individual characteristics and circumstances.

The development of techniques such as testicular sperm extraction (TESE) and microdissection-TESE (m-TESE) has allowed for the retrieval of sperm directly from the testes, expanding the options for NOA patients [3, 70]. Apart from advances in surgical techniques to extract spermatozoa from testes, laboratory techniques to process surgically retrieved sperm have contributed significantly to the success of assisted reproduction cycles using these samples. More meticulous methods of searching for sperm in testicular samples have improved sperm retrieval rates. These include enhanced sperm selection methods such as morphology-based selection, DNA integrity assessment, and advanced imaging technologies [67, 68, 69]. Moreover, the knowledge, skill, and experience of embryologists during sperm separation from testicular tissue and selecting the best sperm have developed over the decades, further boosting success rates.

While challenges remain, ongoing research and technological advancements continue to drive progress. By combining clinicians' expertise, advancements in laboratory techniques, and a patient-centered approach, the field of assisted reproduction in NOA patients is poised to continue improving outcomes and providing hope for individuals and couples facing infertility.

References

1. Achermann APP, Pereira TA, Esteves SC. Microdissection testicular sperm extraction (micro-TESE) in men with infertility due to nonobstructive azoospermia: summary of current literature. Int Urol Nephrol. 2021;53(11):2193–210. https://doi.org/10.1007/s11255-021-02979-4.
2. Aydos K, Aydos OS. Sperm selection procedures for optimizing the outcome of icsi in patients with noa. J Clin Med. 2021;10(12) https://doi.org/10.3390/jcm10122687.
3. Schlegel PN. Testicular sperm extraction: microdissection improves sperm yield with minimal tissue excision. Hum Reprod. 1999;14(1):131–5. https://doi.org/10.1093/humrep/14.1.131.
4. Ishikawa T. Surgical recovery of sperm in non-obstructive azoospermia. Asian J Androl. 2012;14(1):109–15. https://doi.org/10.1038/aja.2011.61. Epub 2011 Nov 28. PMID: 22120931; PMCID: PMC3735145
5. Esteves SC, Miyaoka R, Orosz JE, Agarwal A. An update on sperm retrieval techniques for azoospermic males. Clinics (Sao Paulo). 2013;68(Suppl 1):99–110. https://doi.org/10.6061/clinics/2013(sup01)11. PMID: 23503959; PMCID: PMC3583154
6. Ogouma L, Berthaut I, Lévy R, Hamid RH, Prades M, Audouin M, Sermondade N, Dupont C. Testicular sperm extraction (TESE) outcomes in the context of malignant disease: a systematic review. Asian J Androl. 2022;24(6):584–90. https://doi.org/10.4103/aja2021129. PMID: 35259785; PMCID: PMC9809488
7. Westlander G. Utility of micro-TESE in the most severe cases of non-obstructive azoospermia. Ups J Med Sci. 2020;125(2):99–103. https://doi.org/10.1080/03009734.2020.1737600. Epub 2020 Apr 1. PMID: 32233715; PMCID: PMC7721032
8. Liu J, Tsai YL, Katz E, Compton G, Garcia JE, Baramki TA. Outcome of in-vitro culture of fresh and frozen-thawed human testicular spermatozoa. Hum Reprod. 1997;12(8):1667–72. https://doi.org/10.1093/humrep/12.8.1667.
9. Crabbé E, Verheyen G, Tournaye H, Van Steirteghem A. The use of enzymatic procedures to recover testicular germ cells. Hum Reprod. 1997;12(8):1682–7. https://doi.org/10.1093/humrep/12.8.1682. PMID: 9308793
10. Flannigan RK, Schlegel PN. Testicular sperm extraction by microdissection: preoperative optimization of the patient, surgical technique, and tissue processing. Fertil Steril, March 2019;111(3):420–426. https://doi.org/10.1016/j.fertnstert.2019.01.003. PMID308227516.
11. Oates RD, Mulhall J, Burgess C, Cunningham D, Carson R. Fertilization and pregnancy using intentionally cryopreserved testicular tissue as the sperm source for intracytoplasmic sperm injection in 10 men with non-obstructive azoospermia. Hum Reprod. 1997;12(4):734–9.
12. Fishel S, Green S, Hunter A, Lisi F, Rinaldi L, Lisi R, McDermott H, Human Fertilization with round and elongated spermatids. Human Reprod. 1997 Feb;12(2):336–40. https://doi.org/10.1093/humrep/12.2.336. PMID: 9070722
13. Mangoli V, Mangoli R, Dandekar S, Suri K, Desai S. Selection of viable spermatozoa from testicular biopsies: a comparative study between pentoxifylline and hypoosmotic swelling test. Fertil Steril. 2011;95(2):631–4. https://doi.org/10.1016/j.fertnstert.2010.10.007.
14. Nagy ZP, Devroey P, Verheyen G, Van Steirteghem AC, Tournaye H. An improved treatment procedure for testicular biopsy specimens offers more efficient sperm recovery: case series. Fertil Steril. 1997;68(2):376-9. https://doi.org/10.1016/S0015-0282(97)81534-8.
15. Jow W, Steckel J, Schlegel PN, Magid MS, Goldstein M. Motile sperm in human testis specimens. J Androl. 1993;14(3):194–8.
16. Balaban B, Urman B, Sertac A, Alatas C, Aksoy S, Mercan R, Nuhoglu A. In-vitro culture of spermatozoa induces motility and increases implantation and pregnancy rates after testicular sperm extraction and intracytoplasmic sperm injection. Hum Reprod. 1999;14:2808–11. https://doi.org/10.1093/humrep/14.11.2808.
17. Salzbrunn A, Benson DM, Holstein AF, Schulze W. A new concept for the extraction of testicular spermatozoa as a tool for assisted fertilization (ICSI). Hum Reprod. 1996;11(4):752–5. https://doi.org/10.1093/oxfordjournals.humrep.a019248.

18. Fujii Y, Motoyama H, Hiraguchi K, Kobashi C, Kunitomi K. A simple method for recovering the motile spermatozoa from extremely low quality sperm samples. Hum Reprod. 1997;12(6):1218–21. https://doi.org/10.1093/humrep/12.6.1218. PMID: 9222004
19. Aboukhshaba A, Punjani N, Doukakis S, Zaninovic N, Palermo G, Schlegel PN. Testicular sperm characteristics in men with nonobstructive azoospermia and their impact on intracytoplasmic sperm injection outcome. Fertil Steril. 2022;117(3):522–7. https://doi.org/10.1016/j.fertnstert.2021.09.024.
20. James ER, Carrell DT, Aston KI, Jenkins TG, Yeste M, Salas-Huetos A. The role of the epididymis and the contribution of epididymosomes to mammalian reproduction. Int J Mol Sci. 2020;21(15):1–17. https://doi.org/10.3390/ijms21155377.
21. Taşdemir I, Taşdemir M, Tavukçuoğlu S. Effect of pentoxifylline on immotile testicular spermatozoa. J Assist Reprod Genet. 1998;15(2):90–2. https://doi.org/10.1007/BF02766832.
22. Marques de Oliveira N, Sánchez RV, Rodriguez Fiesta S, Lopez Salgado T, Rodríquez R, Bethencourt JCA, Zamora RB. Pregnancy with frozen-thawed and fresh testicular biopsy after motile immotile sperm microinjection, using the mechanical touch technique to assess viability. Hum Reprod. 2004;19(2):262–5. https://doi.org/10.1093/humrep/deh083.
23. Jayendran RS, Van Der Ven HH, Perez-Pelaez M, Crabo BG, Zaneveld LJD. Development of an assay to assess the functional integrity of the human sperm membrane and its relationship to other semen characteristics. J Reprod Fertil. 1984;70(1):219–28. https://doi.org/10.1530/jrf.0.0700219.
24. Sallam HN, Farrag A, Agameya A-F, El-Garem Y, Ezzeldin F. The use of the modified hypo-osmotic swelling test for the selection of immotile testicular spermatozoa in patients treated with ICSI: a randomized controlled study. Hum Reprod. 2005;20(12):3435–40. https://doi.org/10.1093/humrep/dei249.
25. Kızılay F, Altay B. Sperm function tests in clinical practice. Turk J Urol. 2017;43(4):393–400. https://doi.org/10.5152/tud.2017.96646.
26. Nixon B, Schjenken JE, Burke ND, Skerrett-Byrne DA, Hart HM, De Iuliis GN, Martin JH, Lord T, Bromfield EG. New horizons in human sperm selection for assisted reproduction. Front Endocrinol. 2023;14(February):1–15. https://doi.org/10.3389/fendo.2023.1145533.
27. Mangoli E, Khalili MA. The beneficial role of intra cytoplasmic morphologically selected sperm injection (IMSI) in assisted reproduction. J Reprod Infertil. 2020;21(1):3–10. PMID: 32175260; PMCID: PMC7048693
28. Hershko-Klement A, Sukenik-Halevy R, Biron Shental T, Miller N, Berkovitz. Intracytoplasmic morphologically selected sperm injection and congenital birth defects: a retrospective cohort study A. Andrology. 2016;4(5):887–93. https://doi.org/10.1111/andr.12221.
29. Ai L, et al. Intracytoplasmic morphologically selected sperm injection of testicular sperm: clinical outcome in azoospermia patients. Zhonghua Nan Ke Xue. 2010 Sep;16(9):824-8. Chinese. PMID: 21050644. https://doi.org/10.3760/cma.j.issn.1009-3591.2010.09.011.
30. Keskintepe L, Beyhan Z, Dayal M, Hart J, Keskintepe M. Intracytoplasmic morphologically selected sperm injection (IMSI) does not improve clinical outcomes and embryo ploidy in assisted reproductive cycles. Fertil Steril. 2016;106(3):e163. https://doi.org/10.1016/j.fertnstert.2016.07.480.
31. Souza Setti A, Ferreira RC, Paes de Almeida Ferreira Braga D, de Cássia Sávio Figueira R, Iaconelli A Jr, Borges E Jr. Intracytoplasmic sperm injection outcome versus intracytoplasmic morphologically selected sperm injection outcome: a meta-analysis. Reprod Biomed Online. 2010;21(4):450–5. https://doi.org/10.1016/j.rbmo.2010.05.017. Epub 2010 Jun 19. PMID: 20800549
32. Teixeira DM, Barbosa MA, Ferriani RA, Navarro PA, Raine-Fenning N, Nastri CO, Martins WP. Regular (ICSI) versus ultra-high magnification (IMSI) sperm selection for assisted reproduction. Cochrane Database Syst Rev. 2013;25(7):CD010167. https://doi.org/10.1002/14651858.CD010167.pub2. PMID: 23884963

33. Oliveira JB, Cavagna M, Petersen CG, Mauri AL, Massaro FC, Silva LF, et al. Pregnancy outcomes in women with repeated implantation failures after intracytoplasmic morphologically selected sperm injection (IMSI). Reprod Biol Endocrinol. 2011;9:99.
34. Lo Monte G, Murisier F, Piva I, Germond M, Marci R. Focus on intracytoplasmic morphologically selected sperm injection (IMSI): a mini-review. Asian J Androl. 2013;15(5):608–15. https://doi.org/10.1038/aja.2013.54. Epub 2013 Jul 8. PMID: 23832017; PMCID: PMC3881647
35. Lukaszuk K, Jakiel G, Wocławek Potocka I, Kiewisz J, Olszewska J, Sieg W, Podolak A, Pastuszek E, Wdowiak A. IMSI-guidelines for sperm quality assessment. Diagnostics (Basel). 2022;12(1):192. https://doi.org/10.3390/diagnostics12010192. PMID: 35054359; PMCID: PMC8774575
36. Alahmar AT, Singh R, Palani A. Sperm DNA fragmentation in reproductive medicine: a review. J Hum Reprod Sci. 2022;15(3):206–18. https://doi.org/10.4103/jhrs.jhrs_82_22.
37. Zhang Z, Dai C, Shan G, Chen X, Liu H, Abdalla K, Kuznyetsova I, Moskovstev S, Huang X, Librach C, Jarvi K, Sun Y. Quantitative selection of single human sperm with high DNA integrity for intracytoplasmic sperm injection. Fertil Steril. 2021;116(5):1308–18. https://doi.org/10.1016/j.fertnstert.2021.06.016.
38. Goss DM, Vasilescu SA, Vasilescu PA, Cooke S, Kim SH, Sacks GP, Gardner DK, Warkiani ME. Evaluation of an artificial intelligence-facilitated sperm detection tool in azoospermic samples for use in ICSI. Reprod Biomed Online. 2024;49(1):103910. https://doi.org/10.1016/j.rbmo.2024.103910. Epub 2024 Feb 22. PMID: 38652944
39. Wu DJ, Badamjav O, Reddy VV, Eisenberg M, Barry B. A preliminary study of sperm identification in microdissection testicular sperm extraction samples with deep convolutional neural networks. Asian J Androl. 2021;23:135–9. https://doi.org/10.4103/aja.aja.
40. Jiang T, Gradus JL, Rosellini AJ. Supervised machine learning: a brief primer. Behav Ther. 2020;51(5):675–87. https://doi.org/10.1016/j.beth.2020.05.002.
41. Chen F, De Neubourg D, Debrock S, Peeraer K, D'Hooghe T, Spiessens C. Selecting the embryo with the highest implantation potential using a data mining based prediction model. Reprod Biol Endocrinol. 2016;14(1) https://doi.org/10.1186/s12958-016-0145-1.
42. Bachelot G, Dhombres F, Sermondade N, Hamid RH, Berthaut I, Frydman V, Prades M, Kolanska K, Selleret L, Mathieu-D'Argent E, Rivet-Danon D, Levy R, Lamazière A, Dupont C. A machine learning approach for the prediction of testicular sperm extraction in non-obstructive azoospermia: algorithm development and validation study. J Med Internet Res. 2023;25(e44047):1–14. https://doi.org/10.2196/44047.
43. Esteves SC, Varghese AC. Laboratory handling of epididymal and testicular spermatozoa: what can be done to improve sperm injections outcome. J Hum Reprod Sci. 2012;5(3):233–43. https://doi.org/10.4103/0974-1208.106333.
44. Lee J, Yoo JH, Lee JH, Ahn HS, Hwang KJ, Kim M. Effect of in vitro testicular spermatozoa culture on pregnancy outcomes: an experience at a single university hospital. Yeungnam Univ J Med. 2021;38(1):53–9. https://doi.org/10.12701/yujm.2020.00773.
45. Nabi A, Khalili MA, Halvaei I, Roodbari F. Prolonged incubation of processed human spermatozoa will increase DNA fragmentation. Andrologia. 2014;46(4):374–9.
46. Hosseini A, Khalili MA. Improvement of motility after culture of testicular spermatozoa: the effects of incubation timing and temperature. Transl Androl Urol. 2017;6:271–6. https://doi.org/10.21037/tau.2017.03.43.
47. Wu B, Wong D, Lu S, Dickstein S, Silva M, Gelety TJ. Optimal use of fresh and frozen-thawed testicular sperm for intracytoplasmic sperm injection in azoospermic patients. J Assist Reprod Genet. 2005;22(11–12):389–94. https://doi.org/10.1007/s10815-005-7481-y. PMID: 16331535
48. Coetzee K, Ozgur K, Berkkanoglu M, Bulut H, Isikli A. Reliable single sperm cryopreservation in cell sleepers for azoospermia management. Andrologia. 2016;48(2):203–10. https://doi.org/10.1111/and.12434.

49. Karacan M, Alwaeely F, Erkan S, Çebi Z, Berberoğlugil M, Batukan M, Uluğ M, Arvas A, Çamlıbel T. Outcome of intracytoplasmic sperm injection cycles with fresh testicular spermatozoa obtained on the day of or the day before oocyte collection and with cryopreserved testicular sperm in patients with azoospermia. Fertil Steril. 2013;100(4):975–80. https://doi.org/10.1016/j.fertnstert.2013.06.031.
50. Grynberg M, Chevalier N, Mesner A, Rocher L, Prisant N, Madoux S, Feyereisen E, Ferlicot S, Fanchin R, Frydman R, Frydman N, Izard V. Non-obstuctive azoospermia: option of the testicular sperm extraction performed on the day of oocyte retrieval. J Gynecol Obstet Biol Reprod (Paris). 2010;
51. Eliveld J, van Wely M, Meißner A, Repping S, van der Veen F, van Pelt AMM. The risk of TESE-induced hypogonadism: a systematic review and meta-analysis. Hum Reprod Update. 2018;24(4):442–54. https://doi.org/10.1093/humupd/dmy015.
52. Mauri AL, Petersen CG, Baruffi RL, Ferreira RC, Franco JG Jr. Comparison of the cryopreservation of human embryos obtained after intracytoplasmic sperm injection with a slow cooling or an ultrarapid cooling procedure. J Assist Reprod Genet. 2001;18(5):257–61. https://doi.org/10.1023/a:1016630721045. PMCID: PMC3455333
53. Schiewe MC, Rothman C, Spitz A, Werthman PE, Zeitlin SI, Anderson RE. Validation-verification of a highly effective, practical human testicular tissue in vitro culture-cryopreservation procedure aimed to optimize pre-freeze and post-thaw motility. J Assist Reprod Genet. 2016;33(4):519–28. https://doi.org/10.1007/s10815-016-0659-7. Epub 2016 Feb 4. PMID: 26847133
54. Zhou D, Wang XM, Li RX, Wang YZ, Chao YC, Liu ZZ, Huang ZH, Nie HC, Zhu WB, Tan YQ, Fan LQ. Improving native human sperm freezing protection by using a modified vitrification method. Asian J Androl. 2021;23(1):91–6. https://doi.org/10.4103/aja.aja_29.
55. Keskintepe L, Eroglu A. Freeze-drying of mammalian sperm. Methods Mol Biol. 2015;1257:489–97. https://doi.org/10.1007/978-1-4939-2193-5_25. PMID: 25428025
56. Cohen J, Garrisi GJ, Congedo-Ferrara TA, Kieck KA, Schimmel TW, Scott RT. Cryopreservation of single human spermatozoa. Hum Reprod. 1997;12(5):994–1001.
57. Gil Salom M, Romero J, Rubio C, Ruiz A, Remohi J, Pellicer A. Intracytoplasmic sperm injection with cryopreserved testicular spermatozoa. Mol Cell Endocrinol. 2000;169(1–2):15–9.
58. Just A, Gruber I, Wöber M, Lahodny J, Obruca A, Strohmer H. Novel method for the cryopreservation of testicular sperm and ejaculated spermatozoa from patients with severe oligospermia: a pilot study. Fertil Steril. 2004;82(2):445–7. https://doi.org/10.1016/j.fertnstert.2003.12.050. PMID: 15302297
59. Isaev D, Zaletov S, Zaeva V, Zakharova E, Shafei R, Krivokharchenko I. Artificial microcontainers for cryopreservation of solitary spermatozoa. 2007. https://doi.org/10.13140/2.1.3645.9523.
60. Desai N, Culler C, Goldfarb J. Cryopreservation of single sperm from epidydimal and testicular samples on cryoloops: preliminary case report. Hum Reprod. 2004;82(September):264–5.
61. Mangoli RV, Mangoli VS, Desai SK, Poojary B, Suri K. PP-022 – vitrification of low number of sperms – an effective option. Reprod Biomed Online. 2016;32:S10–1. https://doi.org/10.1016/s1472-6483(16)30157-2.
62. Berkovitz A, Miller N, Silberman M, Belenky M, Itsykson P. A novel solution for freezing small numbers of spermatozoa using a sperm vitrification device. Hum Reprod. 2018;33(11):1975–83. https://doi.org/10.1093/humrep/dey304.
63. Hezavehei M, Sharafi M, Kouchesfahani HM, Henkel R, Agarwal A, Esmaeili V & Shahverdi A 2018 Sperm cryopreservation: a review on current molecular cryobiology and advanced approaches. Reproductive Biomedicine Online 37 327–339. https://doi.org/10.1016/j.rbmo.2018.05.012.
64. Aizpurua J, Medrano L, Enciso M, Sarasa J, Romero A, Fernández MA, Gómez-Torres MJ. New permeable cryoprotectant-free vitrification method for native human sperm. Hum Reprod. 2017;32(10):2007–15. https://doi.org/10.1093/humrep/dex281.

65. Ohno M, Tanaka A, Nagayoshi M, Yamaguchi T, Takemoto Y, Tanaka I, Watanabe S, Itakura A. Modified permeable cryoprotectant-free vitrification method for three or fewer ejaculated spermatozoa from cryptozoospermic men and 7-year follow-up study of 14 children born from this method. Hum Reprod. 2020;35(5):1019–28. https://doi.org/10.1093/humrep/deaa072.
66. Esteves SC, Roque M, Bedoschi G, Haahr T, Humaidan P. Intracytoplasmic sperm injection for male infertility and consequences for offspring. Nat Rev Urol. 2018;15(9):535–62. https://doi.org/10.1038/s41585-018-0051-8.
67. Simon L, Murphy K, Shamsi MB, Liu L, Emery B, Aston KI, Hotaling J, Carrell DT. Paternal influence of sperm DNA integrity on early embryonic development. Hum Reprod. 2014;29(11):2402–12. https://doi.org/10.1093/humrep/deu228.
68. Bartoov B, Berkovitz A, Eltes F, Kogosowski A, Menezo Y, Barak Y. Real-time fine morphology of motile human sperm cells is associated with IVF-ICSI outcome. J Androl. 2002;23(1):1–8. https://doi.org/10.1002/j.1939-4640.2002.tb02595.x.
69. Esteves SC. Novel concepts in male factor infertility: clinical and laboratory perspectives. J Assist Reprod Genet. 2016;33(10):1319–35. https://doi.org/10.1007/s10815-016-0763-8.
70. Amer M, Ateyah A, Hany R, Zohdy W. Prospective comparative study between microsurgical and conventional testicular sperm extraction in non-obstructive azoospermia: follow-up by serial ultrasound examinations. Hum Reprod. 2000;15(3):653–6. https://doi.org/10.1093/humrep/15.3.653.

Chapter 14
Management of Nonobstructive Azoospermia After Prior Failed Treatment

Logan Hubbard, Muslim Dogan Deger, and Amarnath Rambhatla

Introduction

Azoospermia is the complete lack of spermatozoa in two different centrifuged specimens of semen and is categorized as either obstructive (OA) or nonobstructive azoospermia (NOA). Men with OA can achieve biological paternity by sperm retrieval from the testicle or epididymis in conjunction with intracytoplasmic sperm injection (ICSI) or through a surgical procedure to alleviate the obstruction, thus allowing sperm to be present in the ejaculate. Patients with NOA may still be able to genetically father children on their own, even though they do not have sperm in their ejaculate, as they often harbor residual, localized foci of spermatogenesis in their testes. Conventionally, the anatomical location of the cause—pre-testicular or testicular—is used to classify the etiology of NOA. Pre-testicular NOA, also known as secondary hypogonadism, results from an imbalance in hormones regulating the hypothalamic–pituitary–testicular (HPT) axis that prevents a physically normal testis from being adequately stimulated to create sperm [1]. On the other hand, primary hypogonadism is due to testicular failure and can arise from a multitude of causes, including extrinsic damage to the testicular parenchyma or from more insidious genetic or idiopathic etiologies.

NOA represents one of the most challenging scenarios in male factor infertility. The main treatment option for men with NOA who wish to have biological offspring is microscopic testicular sperm extraction (mTESE) in conjunction with

L. Hubbard (✉)
Department of Urology, University of Minnesota, Minneapolis, MN, USA

M. D. Deger
Department of Urology, Tekirdag City Hospital, Tekirdag, Turkey

A. Rambhatla
Vattikuti Urology Institute, Henry Ford Hospital, Detroit, MI, USA
e-mail: arambha1@hfhs.org

W. Zohdy et al. (eds.), *Non-Obstructive Azoospermia*,
https://doi.org/10.1007/978-3-031-99431-9_14

ICSI, with or without medical/hormonal modulation. The success rates for surgical sperm retrieval (SSR) in NOA often range from 20% to 60%, which can be dependent on multiple factors [2]. For example, the results of SSR in patients with subnormal vs normal testosterone levels showed that patients with normal testosterone levels had a much higher likelihood of SSR than patients with low testosterone levels [3]. Additionally, individuals with NOA who have a clinical varicocele may have varicocele correction performed prior to SSR, as this might lead to improved outcomes or the identification of ejaculated sperm. It is hence the goal of this chapter to address options for optimizing and treating arguably the most difficult to manage population in all of male infertility: patients who have previously failed a mTESE procedure but have a continued desire to bear biologic progeny.

Options for Surgical Sperm Retrieval in NOA

Before one can fully understand the complex options available to men in the salvage setting, a complete and thorough understanding of first-line treatments is mandatory. Beginning with the least invasive option, percutaneous aspiration of the sperm is accomplished by inserting a small or large-diameter needle into the testis via the scrotal skin with careful attention to the avoidance of vascular structures. The needle tip may be inserted and withdrawn several times into the testicle to reach different areas while applying suction. Jensen et al. conducted a study, performing testicular sperm aspiration (TESA) on 125 men with NOA with an SSR rate of 30.4%. Among nine men with NOA in whom TESA was negative, only one showed positive SSR on mTESE [4]. The key benefits of the TESA procedure are its simplicity, low cost, minimal invasiveness, and diminished patient discomfort. However, aspiration is not completely benign, and there are risks involved with sperm retrieval in this manner. A study in rams assessed testicular changes after testicular biopsy (using both needle aspiration as well as cTESE) as compared to the contralateral control testicle. When comparing testicles subjected to TESA against the contralateral healthy control testicle, there was an increase in microcalcifications, tubular damage with resulting fibrosis, and surrounding areas of seminiferous tubule dilation on histologic analysis [5]. Although not assessed in this animal study, multiple needle biopsies have been shown in rat studies to deposit an increasing amount of scar tissue.

Underlying all sperm retrieval procedures is the requirement of finding sperm able to be utilized in assisted reproductive techniques (ART). Therefore, larger sperm yields are often required, necessitating a scrotal incision and open biopsy of the testes termed conventional TESE (cTESE). In single-arm investigations, reported SSR rates are around 50% [6]. When compared to aspiration and microscopic TESE procedures, cTESE has been associated with a greater risk of complications. Intratesticular hematoma three months after cTESE was found in 51.7% of patients. Investigations into longer-term outcomes found that, at 6-month follow-up, testicular fibrosis was seen in up to 30% of individuals.

Schlegel pioneered the use of an operating optical microscope to analyze seminiferous tubules at a magnification of 20–25x and extract those tubules that were bigger, dilated, and opaque and thus more likely to contain mature sperm [7]. The reasoning behind this procedure was to maximize the likelihood of sperm retrieval with a smaller volume of tissue collected and, as a result, a decreased risk of complications. When cTESE and mTESE were directly compared, the unadjusted SSR rate for cTESE (95% CI 30–40%) was 35%, whereas for mTESE (95% CI 47–58%), it was 52%. SSR in mTESE was 1.5 times more likely to yield sperm when compared with cTESE (95% CI 1.4–1.6) [8]. Another study conducted by Deruyver et al. showed the SSR rate with cTESE ranged from 16.7% to 45% and in the mTESE group from 42.9% to 63% [9].

A refinement of the mTESE technique was first described by Kamal et al. in 2004, demonstrating improved sperm retrieval rates when isolating the most dilated tubule using a microscope, termed single seminiferous tubule sampling [10]. A separate study in men with NOA reported a differential SRR of 84.2% rate when sampling single tubules larger than 300 μm in diameter, compared to 36.3% retrieval rate for tubules smaller than 300 μm, using an operative microscope. Furthermore, a cutoff size of 110 μm was found to have a sensitivity of 86.0% and specificity of 74.4% with positive and negative predictive values of 0.858 and 0.256, respectively [11]. However, regardless of the procedure of choice used for sperm extraction, the fact that a significant percentage of men with NOA will fail their initial TESE procedure remains sobering. Thus, a firm understanding of what constitutes a failed TESE and what are the predictors of success prior to sperm retrieval is vital to the reproductive urologist.

Definitions of Failure and Predictors of Success on Primary MTESE

Failure to retrieve sperm on the initial extraction can, in some cases, merit a repeat TESE procedure. If sperm was retrieved following the initial surgery, Ghalayini et al.'s research showed that 91.5% of patients had successful repeated mTESE trials [12]. Salvage TESE implies multiple failures and therefore multiple procedures beyond just a repeat TESE. In 34 males with NOA, Westlander et al. investigated the viability of recurrent testicular sperm aspiration. They discovered that it was possible to repeat the process several times (up to the sixth try in one patient) without deleterious effects to the patient, the fertilization rate (range of 40.2–65.4%), or the couple's pregnancy outcomes [13]. Importantly the fertility numbers did show a downward trend with subsequent TESA procedures. Xu et al. conducted a study of 52 NOA males who underwent salvage mTESE and conducted multivariate logistic regression to generate a likelihood ratio and predictive formula for sperm retrieval probability based on testicular histopathology and total testosterone. A predicted probability of more than 71% was established for the formula as the cut-off value in predicting sperm retrieval based on receiver operator characteristics [14].

Although there are options for those failing initial management for NOA, much effort has been invested into determining whether a TESE procedure will be successful. Unfortunately, as of this moment, it is still not possible to use clinical noninvasive measures to predict the mTESE result in NOA. Reproductive hormone levels—testosterone, LH, inhibin B, and FSH—have been investigated as possible indicators of mTESE effectiveness. However, their predictive power has proven to be low. Even in patients with high FSH levels and low testosterone levels, there are areas that harbor intact spermatogenesis [12]. Nonetheless, there is no clear consensus on this issue.

Y-chromosome microdeletion and karyotype analyses are important genetic factors in the setting of NOA. Patients with Klinefelter syndrome showed lower SSR rates (31.4%). While acceptable SSR rates were detected in azoospermia factor-c (AZFc) deletions (70.4%), sperm was rarely detected in AZFa and AZFb deletions [15]. Regardless of the technique used for sperm retrieval, there remains a question of what the optimal timeframe is to perform a repeat TESE. For up to 6 months following TESE, transient negative physiological effects are frequently observed in the testes. Moreover, it takes time for men with NOA to recover testicular and spermatogenic function after an initial procedure; thus, it is recommended to wait at least 6 months following mTESE before contemplating repeat surgery. Yet, despite the logic inherent, studies have found that the amount of time between sperm retrieval operations has little bearing on the likelihood of procuring testicular sperm [16].

Of all the factors that have been reviewed, mTESE success rates were influenced the most by the major testicular histologic subtype. Ghalayini et al. evaluated sperm retrieval success by mTESE based on histopathology outcomes, including 134 men with NOA. They found SSR rates in maturation arrest to be 40.9%, Sertoli-cell-only syndrome (SCOS) 31.5%, and hypospermatogenesis 94.8% [12]. In a separate study, 365 NOA patients' SSR rates by mTESE were evaluated. Compared to individuals with SCOS (19.5%), those with maturation arrest (40.3%) had a greater sperm retrieval. Patients with hypospermatogenesis showed better SSR than the other two groups (SSR = 100.0%; $P < 0.001$) [17]. Although histopathology provides accurate information on the state of spermatogenesis in men with NOA, the evidence correlating histopathology and SSR is highly variable, as described above. This has led to the guideline statements that testicular biopsy should only be performed concurrently with a surgical sperm retrieval to avoid unnecessary procedures in infertile males [18].

Treatment, Optimization, and Outcomes Following Failed Testicular Sperm Extraction

Success and failure rates of TESE procedures can be related to patient factors and whether cTESE or mTESE were performed initially. Men failing cTESE or TESA may benefit from an mTESE. As aforementioned, there have been several studies showing improved SSR when comparing mTESE to cTESE, including one large meta-analysis showing a difference of 52% versus 32% [8]. Head-to-head studies have also shown mTESE to be superior in terms of SSR; however, these studies have been performed as the primary procedure, and therefore cannot be fully extrapolated to failed initial treatments. However, based on the inherent numerical advantage provided by mTESE, this would appear to be a logical option after an initial failed cTESE or TESA. When considering salvage mTESE specifically after failed cTESE or TESA, no large-scale or randomized trials have been performed, and the SSR has a high level of variance in the literature. Kalsi et al. looked at men undergoing salvage mTESE after either failed cTESE or TESA, finding an SSR rate of 46.5% with maturation arrest and SCOS accounting for the lowest rates among histological variants [19]. On the other hand, in a study of 125 hormonally optimized men who had a negative mTESE for their first sperm retrieval procedure, a repeat mTESE successfully recovered sperm in 23 men (18.4%) [20]. Given the variable SSR rates, which are largely dependent on the initial procedure performed on the patient, the decision as to whether to proceed with a repeat TESE procedure should be individualized with a frank discussion of risks, benefits, and expectations of not only the infertile male but also their female partner.

Surgical and Lifestyle Optimization

Yet, successful sperm retrieval does not occur in a vacuum, and there are many factors that can be corrected and/or optimized to improve upon the diminished SSR aforementioned. Varicoceles may represent a modifiable risk factor of azoospermia that can be corrected prior to an initial TESE as well as in cases of salvage mTESE. While varicocele repair has, in general, remained a controversial topic, multiple studies, including a recent large meta-analysis, have demonstrated improvements in conventional semen parameters after varicocelectomy [21]. Correction of varicocele prior to sperm retrieval in men with NOA is a controversial topic, but some studies have shown benefit. Kirby et al. looked more specifically at azoospermic and severely oligospermic men and found varicocelectomy to confer some improvements in SSR (OR 2.509), pregnancy, and live birth rates [22]. Conversely, a few small studies looking specifically at varicocelectomy prior to salvage mTESE did not find a significant difference in SSR; however, these studies were heterogeneous and underpowered to make such a distinction, thus requiring a nuanced and personalized discussion with each infertile couple [23]. Post-varicocelectomy spermatogenesis also seems to have a correlation to pre-procedure histopathology. A systematic review studying outcomes after varicocele repair in men with NOA found that 62.9% of men with hypospermatogenesis post-varicocelectomy had the presence of sperm in semen versus 26.3% of patients with maturation arrest and 7.3% with SCOS. Furthermore, post-varicocele repair sperm extraction in men with NOA was 48.9% versus 32.1% in untreated men, with an average spontaneous pregnancy rate of 5.24% [24]. Thus, there seems to be some evidence in favor of varicocele repair prior to proceeding with further sperm extraction procedures in the setting of a failed previous mTESE for men with NOA and varicocele, especially with certain testicular histopathologies. However, while varicoceles remain a contributing factor to male infertility, their presence is likely one of several factors associated with a patient's azoospermia and not the sole determinant. Although correcting a varicocele prior to repeat TESE is unlikely to improve a patient from azoospermia to sperm appearing in the ejaculate, even small improvements to the testicular microenvironment may provide benefit in patients undergoing repeat TESE procedures and merit discussion and counseling with the infertile couple.

Obesity represents another infertility and health risk factor that can be readily optimized prior to any salvage sperm retrieval procedure. There is clinical and basic science evidence demonstrating obesity's adverse effects on testosterone, conventional semen parameters, embryo quality, epigenetic remodeling, and changes in non-coding mRNA expression [25, 26, 27]. A retrospective study by Li et al. was unable to clearly demonstrate an association of elevated body mass index (BMI) with lower SSR, embryo quality, or clinical outcomes. However, in obese men with NOA undergoing TESA-ICSI cycles, obese men had lower T and estradiol (E2) levels [28]. Although evidence linking weight loss directly to improved sperm retrieval rates is limited, its potential benefits on hormonal profiles and other previously discussed parameters—as well as general health advantages—make it an important topic to discuss before undergoing repeat or salvage TESE.

Hormonal Optimization

Just as obesity can have a potent effect on the gonadal axis, there is mounting evidence that a primary TESE procedure precipitates a transient but potentially impactful hypogonadal state. Disruption of the seminiferous tubules, hematoma, and scar tissue formation has been shown to cause a decrease in both systemic and intratesticular testosterone that, in general, seems to resolve in 18–26 months on average. Additionally, a reduction in testicular volume of at least 2 mL was seen in 25% of men following cTESE and 2.5% of men following mTESE [29]. A meta-analysis performed by Eliveld et al. demonstrated a 2.7 nmol/L decrease in total testosterone 6 months (often with symptomatic hypogonadism) after TESE, which almost universally resolved by 18 months' time [30]. However, other studies have suggested that the transient adverse effects on the testicle last around 6 months [7]. The optimal timing for a repeat TESE procedure has not been established, but some studies have suggested that repeat sperm extraction procedures are more successful if performed after 6 months [12].

Studies in animal models have shown that pulsatile hormonal stimulation using human chorionic gonadotropin (hCG) can stimulate Leydig cells (even under hypergonadotropic conditions) and restore their function, thus improving intratesticular testosterone and the chances for sperm retrieval [31]. Two small clinical studies have shown a benefit of hormonally optimizing patients—using a combination of hCG and recombinant FSH—prior to salvage mTESE, yielding an SSR rate ranging from 10% to 20% when compared against untreated controls [32, 33]. There is evidence from large-scale meta-analyses that eugonadotropic men may have better chances of sperm retrieval during the primary mTESE procedure than hypergonadotropic men. A higher SSR rate was found in hormonally optimized men (OR 1.96, 95% CI: 1.08–3.56, $P = 0.03$) in general, and on subgroup analysis the likelihood of sperm retrieval was shown to favor eugonadal (OR 2.13, 95% CI: 1.10–4.14, $P = 0.02$) men over hypergonadotropic men (OR 1.73, 95% CI: 0.44–6.77, $P = 0.43$) with the authors discouraging upfront hormonal therapy from being universally applied [34]. One can therefore argue that, given this evidence, hormonal therapy in hypergonadotropic men may have minimal benefit in patients undergoing repeat mTESE. Supporting this point in the salvage setting, a recent meta-analysis found that lower levels of FSH (standard mean difference: −0.86, 95% CI: −1.18 to −0.54) and LH (standard mean difference: −0.68, 95% CI: −1.16 to −0.19) were strong predictors of sperm retrieval rates in men failing their initial TESE procedure [23]. Though promising, this data remains limited and, as reflected in societal guideline statements, should not be considered the standard of care. Therefore, the decision to begin hormonal therapy before repeat mTESE should be nuanced, especially given the potential adverse effects of hormonal and surgical therapy, as well as the significant financial burden affecting conservatively upward of 50% of men undergoing fertility care [35].

A group of NOA patients that bear special mention in the setting of repeated mTESE procedures are Klinefelter syndrome (KS) patients. Sperm retrieval rates at initial mTESE in men with KS range from 45% to 50% based on the available data. There is predictably less evidence pertaining to salvage mTESE; a small study found that of 18 non-mosaic KS men experiencing unsuccessful index TESE, only 3 men (16.7%) had successful sperm retrieval on repeat mTESE. However, it bears noting that this percentage represents non-mosaic KS cohorts who have been traditionally viewed as sterile. Spermatogenesis can be largely dependent on mosaic variants of KS, in which 50% of mosaic men had sperm in the ejaculate versus only 7% non-mosaic KS men, with traditionally higher fertilization rates versus non-mosaic patients [36, 37, 38]. This has obvious and profound implications regarding the reproductive urologist's decision for salvage mTESE, since, by nature of the genetic mutation, there is a higher likelihood of finding areas of spermatogenesis on either index or repeat TESE than non-mosaic variants. This is evidenced by work from Tsukamoto et al., whose group found that in men with KS undergoing sperm retrieval, men in the sperm-found group had a significantly lower mosaic ratio (4.3% versus 38.6%) compared with men where no sperm was found. This implies men with more 46 XY cells had a greater likelihood of finding sperm on mTESE. However, the overall rates of sperm retrieval in the groups did not differ to a large degree with the non-mosaic group having a sperm retrieval rate of 46.5% and the mosaic group having a rate of 50% ($P = 0.82$). Their study additionally found that their mosaic KS group had better ICSI outcomes, thought to be due to the high utilization of motile sperm [39]. While these margins are admittedly small, in situations of repeat or salvage TESE, these could potentially be meaningful differences to counsel patients who may be considering repeat procedures.

Heat Mapping and Sperm Preservation

Fine needle aspiration (FNA) mapping after a failed mTESE has been suggested as a method of "mapping" the testes to decide whether a repeat mTESE is worthwhile, and also to identify which region is most likely to have sperm. It involves multiple percutaneous aspirations of testicular contents using a small-gauge needle, with the aspirates being stained and examined later. In the only study looking at FNA after failed index TESE, 82 men met criteria, with 24 of those men (29.3%) finding sperm—predominantly in the periphery of the testis—on FNA after failed TESE. Fifteen men went on to repeat mTESE, with successful sperm retrieval in all 15 cases [40]. Though this represents promising data, several important details should be considered. A randomized trial comparing FNA to salvage mTESE would be useful to determine if FNA provides superior detection over mTESE alone. This question becomes amplified when realizing that the patient must in turn undergo another separate procedure with all the associated risks and benefits previously discussed. Additionally, samples identified in mapping are essentially discarded in situations where even a single sperm is extremely valuable; hence, FNA should only be considered after careful patient counseling.

Another intricacy worth considering centers around what to do with retrieved biopsies and sperm obtained from the salvage mTESE. There remains controversy in the field as to whether fresh or cryopreserved sperm is suitable. Based on current guidelines, there was found to be a calculated 92.2% rate of finding usable sperm for ART after a freeze–thaw cycle [41]. This is admittedly a low probability of being unable to find suitable sperm for ART, meaning most couples would likely benefit from cryopreservation. Yet, despite this fact, it was found that the live birth rate had a relative risk of 0.77 when compared to using fresh sperm, demonstrating a small but measurable difference between the two [41]. Additionally, the method used for sperm preservation seems to play a role in outcomes, with recent advances in vitrification showing great promise in the field of ART. Vitrification involves rapidly plunging samples into liquid nitrogen, compared to conventional slow freezing. A recent meta-analysis comparing conventional cryopreservation to vitrification found significantly higher post-thaw rates of motility and progressive motility, but similar rates of DNA fragmentation indices and morphology between vitrification and conventional freezing methods [42]. Although there is a likely benefit in these sperm parameters with vitrification, there was significant heterogeneity among the studies in their vitrification protocols; therefore, more research regarding ideal protocols, as well as inclusion of pregnancy rates, is required. Yet, when considering salvage mTESE, these small details should be strongly considered by the reproductive urologist and the infertile couple, as they provide tangible benefits in situations where incremental improvements may prove vital.

Fertility Outcomes After Salvage mTESE

As previously discussed, the overall SSR upon salvage mTESE is dependent on a multitude of factors. However, as with most questions in fertility, the truest endpoints are pregnancy and live birth. Among patients undergoing a first-time TESE, the fertilization rate with ICSI ranged from 47% to 67%. The pooled clinical pregnancy rate with index TESE procedures was found to be approximately 39% while the mean subsequent live birth rate per 100 embryo transfer cycles was 24% (with a wide range of 12–62%) [43, 44]. Data regarding ART and live birth rates in repeat or salvage mTESE are very limited. Karacan et al. studied a small cohort of 39 men with prior unsuccessful cTESE; out of those men, only 6 (15.3%) had spermatozoa found on repeat mTESE. Clinical pregnancy rates were 16.6% on the repeat TESE group, with an implantation rate of 9% and a miscarriage rate of 8.3%. The live birth rate in the study was found to be just 1 out of 39 men, or 2.5% when azoospermia was encountered on the index TESE procedure [45]. While the overall SRR of TESE procedures is more familiar to reproductive physicians, at the end of the day the ultimate bar by which success is measured is live births for the infertile couple. Though this data is largely retrospective in nature, it provides valuable information for those seeking counsel on repeated procedures and their chances of conception.

Future Directions and Emerging Technology

Ultrasonography

Scrotal ultrasound is a familiar modality to all reproductive urologists; its ease, cost, and minimally invasive nature make it ideal to answer numerous infertility questions. Utilizing ultrasonography with a seminiferous tubule size cutoff of >250 μm, there was a 77% sensitivity and 81% specificity (AUC > 0.82) for detecting sperm on corresponding mTESE [46]. It is clear that this could provide a minimally invasive method of determining areas of likely spermatogenesis and in turn allow a more targeted approach to those deciding to undergo salvage mTESE. Other interesting uses of ultrasound in men with NOA have utilized power and color Doppler to assess the impact of testicular perfusion on SRR and found that in men with 3 or more detectable intratesticular vessels 60% of the men with NOA required <3 biopsies for successful sperm retrieval versus just 18% in men with no detectable vessel on ultrasound. There was also a significant correlation between the presence of a vessel on ultrasound and the probability of successful sperm extraction during sampling of that specific segment [47].

MRI and Spectroscopy

Recent studies in functional magnetic resonance imaging (fMRI) have looked at the random Brownian diffusion of water through tissues via a function called apparent diffusion coefficient (ADC), whereby increased diffusion across a surface area correlates to diminished cellularity, normally restricting fluid motion. ADC was associated with increased rates of NOA in men versus healthy controls—indicating a loss of seminiferous tubule density, germ cells, Sertoli and Leydig cells, and overall decrease in cellularity normally restricting fluid diffusion—with a cutoff of 1.1×10^{-3} mm^2/s as a cutoff differentiating NOA testis with normal versus abnormal spermatogenesis [48]. In the same study, ADC and magnetization transfer ratio (another measure of fluid diffusion) were both significantly elevated in NOA testicles who underwent a negative mTESE.

MRI spectroscopy has also emerged as a promising technology as a method of identifying spermatogenic function in men with NOA. Choline, in particular, has been found to be higher in men with normal spermatogenic function [49]. A prospective study by Said et al. examined 120 men, including 60 with NOA, who underwent scrotal MRI with spectroscopy. Low levels of choline on MRI spectroscopy in the NOA group (representing impaired sperm integrity) were predictive of sperm retrieval rates on TESE with an area under the curve of 0.923, with a sensitivity of 90.2% and a specificity of 84.2% [50]. These local changes in choline density can therefore offer a heat map of areas likely to harbor intact spermatogenesis and could prove useful in surgical planning for a potential repeat or salvage mTESE.

Sperm Biomarkers

Biomarkers for male infertility have also been extensively studied in recent years and may also provide a way to determine the likelihood of a successful mTESE in either the index or salvage setting. There has been significant research in the area of RNA and RNA subgroups in male infertility, especially NOA and idiopathic infertility. A group investigating PIWI-interacting RNA (a subgroup of RNA expressed specifically in mammalian germ cells) in 10 men with NOA found a differential pattern of mRNA expression in men with unsuccessful sperm retrieval versus those with successful sperm retrieval [51]. Although still in its nascency, this could provide biomarkers predictive of focal spermatogenesis and therefore the likelihood of finding sperm with a mTESE or salvage mTESE.

Cellular Therapy and Gene Therapy

Beyond simply determining spermatogenic potential or the probability of finding sperm on an extraction procedure, there has been continuing research as to whether spermatogenic function can be augmented or even completely restored prior to a salvage TESE. One area of intense research is the use of cellular therapy and stem cells to aid in spermatogenic recovery. Spermatogenesis, at its most elemental level, is a stem cell-driven process; therefore, it is reasonable to suggest that the pluripotency of spermatogonial stem cells (SSCs) could potentially replenish the depleted pool of sperm precursors—often referred to as "artificial sperm." There is currently active research into other various types of stem cells, including mesenchymal and adipose-derived stem cells; however, these approaches are still in their infancy and face similar challenges, ranging from the efficiency of cryopreservation to societal and cultural attitudes toward the science as a whole [52]. Yet, the prospect of replacing lost spermatogonial precursors and potentially re-stimulating native sperm production prior to a repeat mTESE highlights the promise of stem cell research as a worthwhile avenue to explore in men who have failed an initial TESE.

Recent advances in genetics have augmented our understanding of its role in male infertility and azoospermia. Of particular interest are mutations—such as the cohesin protein coding region stromal antigen 3 (STAG3)—important for meiosis and whose loss results in meiotic arrest [53]. Using clustered regularly interspaced short palindromic repeats (CRISPR)- associated endonucleases (Cas9), the underlying genetic mutation was repaired, leading to the restoration of wild-type SSC lines as confirmed by whole-genome sequencing [54]. Furthermore, males with repaired SSC lineages were able to spontaneously reproduce at an acceptable rate. There are multiple other gene mutations that are being investigated that are thought to be responsible for meiotic arrest and hypospermatogenesis; however, these studies remain in vitro and there still remains substantial work before it is practical clinically.

Concluding Remarks

Nonobstructive azoospermia has remained a clinical and scientific dilemma in the field of infertility; however, perhaps no patient population is as challenging to manage as those who have failed initial treatment. Although the advent of mTESE has offered men who were previously deemed sterile a viable surgical option for finding sperm, it is far from a perfect solution to the problem of NOA. For men who undergo an initial TESE procedure, the chances of finding sperm come down to essentially a coin flip. However, this still leaves a significant portion of men undergoing invasive sperm extraction procedures without an obvious recourse. Although there is no current standard of care for men who have failed initial SSR, recent advances in the understanding of surgical optimization prior to repeat TESE (management of obesity, hypogonadism), as well as developments in different surgical techniques and cryopreservation, offer immediate hope to those with NOA failing initial management. However, exciting developments in imaging for the identification of spermatogenesis, spermatogonial stem cell and gene therapies, and semen biomarkers are now offering fresh potential for biological paternity in men with NOA who have failed index treatments—an outcome previously thought to be impossible.

References

1. Cocuzza M, Alvarenga C, Pagani R. The epidemiology and etiology of azoospermia. Clinics (Sao Paulo). 2013;68(Suppl 1):15–26.
2. Enatsu N, Chiba K, Fujisawa M. The development of surgical sperm extraction and new challenges to improve the outcome. Reprod Med Biol. 2016;15(3):137–44.
3. Caroppo E, Colpi GM. Hormonal treatment of men with nonobstructive azoospermia: what does the evidence suggest? J Clin Med. 2021;10(3)
4. Jensen CF, Ohl DA, Hiner MR, Fode M, Shah T, Smith GD, Sonksen J. Multiple needle-pass percutaneous testicular sperm aspiration as first-line treatment in azoospermic men. Andrology. 2016;4(2):257–62.
5. Fedder J, Marcussen N, Fedder MDK, Engvad B. Testicular damage following testicular sperm retrieval: a Ram model study. Biomed Res Int. 2017;2017:2472805.
6. Fraietta R. Microdissection is the best way to perform sperm retrieval in men with non-obstructive azoospermy? | Opinion: Yes. Int Braz J Urol. 2018;44(6):1063–6.
7. Schlegel PN. Testicular sperm extraction: microdissection improves sperm yield with minimal tissue excision. Hum Reprod. 1999;14(1):131–5.
8. Bernie AM, Mata DA, Ramasamy R, Schlegel PN. Comparison of microdissection testicular sperm extraction, conventional testicular sperm extraction, and testicular sperm aspiration for nonobstructive azoospermia: a systematic review and meta-analysis. Fertil Steril. 2015;104(5):1099–103. e1091–3
9. Deruyver Y, Vanderschueren D, Van der Aa F. Outcome of microdissection TESE compared with conventional TESE in non-obstructive azoospermia: a systematic review. Andrology. 2014;2(1):20–4.
10. Kamal A, Fahmy I, Mansour RT, Abou-Setta AM, Serour GI, Aboulghar MA. Selection of individual testicular tubules from biopsied testicular tissue with a stereomicroscope improves sperm retrieval rate. J Androl. 2004;25(1):123–7.
11. Amer M, Zohdy W, Abd El Naser T, Hosny H, Arafa M, Fakhry E. Single tubule biopsy: a new objective microsurgical advancement for testicular sperm retrieval in patients with nonobstructive azoospermia. Fertil Steril. 2008;89(3):592–6.
12. Ghalayini IF, Alazab R, Halalsheh O, Al-Mohtaseb AH, Al-Ghazo MA. Repeated microdissection testicular sperm extraction in patients with non-obstructive azoospermia: outcome and predictive factors. Arab J Urol. 2022;20(3):137–43.
13. Westlander G, Rosenlund B, Soderlund B, Wood M, Bergh C. Sperm retrieval, fertilization, and pregnancy outcome in repeated testicular sperm aspiration. J Assist Reprod Genet. 2001;18(3):171–7.

14. Xu T, Peng L, Lin X, Li J, Xu W. Predictors for successful sperm retrieval of salvage microdissection testicular sperm extraction (TESE) following failed TESE in nonobstructive azoospermia patients. Andrologia. 2017;49(4)
15. Kızılay F, Semerci B, Şimşir A, Kalemci S, Altay B. Analysis of factors affecting repeat microdissection testicular sperm extraction outcomes in infertile men. Turk J Urol. 2019;45(Supp. 1):S1–6.
16. Tai MC, Huang IS, Huang CY, Huang WJ. Feasibility of repeat microdissection testicular sperm extraction within 6 months for nonobstructive azoospermia. J Chin Med Assoc. 2023;86(3):300–5.
17. Esteves SC, Prudencio C, Seol B, Verza S, Knoedler C, Agarwal A. Comparison of sperm retrieval and reproductive outcome in azoospermic men with testicular failure and obstructive azoospermia treated for infertility. Asian J Androl. 2014;16(4):602–6.
18. EAU Guidelines. Edn. presented at the EAU Annual Congress Milan 2023. ISBN 978-94-92671-19-6.
19. Kalsi JS, Shah P, Thum Y, Muneer A, Ralph DJ, Minhas S. Salvage micro-dissection testicular sperm extraction; outcome in men with non-obstructive azoospermia with previous failed sperm retrievals. BJU Int. 2015;116(3):460–5.
20. Özman O, Tosun S, Bayazıt N, Cengiz S, Bakırcıoğlu ME. Efficacy of the second micro-testicular sperm extraction after failed first micro-testicular sperm extraction in men with non-obstructive azoospermia. Fertil Steril. 2021;115(4):915–21.
21. Agarwal A, Cannarella R, Saleh R, Boitrelle F, Gül M, Toprak T, Salvio G, Arafa M, Russo GI, Harraz AM, Singh R, Garrido N, Hamoda TAA, Rambhatla A, Kavoussi P, Kuroda S, Çalik G, Saini P, Ceyhan E, Dimitriadis F, Henkel R, Crafa A, Palani A, Duran MB, Maziotis E, Saïs É, Bendayan M, Darbandi M, Le TV, Gunes S, Tsioulou P, Sengupta P, Hazir B, Çeker G, Darbandi S, Durairajanayagam D, Aghamajidi A, Alkhalidi N, Sogutdelen E, Leisegang K, Alarbid A, Ho CCK, Malhotra V, Finocchi F, Crisóstomo L, Kosgi R, ElBardisi H, Zini A, Birowo P, Colpi G, Park HJ, Serefoglu EC, Nguyen Q, Ko E, de la Rosette J, Pinggera GM, Nguyen HVP, Kandil H, Shah R. Impact of varicocele repair on semen parameters in infertile men: a systematic review and meta-analysis. World J Mens Health. 2023;41(2):289–310.
22. Kirby EW, Wiener LE, Rajanahally S, Crowell K, Coward RM. Undergoing varicocele repair before assisted reproduction improves pregnancy rate and live birth rate in azoospermic and oligospermic men with a varicocele: a systematic review and meta-analysis. Fertil Steril. 2016;106(6):1338–43.
23. Zhang F, Dai M, Yang X, Cheng Y, Ye L, Huang W, Chen X, Yin T, Sha Y. Predictors of successful salvage microdissection testicular sperm extraction (mTESE) after failed initial TESE in patients with non-obstructive azoospermia: a systematic review and meta-analysis. Andrology. 2024;12(1):30–44.
24. Jensen S, Ko EY. Varicocele treatment in non-obstructive azoospermia: a systematic review. Arab J Urol. 2021;19(3):221–6.
25. Jiang Y, Shen Z, Xu J, Zhu J, Wang H, Chen W, Sun Y, Yang Q. The impact of female BMI on sperm DNA damage repair ability of oocytes and early embryonic development potential in intracytoplasmic sperm injection cycles. Front Endocrinol (Lausanne). 2023;14:1168010.
26. Marcho C, Oluwayiose OA, Pilsner JR. The preconception environment and sperm epigenetics. Andrology. 2020;8(4):924–42.
27. Wang S, Sun J, Wang J, Ping Z, Liu L. Does obesity based on body mass index affect semen quality?-A meta-analysis and systematic review from the general population rather than the infertile population. Andrologia. 2021a;53(7):e14099.
28. Li F, Yang Q, Shi H, Xin H, Luo X, Sun Y. Effects of obesity on sperm retrieval, early embryo quality and clinical outcomes in men with nonobstructive azoospermia undergoing testicular sperm aspiration-intracytoplasmic sperm injection cycles. Andrologia. 2019a;51(6):e13265.
29. Billa E, Kanakis GA, Goulis DG. Endocrine follow-up of men with non-obstructive azoospermia following testicular sperm extraction. J Clin Med. 2021;10(15)

30. Eliveld J, van Wely M, Meißner A, Repping S, van der Veen F, van Pelt AMM. The risk of TESE-induced hypogonadism: a systematic review and meta-analysis. Hum Reprod Update. 2018;24(4):442–54.
31. Wistuba J, Luetjens CM, Stukenborg JB, Poplinski A, Werler S, Dittmann M, Damm OS, Hämäläinen T, Simoni M, Gromoll J. Male 41, XXY* mice as a model for klinefelter syndrome: hyperactivation of leydig cells. Endocrinology. 2010;151(6):2898–910.
32. Amer MK, Ahmed HEH, GamalEl Din SF, Fawzy Megawer A, Ahmed AR. Evaluation of neoadjuvant gonadotropin administration with downregulation by testosterone prior to second time microsurgical testicular sperm extraction: a prospective case-control study. Urologia. 2020;87(4):185–90.
33. Shiraishi K, Ohmi C, Shimabukuro T, Matsuyama H. Human chorionic gonadotrophin treatment prior to microdissection testicular sperm extraction in non-obstructive azoospermia. Hum Reprod. 2012;27(2):331–9.
34. Tharakan T, Corona G, Foran D, Salonia A, Sofikitis N, Giwercman A, Krausz C, Yap T, Jayasena CN, Minhas S. Does hormonal therapy improve sperm retrieval rates in men with non-obstructive azoospermia: a systematic review and meta-analysis. Hum Reprod Update. 2022;28(5):609–28.
35. Strasser MO, Dupree JM. Care delivery for male infertility: the present and future. Urol Clin North Am. 2020;47(2):193–204.
36. Harari O, Bourne H, Baker G, Gronow M, Johnston I. High fertilization rate with intracytoplasmic sperm injection in mosaic Klinefelter's syndrome. Fertil Steril. 1995;63(1):182–4.
37. Samplaski MK, Lo KC, Grober ED, Millar A, Dimitromanolakis A, Jarvi KA. Phenotypic differences in mosaic Klinefelter patients as compared with non-mosaic Klinefelter patients. Fertil Steril. 2014;101(4):950–5.
38. Schiff JD, Li PS, Goldstein M. Correlation of ultrasound-measured venous size and reversal of flow with Valsalva with improvement in semen-analysis parameters after varicocelectomy. Fertil Steril. 2006;86(1):250–2.
39. Tsukamoto J, Enatsu N, Nakahara E, Furuhashi K, Chiba K, Enatsu Y, Mizusawa Y, Okamoto E, Kokeguchi S, Shiotani M. Differences in clinical outcomes between men with mosaic Klinefelter syndrome and those with non-mosaic Klinefelter syndrome. Reprod Med Biol. 2024;23(1):e12579.
40. Jarvis S, Yee HK, Thomas N, Cha I, Prasad KC, Ramsay JWA, Turek PJ. Sperm fine-needle aspiration (FNA) mapping after failed microdissection testicular sperm extraction (TESE): location and patterns of found sperm. Asian J Androl. 2018;21(1):50–5.
41. Flannigan R, Tadayon Najafabadi B, Violette PD, Jarvi K, Patel P, Bach PV, Domes T, Zini A, Grober E, Mak V, Fischer MA, Chan P, Lo K, Chow V, Wu C, Grantmyre J, Patry G, Schlegel PN, Roberts M. 2023 Canadian Urological Association guideline: evaluation and management of azoospermia. Can Urol Assoc J. 2023;17(8):228–40.
42. Li YX, Zhou L, Lv MQ, Ge P, Liu YC, Zhou DX. Vitrification and conventional freezing methods in sperm cryopreservation: a systematic review and meta-analysis. Eur J Obstet Gynecol Reprod Biol. 2019b;233:84–92.
43. Achermann APP, Pereira TA, Esteves SC. Microdissection testicular sperm extraction (micro-TESE) in men with infertility due to nonobstructive azoospermia: summary of current literature. Int Urol Nephrol. 2021;53(11):2193–210.
44. Almekaty K, Abomelha S, Thum Y, Nicopoullos J, Bracewell-Milnes T, Yap T, Minhas S. Reporting on longitudinal live birth rates and cumulative delivery rates are more realistic outcome measures than sperm retrieval rates in couples undergoing mTESE-ICSI. Hum Fertil (Camb). 2019;22(2):139–44.
45. Karacan M, Ulug M, Arvas A, Cebi Z, Erkan S, Camlıbel T. Live birth rate with repeat microdissection TESE and intracytoplasmic sperm injection after a conventional testicular biopsy in men with nonobstructive azoospermia. Eur J Obstet Gynecol Reprod Biol. 2014;183:174–7.

46. Nariyoshi S, Nakano K, Sukegawa G, Sho T, Tsuji Y. Ultrasonographically determined size of seminiferous tubules predicts sperm retrieval by microdissection testicular sperm extraction in men with nonobstructive azoospermia. Fertil Steril. 2020;113(1):97–104. e102
47. Nowroozi MR, Ayati M, Amini E, Radkhah K, Jamshidian H, Delpazir A, Ghasemi F, Rajabzadeh Kanafi A. Assessment of testicular perfusion prior to sperm extraction predicts success rate and decreases the number of required biopsies in patients with non-obstructive azoospermia. Int Urol Nephrol. 2015;47(1):53–8.
48. Ntorkou A, Tsili AC, Goussia A, Astrakas LG, Maliakas V, Sofikitis N, Argyropoulou MI. Testicular apparent diffusion coefficient and magnetization transfer ratio: can these MRI parameters be used to predict successful sperm retrieval in nonobstructive azoospermia? AJR Am J Roentgenol. 2019;213(3):610–8.
49. Baleato-González S, García-Figueiras R, Santiago-Pérez MI, Requejo-Isidro I, Vilanova JC. Usefulness of 1H magnetic resonance spectroscopy in human testes: preliminary study. Clin Radiol. 2015;70(9):1026–31.
50. Hesham Said A, Ragab A, Zohdy W, Ibrahim AS, Abd El Basset AS. Diffusion-weighted magnetic resonance imaging and magnetic resonance spectroscopy for non-invasive characterization of azoospermia: a prospective comparative single-center study. Andrology. 2023;11(6):1096–106.
51. Cao C, Wen Y, Wang X, Fang N, Yuan S, Huang X. Testicular piRNA profile comparison between successful and unsuccessful micro-TESE retrieval in NOA patients. J Assist Reprod Genet. 2018;35(5):801–8.
52. Abdelaal NE, Tanga BM, Abdelgawad M, Allam S, Fathi M, Saadeldin IM, Bang S, Cho J. Cellular therapy via spermatogonial stem cells for treating impaired spermatogenesis, non-obstructive azoospermia. Cells. 2021;10(7)
53. van der Bijl N, Röpke A, Biswas U, Wöste M, Jessberger R, Kliesch S, Friedrich C, Tüttelmann F. Mutations in the stromal antigen 3 (STAG3) gene cause male infertility due to meiotic arrest. Hum Reprod. 2019;34(11):2112–9.
54. Wang YH, Yan M, Zhang X, Liu XY, Ding YF, Lai CP, Tong MH, Li JS. Rescue of male infertility through correcting a genetic mutation causing meiotic arrest in spermatogonial stem cells. Asian J Androl. 2021b;23(6):590–9.

Chapter 15
Emotional and Psychological Impact of Nonobstructive Azoospermia (NOA)

Mohammed Nasreldin Sadek, Wael Zohdy, and Murat Gül

Introduction

Infertility is significantly prevalent among couples worldwide, affecting one in eight couples. Infertility has reproductive aspect as well as mental and social aspects [1]. Being unable to conceive is a stressful life situation for couples and it has its psychological consequences [2]. The desire of man for reproduction to set up a family is a strong psychological need and an important pillar of social life. Therefore, infertility has a wide range of psychological consequences ranging from normal, simple reactions to stress to complex psychiatric symptoms or disorders [2]. Moreover, unsuccessful treatment often leads to a prolonged grief response and highlights the need for post-treatment psychological support [3]. In this chapter, we evaluate the emotional and psychological impact of infertility, especially non-obstructive azoospermia (NOA), in men.

M. N. Sadek (✉)
Department of Psychiatry, Cairo University, Giza, Egypt

W. Zohdy
Department of Andrology, Cairo University, Giza, Egypt

M. Gül
Department of Urology, Selçuk University School of Medicine, Konya, Türkiye

Department of Andrology, Selçuk University School of Medicine, Konya, Türkiye

W. Zohdy et al. (eds.), *Non-Obstructive Azoospermia*,
https://doi.org/10.1007/978-3-031-99431-9_15

Psychological Aspects of NOA

Psychological Impact of Infertility

When a couple is diagnosed with infertility, they commonly experience a variety of stressors. These stressors include, but are not limited to, disruptions in a couple's personal life and relationships with others, changes in the quality of couples' emotional and sexual relationship, and alteration in couple's relationships with co-workers, family, and friends [4, 5, 6, 7].

These feelings of distress combined with the lack of social support may lead to physiological and psychological symptoms such as anxiety, depression, and bereavement [8, 9]. Stress levels influence the outcome of infertility treatment, as well as contribute to patients' decisions to continue treatment [10].

a. **Psychiatric Disorders and Infertility**

   The diagnosis of infertility or prolonged, unsuccessful efforts to have a baby can cause stress, anxiety, and depression at levels equal to those found in women diagnosed with heart disease, metastatic cancer, or HIV infection. The reproductive hormones are negatively affected by the stress, making it more difficult for couples to conceive [11, 12].

   Major depressive disorder is significantly prevalent in infertile couples than in fertile controls, with estimates ranging from 15% to 54%. Anxiety has also been shown to be significantly higher in infertile couples when compared to the general population, with 8–25% of infertile couples reporting clinically significant anxiety [13, 14].

b. **Stress Response to Infertility**

   The chronic stress associated with infertility triggers a stress response like one triggered by physical or emotional stress. Stress activates both the hypothalamic–pituitary–adrenal axis (HPA) and the sympathetic arm of the autonomic nervous system to release "stress hormones." These stress hormones, which include cortisol, ACTH, norepinephrine, and epinephrine, shift behavior and physiology to increase the odds of survival in the face of an immediate threat. Stress hormones increase heart rate, blood pressure, respiration rate, blood flow to muscles, and metabolic rate. These same hormones shut down systems not needed for the response to an immediate threat, such as reproduction, digestion, and growth [15, 16].

   When stress diminishes, the stress response turns off, stress hormone levels fall, and the body quickly recovers and returns to balance (homeostasis). However, chronic stress associated with infertility leads to sustained release of stress hormones with negative effects on health and reproduction [17].

   Stress hormones disrupt hormone release from each level of the reproductive HPA. In men, stress hormones disrupt testosterone and sperm production, decrease the desire to reproduce, and make it more difficult for men to get erections. In women, stress hormones disrupt egg maturation, ovulation, and the physiological changes that support embryo implantation, placenta formation, pregnancy, and childbirth, as well as reducing the desire to reproduce [17].

c. **Stigma and Infertility**

Perhaps what may be of concern is that even after successful treatment and pregnancies and the time that had passed, some women who receive treatment for infertility maintain a view of themselves as wounded by the process and have still to come to terms with the intense distress experienced at that time. The needs of all couples should be addressed, and those with higher levels of psychological distress may need continuing care and follow-up [18, 19].

Psychological Distress and Infertility Treatment

Experiencing infertility is described as a time of emotional uncertainty and hope. The experience itself is determined by a routine of activities focused on the possibility of the pregnancy, including frequent visits to physicians, examinations, and treatment procedures [20].

In men with NOA, sperm retrieval may fail in almost 50% of cases [21, 22]. Consequently, women reported experiencing challenges in accepting that their infertility would remain unresolved. Many felt that they had started with unrealistic expectations of treatment success and felt vulnerable to the pressures of both the media and society. Peddie et al., in their semi-structured interviews of 25 women with unsuccessful in vitro fertilization (IVF) cycles, and who decided to discontinue the treatment, concluded that significant limitations in the quality of communication and in the provision of post-treatment support exist [18]. Women who are prepared for egg collection and ICSI on the same day of sperm retrieval in men with NO are subjected to a tremendous pressure and anxiety as measured by the state-trait anxiety inventory and perceived stress scale [23]. Such anxiety may be exaggerated in countries where sperm donation is prohibited or unethical [24].

Men and women referred for IVF may face additional stress undergoing this treatment, as it is physically rigorous, expensive, and frequently uncovered by insurance [25]. Factors such as age and frustrating IVF attempts can be associated with emotional instability, anxiety, and depression [26].

When studying men undergoing their first IVF or ICSI treatment with daily monitoring, a small study found that the men's psychological reactions were similar, except that ICSI patients showed marginally more anticipatory anxiety on the days prior to oocyte retrieval, possibly attributable to the uncertainty of fertilization [27].

In light of the discrepancy in the results, there has been increasing interest in the factors that contribute to dropout from infertility treatment since this population is often not included or declines to participate in studies. Whereas cost or refusal of physicians to continue treatment have been cited as reasons for discontinuing treatment, research suggests that one-quarter of dropouts are due to psychological factors [28].

Gender Differences in Experiencing Infertility

Although most psychosocial infertility studies include both partners, few studies in this field actually focus on men's experience of infertility. A considerable body of literature examines the impact of treatment and addresses the negative influence of infertility on women's self-esteem, marital relations, sexual satisfaction, and psychological well-being, with women reporting more difficulty with these aspects than their male partners [29].

Even though men are not immune to psychological distress associated with infertility, women seem to carry a heavier burden and appear to be more vulnerable to its negative social and environmental consequences [30].

It was found that infertile men activate coping strategies less often than men with idiopathic, female, or mixed infertility, but the study concluded that gender and role expectations can make the women become the primary sufferers in the context of this type of treatment [31].

It is reported that there is more stress, and more social and sexual concern, in both men and women, in couples with male infertility than in couples with female infertility, but also that women experience greater global stress than men [5].*

Caveat: Research on stress and coping strategies is culture dependent, and generalizations should be made with caution.

Coping with Infertility

(a) **Need for Coping**

As infertility is an unplanned and unexpected stress, couples typically lack the knowledge and skill set to adequately manage infertility stress. As a result, couples engage in a variety of coping strategies in an attempt to regain control over their lives and rebalance the disruptions they have experienced in their personal, marital, and social relationships. Coping is formally defined as cognitive or behavioral efforts used to manage and control the stress in situations where a stressor exceeds a couple's perceived or actual resources [32].

Infertility is a stressor that often affects a couple's personal and relational resources, and coping strategies are a natural outgrowth of the experience. As men and women find themselves in an unfamiliar situation, they find many ways to cope with infertility [33].

(b) **Types of Coping Strategies**

Four primary types of coping strategies are known: active-avoidance strategies (e.g., avoiding pregnant women or children), active-confronting strategies (e.g., showing feelings, asking others for advice), passive-avoidance strategies (e.g., hoping for a miracle), and meaning-based strategies (e.g., growing as a person in a good way; finding other goals in life) [33].

Previous studies have found that avoidance coping strategies, which are primarily aimed at removing the person or couple from emotionally painful situations, are consistently linked with an increase in infertility stress and psychological distress [34].

Coping strategies such as active-confronting coping (e.g., attempts to modify infertility stress by acting toward problem resolution) and meaning-based coping (e.g., redefining the meaning and implication of infertility) have been linked to successful short- and long-term adaptation to the stress of infertility [35].

(c) **Individual and Partner Coping**

Most studies examining the impact of coping with infertility use the individual as a unit of analysis. Such studies are valuable because men and women cope with infertility in different ways, and highlighting the preferred coping processes of men and women benefits both patients and physicians [36].

A meta-analysis of gender differences in coping with infertility found that while men and women have significant differences in coping strategies, they also show more similarity in coping than was expected [36].

Relative coping scores showed that women tend to use more confrontive coping, accepting responsibility, seeking social support, and escape/avoidance strategies, whereas men use more distancing, self-controlling, and planful problem-solving approaches. These patterns reflect key gender differences in coping with infertility-related stress [34]. These findings highlight that while both men and women use a variety of coping strategies, the preference and effectiveness of these strategies differ by gender. Following their meta-analysis, Jordan and Revenson emphasized the need to reconceptualize coping with infertility as a couple-level stressor, recognizing that both partners are affected by this experience [36].

Research outside of the infertility literature is also recognizing the importance of partner coping effects when examining couples' efforts to cope with life events. This research examines the interactions between partners to assess if an individual's stress levels can be accounted for by a partner's coping strategies. A statistical methodology called the Actor Partner Independence Model (APIM) [37] allows for the simultaneous estimation of both individual effects, referred to as actor effects, and the effects of another closely associated person, referred to as partner effects. Such analysis uses the couple, not the individual, as a unit of analysis. A body of research is accumulating that has used the APIM to examine the impact of partner coping [38]. The value of the APIM is that it provides a complete picture of phenomena that includes both individual and partner effects when coping with stress [34].

Psychological Interventions for Infertility

In light of data suggesting that psychological symptoms may interfere with infertility, the success of infertility treatment, and the ability to tolerate ongoing treatment, interest in addressing these issues during infertility treatment has grown [12]. The attention to emotional distress as a consequence of infertility and its treatment has led worldwide to the recommendation to provide psychosocial interventions for infertile couples. Moreover, a lot of couples themselves have expressed their wish to receive more psychosocial help [39]. However, only 25% of patients take up psychosocial services offered or have the intention to use them [40]. Also, these patients tend to experience more personal, social, and/or marital distress (and marital benefits) than those who do not request counselling or attend support groups (L [40]). Until now, a wide range of psychosocial interventions for infertile couples have been developed [41].

(a) **Social Support**

Involuntary childless people experience the need to share their loss with others [42]. Getting the social support they need may be an important step in dealing with the situation of childlessness. Sufficient social support might even counterbalance the negative effects of an ineffective coping style [35]. However, when these people experience that their grief is not sufficiently acknowledged by their social environment, the social support they get does not fulfill their needs. If getting good social support could protect people from the negative effects of an ineffective coping style, the opposite might also be true. If involuntary childless people are getting no social support, or if they are unsatisfied with the support given, this may result in even more distress [43].

(b) **Psychological Assessment and Psychotherapy**

The emotional processes associated with infertility and assisted reproduction treatments are so important that it is essential for a psychologist to be part of the multidisciplinary team. It has been suggesteds that there is a need for professional participation right from the moment of the infertility diagnosis [44].

Psychological assessment of emotional adjustment helps identify individuals at risk of developing emotional disorders and provides a basis for offering tailored psychological support. The time required for diagnostic medical tests, typically around 3 months, can be utilized to address any maladjustment detected or to psychologically prepare couples with fewer emotional resources for the process of infertility treatment [45].

Some interventions designed to alleviate the symptoms of stress, depression, and anxiety in infertile women and men have been researched. Several studies suggest that cognitive behavioral group psychotherapy and support groups decrease stress and mood symptoms, as well as increase fertility rates. In a study, a 10-week group behavioral treatment program significantly reduced anxiety, depression, and anger [12].

In a year-long follow-up study comparing pregnancy rates among women undergoing assisted reproduction, participants were randomized to receive either group cognitive behavioral therapy (CBT) designed to decrease depression and anxiety, a support group intervention, or to no intervention (control group). The viable pregnancy rates were 55% in the CBT group, 54% in the support group, and 20% in the control group [46].

In a study, the intervention group received couples counseling focused on education and stress management throughout their IVF cycle, while the control group received only routine medical care. Patients in the intervention group reported lower anxiety and depression scores and achieved significantly higher pregnancy rates compared to the control group [47].

Psychiatric Side Effects of Hormonal Treatments for Infertility

Mood fluctuations are experienced in women related to normal hormonal changes during their reproductive cycles [48]. The medications used for infertility target these same hormones in the hypothalamic pituitary ovarian axis and can have similar effects on mood [49].

The commonly used medications in fertility treatment alter levels of thyroid hormone, prolactin, estradiol, progestogens, GnRH, and gonadotrophins. Hyperprolactinemia and hypothyroidism are considered treatable causes of infertility. Also, thyroid replacement hormone reduces depressive symptoms [50].

Dopamine agonists, e.g., bromocriptine and cabergoline, treat infertility secondary to hyperprolactinemic anovulation [51], but unfortunately it may increase the risk of impulse control disorders [52] and psychotic symptoms [53, 54, 55]. In addition, they can also induce dopamine toxicity when combined, especially with antidepressants with dopaminergic properties such as bupropion or venlafaxine [56].

Combination oral contraceptive pills (OCPs) are often utilized to synchronize an IVF cycle to a particular schedule [49]. There is a strong association between mood and swinging in estrogen and progesterone levels [57, 48], with estradiol and progestogens contributing to symptoms of depression, anxiety, and decreased libido [58, 59]. These symptoms are often more clinically impairing in women with a past history of previous depressive episodes or disorders and increase their risk for recurrent episodes of psychiatric illness [60, 61, 58, 62].

Ovarian stimulation, and off-label use in men to increase spermatogenesis, are commonly done by using selective estrogen receptor modulators (SERMs)—such as clomiphene citrate and tamoxifen—and aromatase inhibitors—such as letrozole [63, 64]. Side effects related to these medications are well reported in women and in rare case reports in men [63], and may even include transient psychotic episodes related to clomiphene [53, 65]. Because of their reduction in estrogen, the most commonly experienced side effects of these medications resemble those in menopause—including insomnia, decreased libido, and mood swings [60].

Symptoms of anxiety and depression have been correlated with the use of injectable medications (e.g., GnRH agonists, GnRH antagonists, and gonadotropins like FSH), which are administered to induce the production of multiple follicles during IVF cycles [57]. These medications cause pituitary downregulation, resulting in a hypogonadal state [57, 48, 59]. Hypogonadotropic states are associated with a sense of anhedonia, lack of interest, anxiety, insomnia, decreased libido, fatigue, and depressed mood [57, 48, 59]. The longer the duration of treatment, the more severe the depressive symptoms. Previous failed assisted reproductive treatment cycles and a prior history of psychiatric illness are also considered risk factors for the development of anxiety and depressive symptoms [66, 67].

A second group of injectable medications (e.g., human menopausal gonadotropins (hMG) and human chorionic gonadotropin (hCG)) trigger ovulation and are structurally similar to LH and FSH and may induce symptoms of anxiety [68]. This anxiety may also be amplified in anticipation of the invasive procedure that will follow in the next several hours or days to retrieve the oocytes [66, 69].

Overall, most medications used in treating infertility have mood-destabilizing effects. These symptoms are exacerbated by the realization of high rates of failure in fertility treatments, examinations, tests, the invasive nature of medication administration, and the prolonged pursuit of parenthood, often for years without success [69]. However, detailed studies regarding men suffering from nonobstructive azoospermia (NOA) and their fertile partners are scarce, and the association of other reproductive hormones with mood is not fully understood. It is likely that both androgens and gonadotropins, including follicle-stimulating hormone (FSH) and luteinizing hormone (LH), affect the moods and emotions of men [70, 69].

Psychotropic Medications and Infertility

Psychotropic medications may also alter the protein binding of hormones and metabolism and influence the levels of sex steroids [71]. The reproductive function in both men and women may be influenced by psychotropic medications through their effect on the levels of neurotransmitters, such as serotonin, dopamine, and GABA, which are involved in the physiologic regulation of the male and female reproductive axes [71]. However, a systematic review concluded that clinical studies have not demonstrated a deleterious effect of psychotropic medication on oocytes in terms of retrieval and pregnancy rates [72].

A. **Antidepressants**

Studies reported that the exposure to SSRIs during IVF shows no difference in pregnancy outcomes when compared to the control group [73, 74]. In addition, a recent retrospective cohort analysis showed that patients exposed to SSRIs in vivo did not demonstrate an increased rate of embryo aneuploidy in IVF. IVF outcomes of patients exposed to SSRIs do not differ from those of unexposed patients [75].

Some antidepressants, especially the SSRIs and venlafaxine, can cause sexual dysfunction and negatively impact both female and male fertility [76, 77]. However, as depressive disorder itself can cause decreased libido, the benefits of treating depressive disorder-induced sexual dysfunction versus the risks of antidepressant-induced sexual dysfunction must be weighed on a case-by-case basis. Alternatively, bupropion, mirtazapine, vortioxetine, and vilazodone may be considered as antidepressants that are not associated with decreased libido [76, 77].

B. **Mood Stabilizers and Antipsychotics**

The risk of infertility can be increased by treatment with certain mood stabilizers. Studies show a significantly higher rate of menstrual cycle disorders, hyperandrogenism, and PCOS (which have been associated with infertility) in women receiving prolonged valproate therapy for bipolar disorder. Valproic acid should be avoided in women planning a pregnancy [78].

Also, the risk of psychotropic-induced weight gain should be seriously considered in women planning pregnancy. Among the mood stabilizers, valproic acid, lithium, clozapine, olanzapine, quetiapine, and risperidone have the highest risk of problematic weight gain [79]. Carbamazepine and oxcarbazepine do not appear to cause significant weight gain [79], but they may induce the metabolism of steroid hormones [80], and consequently affect the efficacy of exogenous hormones administered during treatment for infertility.

Also, carbamazepine has been shown to increase the concentration of serum sex hormone binding globulin (SHBG). The increase in serum SHBG levels leads to diminished bioactivity of estradiol, resulting in menstrual disorders and thus reducing fertility [81]. Lamotrigine levels may be decreased by oral contraceptives administered during the initial phase of IVF treatment, and as such should be monitored during this period [82, 80].

C. **Benzodiazepines**

Midazolam is a short-acting benzodiazepine often utilized in conscious sedation protocols during oocyte retrieval [83] [83] and has not been associated with negative reproductive outcomes [84]. In contrast, long-term benzodiazepine use has been found to significantly affect the secretion of pituitary hormones (e.g., gonadotropins and prolactin) [85] and has been associated with a decrease in fertility [86].

Hormonal Abnormalities and Psychological Stress in Men with Klinefelter Syndrome

Morphological and functional studies of the brain demonstrated that KS patients exhibit significant differences in brain structure, including reduced total brain volume as well as decreased gray and white matter volumes compared to the general population. These structural differences have been associated with functional impairments, particularly language abnormalities. Furthermore, a survey conducted in Denmark involving 832 KS patients and 4033 controls revealed an increased risk of hospitalization for psychiatric disorders among KS patients [87].

Other studies reported a high prevalence of depression ranging from 19% to 24% [88]. It has been questioned whether depressive symptoms are specifically associated with genotype alterations in KS or are consequences of physical and emotional traits due to the syndrome [89]. One study reported increased emotional arousal and difficulties in identifying and verbalizing emotions among KS patients [90]. The organic basis for these emotional disturbances may lie in alterations of the amygdala and other limbic structures, which are involved in regulating emotions as well as aggressive and impulsive behaviors [91, 92].

Men with Klinefelter syndrome (KS) have higher anxiety levels during surgical sperm retrieval as compared with men with a normal karyotype. In this context, Yığman and colleagues investigated 20 men with KS and 20 men with NOA and normal karyotypes, all scheduled for TESE under local anesthesia due to azoospermia. The authors used the Spielberger State-Trait Anxiety Inventory (STAI-T and STAI-S) in all patients one hour before surgery. Postoperative pain evaluation was performed at 0, 30, 60, and 120 min with visual analogue scale (VAS). STAI-T inventory was given to the patients again 2 h after the procedure. They observed higher preoperative STAI-S and STAI-T scores and postoperative STAI-T scores of patients in the KS group. Interestingly, there were no significant differences in the postoperative VAS scores between the two groups [93].

Hormonal Abnormalities and Psychological Stress in Men with Other Cryptogenic Anomalies

Stress-induced hormonal changes depend on the severity and nature of the stressor, duration of exposure to the stressor, and the baseline condition of the body. In chronic situations, these may lead to hypogonadotropic hypogonadism. Stress-induced disorders of spermatogenesis are most commonly manifested by reduced sperm concentration and motility and increased percentage of sperm cells of abnormal morphology. The above attempts at generalization must, however, be treated with caution, as the effects of stress are largely dependent on individual responses [94].

Impact of Surgical Sperm Retrieval on Sexual Health, Anxiety, and Mental Health Status

Definitive azoospermia was found to have a negative impact on many aspects of self-esteem, sexual health, and relationship quality. These results suggest the need for better management of men with NOA. These men are frequently lost to follow-up once it has become clear that intra-couple assisted reproductive techniques will not be successful [95].

Some couples give up their efforts to have a child, others turn to adoption procedures, and yet others choose donor sperm programs. It seems necessary to provide patients with clear information about the expected outcome and the impact it may have on their quality of life prior to the TESE procedure. Psychological follow-up should be offered to patients after the TESE procedure, even more so when it has failed. Longer follow-up of these patients would be of value in assessing self-esteem, sex life quality, and relationship quality and, ideally, in helping them to cope with the negative impact of azoospermia and failure of testicular sperm extraction (TESE) [95].

The long-term psychosocial follow-up of azoospermia patients could indeed help to improve their quality of sexual life (erectile function, orgasm, and sexual satisfaction), self-image, and the quality of their relationship. To achieve this, a multidisciplinary approach involving psychological, sexological, and andrological interventions is recommended during the follow-up of infertile men with NOA [95].

Nonobstructive azoospermia particularly affects men in terms of biological, psychological, and social aspects. Topuz and colleagues investigated 40 men with NOA to determine the levels of depression, anxiety, and quality of their lives. They used three questionnaires, the Beck Depression Inventory, the Beck Anxiety Inventory, and the Short Form of the World Health Organization Quality of Life Questionnaire. The authors found 62.5% of patients had minimal depression, 27.5% of patients had mild depression, and 10% of patients had moderate depression. Almost 98% of men had minimal anxiety, and the remaining suffered from severe anxiety. Quality of life scores of the patients were 58.75% for general health status, 70.98% for physical health status, 72.92% for psychological status, 65% for social relations, and 66.25% for environmental status [96].

In addition to the anxiety and depression young infertile couples may face, their frustration has negative effects on the relationships. Bak and coworkers conducted a prospective cross-sectional study on 264 participants, 72 males diagnosed with NOA and their fertile spouses and 60 fertile couples attending a university hospital in South Korea {[70] #3677}. The Beck Anxiety Inventory, Beck Depression Inventory (BDI), and hormone levels were measured during initial and follow-up visits. In NOA men, follicle-stimulating hormone and luteinizing hormone were positively associated with anxiety, in contrast to testosterone, which was inversely associated with anxiety. After the diagnosis of NOA with no testicular sperm, the panic intensity among men increased significantly, whereas their spouses exhibited less panic. By contrast, fertile female partners of NOA men reported higher BDI scores after the initial diagnosis of azoospermia, whereas their partners recorded higher levels of depression after the absence of testicular sperm was discovered. Insomnia was the most common reported complaint for both sexes after the diagnosis of azoospermia. Hormonal abnormalities had a negative effect on the quality of life [70]. The impact on the relationship had been reinforced by Bendayan et al., who used the Dyadic Adjustment Scale (DAS) to measure the relationship between couples. The authors reported that men with NOA and negative TESE may have a negative impact on self-esteem and the quality of the couple's sex life and overall relationship. They recommended that such findings should be borne in mind when counselling men with NOA and their partners to help them cope with and decrease the harmful impacts of azoospermia and negative TESE [95].

In a cohort of 13,000 patients in a national insurance database in the United States, men diagnosed with male factor infertility had a significantly higher risk of adverse health outcomes in the years after an infertility evaluation. Men with azoospermia displayed the highest increased risk of renal disease (HR 2.26, 95% CI 1.20–4.27) and alcohol abuse (HR 1.94, 95% CI 1.11–3.39) compared with testing alone. The hazard ratio for depression after the diagnosis of male factor infertility was 1.19 (95% CI 1.04–1.36), and for anxiety disorders was 1.13 (95% CI 0.98–1.29). The authors recommended additional investigations to understand the association and identify interventions to improve outcomes for these patients [97]. These findings suggest the overall importance of men's reproductive health and warrant additional investigation to understand the association and identify interventions to improve outcomes for these patients.

Sexual dysfunction was assessed in two studies on men with NOA undergoing TESE [98, 99]. Akbal and colleagues evaluated the IIEF-5 in 66 men [100]. The median IIEF-5 scores before mTESE for positive and negative TESE groups were 22 (minimum, 11; maximum, 25) and 23 (minimum, 10; maximum, 25), respectively. After surgical sperm retrieval, IIEF-5 scores for positive and negative TESE were 23.5 (minimum: 10, maximum: 25) and 18 (minimum: 15, maximum: 25), respectively. A significant decrease was evident in men with negative TESE at the end of the follow-up [98]. Eliveld and coworkers reported sexual dysfunctions (hypoactive sexual desire and erectile dysfunction [ED]). Lower libido was reported in one patient out of 55 men with OA (1.8%), and 2/177 (1.1%) in NOA. Erectile dysfunction was observed in 2/177 men with NOA (1.1%). The article did not assess ejaculatory disorders in their cohort [99].

In addition to the IIEF-5, Akbal and colleagues assessed their participants with the Hospital Anxiety and Depression Scale [101]. Men who reported new-onset ED 6 months after surgery had a significant increase in FSH with insignificant elevation in LH levels, while the mean TT levels dropped significantly. Men who reported new-onset ED also reported both depression and anxiety. The authors concluded that failed testicular sperm extraction negatively affects erectile function due to hypogonadism, depression, and anxiety. The higher probability of hypogonadism in men with unsuccessful retrieval attempts could be due to more harvested testicular tissue samples. However, the authors did not report the figures [98]. Eliveld and coworkers reported sexual dysfunctions (hypoactive sexual desire and ED) in 4/177 (2.3%) of men with NOA and in one out of 11 men with KS (9.0%). The authors linked the sexual symptoms to profound hypogonadism in the KS patients (4/11, 36.4%) [99]. Psychological aspects and sexual symptoms in men with azoospermia are summarized in Table 15.1.

Table 15.1 Psychological aspects in infertile men and in patients with azoospermia: summary of tools and findings

Article	Population	Aim	Tools	Main findings
Topuz et al. [96]	40 men with NOA	To determine the levels of depression, anxiety, and quality of life	Beck depression inventory Beck anxiety inventory Short form of the World Health Organization quality of life questionnaire	Around 38% mild to moderate depression Almost 98% of men had minimal anxiety and the remaining suffered from mild anxiety Quality of life scores of the patients were 58.75% for general health status, 70.98% for physical health status, 72.92% for psychological status, 65% for social relations, and 66.25% for environmental status
Bak et al. [70]	72 men with NOA and 60 fertile couples	To study the effects on the relationships	Beck anxiety inventory Beck Depression Inventory (BDI) Hormone levels	FSH and LH were positively associated with anxiety Testosterone was inversely associated with anxiety Negative TESE is associated with a significant increase in the panic intensity Fertile female partners of NOA men reported higher BDI scores after the diagnosis of azoospermia, whereas their partners recorded higher levels of depression after negative surgical sperm retrieval
Bendayan et al. [95]	24 positive TESE 20 negative TESE	To study the effects on the relationships	The Cooper–Smith self-esteem inventory Dyadic Adjustment Scale (DAS) The IIEF-15	Men with NOA, and negative TESE may have a negative impact on the following: Self-esteem Quality of the couple's sex life Overall relationship
Eisenberg et al. [97]	13,027 infertile men and 23,860 receiving only fertility testing	To determine the incidence of chronic medical conditions in men with infertility[a]	International Classification of Diseases, ninth edition, Clinical Modification [ICD9]	The HR of depression after the diagnosis of male factor infertility was 1.19 (95% CI 1.04–1.36), and for anxiety disorders was 1.13 (95% CI 0.98–1.29) Alcohol abuse (HR 1.94, 95% CI 1.11–3.39) compared with testing alone

(continued)

Table 15.1 (continued)

Article	Population	Aim	Tools	Main findings
Akbal et al. [98]	66 men with NOA	Sexual dysfunction causes after surgical sperm retrieval	IIEF-5 and the Hospital Anxiety and Depression Scale Testosterone, FSH, and LH levels	TT levels dropped significantly after surgical sperm retrieval Men who reported new-onset ED reported both depression and anxiety
Eliveld et al. [99]	55 men with OA, 177 NOA, 11 KS	Sexual dysfunction after surgical sperm retrieval	Sexual History[b], FSH, LH, and serum testosterone	Hypoactive sexual desire and erectile dysfunction; lower libido was reported in one patient out of 55 men with OA (1.8%), and 2/177 (1.1%) in NOA; erectile dysfunction was observed in 2/177 men with NOA (1.1%) Sexual symptoms in KS men are due to profound hypogonadism (4/11, 36.4%)

FSH follicle-stimulating hormone, *HR* hazard ratio, *LH* luteinizing hormone, *KS* Klinefelter Syndrome

[a]Chronic medical conditions were evaluated; however, only psychological issues were selected in our review

[b]Ejaculatory functions were not assessed

References

1. Noorbala AA, Ramezanzadeh F, Abedinia N, Naghizadeh MM. Psychiatric disorders among infertile and fertile women. Soc Psychiatry Psychiatr Epidemiol. 2009;44(7):587–91. https://doi.org/10.1007/s00127-008-0467-1.
2. Kohan S, Ghasemi Z, Beigi M. Exploring infertile women's experiences about sexual life: a qualitative study. Iran J Nurs Midwifery Res. 2015;20(1):34–9.
3. Gameiro S, Finnigan A. Long-term adjustment to unmet parenthood goals following ART: a systematic review and meta-analysis. Hum Reprod Update. 2017;23(3):322–37. https://doi.org/10.1093/humupd/dmx001.
4. Greil AL. Infertility and psychological distress: a critical review of the literature. Soc Sci Med. 1997;45(11):1679–704. https://doi.org/10.1016/s0277-9536(97)00102-0.
5. Newton CR, Sherrard W, Glavac I. The fertility problem inventory: measuring perceived infertility-related stress. Fertil Steril. 1999;72(1):54–62. https://doi.org/10.1016/s0015-0282(99)00164-8.
6. Peterson BD, Newton CR, Feingold T. Anxiety and sexual stress in men and women undergoing infertility treatment. Fertil Steril. 2007;88(4):911–4. https://doi.org/10.1016/j.fertnstert.2006.12.023.
7. Schmidt L. Infertility and assisted reproduction in Denmark. Epidemiology and psychosocial consequences. Dan Med Bull. 2006;53(4):390–417.
8. Berghuis JP, Stanton AL. Adjustment to a dyadic stressor: a longitudinal study of coping and depressive symptoms in infertile couples over an insemination attempt. J Consult Clin Psychol. 2002;70(2):433–8. https://doi.org/10.1037/0022-006x.70.2.433.
9. van den Akker OB. Coping, quality of life and psychological symptoms in three groups of sub-fertile women. Patient Educ Couns. 2005;57(2):183–9. https://doi.org/10.1016/j.pec.2004.05.012.

10. Campagne DM. Should fertilization treatment start with reducing stress? Hum Reprod. 2006;21(7):1651–8. https://doi.org/10.1093/humrep/del078.
11. Cousineau TM, Domar AD. Psychological impact of infertility. Best Pract Res Clin Obstet Gynaecol. 2007;21(2):293–308. https://doi.org/10.1016/j.bpobgyn.2006.12.003.
12. Domar AD, Zuttermeister PC, Seibel M, Benson H. Psychological improvement in infertile women after behavioral treatment: a replication. Fertil Steril. 1992;58(1):144–7.
13. Chen TH, Chang SP, Tsai CF, Juang KD. Prevalence of depressive and anxiety disorders in an assisted reproductive technique clinic. Hum Reprod. 2004;19(10):2313–8. https://doi.org/10.1093/humrep/deh414.
14. Parikh F, Madon P, Athalye A, Soonawala R. 46, XX/46, XY karyotype in a phenotypically female abortus. Paper presented at the American Journal of Human Genetics. 2000.
15. Chrousos GP, Torpy DJ, Gold PW. Interactions between the hypothalamic-pituitary-adrenal axis and the female reproductive system: clinical implications. Ann Intern Med. 1998;129(3):229–40. https://doi.org/10.7326/0003-4819-129-3-199808010-00012.
16. Wingfield JC, Sapolsky RM. Reproduction and resistance to stress: when and how. J Neuroendocrinol. 2003;15(8):711–24. https://doi.org/10.1046/j.1365-2826.2003.01033.x.
17. Kalantaridou SN, Makrigiannakis A, Zoumakis E, Chrousos GP. Stress and the female reproductive system. J Reprod Immunol. 2004;62(1–2):61–8. https://doi.org/10.1016/j.jri.2003.09.004.
18. Peddie VL, van Teijlingen E, Bhattacharya S. A qualitative study of women's decision-making at the end of IVF treatment. Hum Reprod. 2005;20(7):1944–51. https://doi.org/10.1093/humrep/deh857.
19. Slade P, Emery J, Lieberman BA. A prospective, longitudinal study of emotions and relationships in in-vitro fertilization treatment. Hum Reprod. 1997;12(1):183–90. https://doi.org/10.1093/humrep/12.1.183.
20. Leite RC, Makuch MY, Petta CA, Morais SS. Women's satisfaction with physicians' communication skills during an infertility consultation. Patient Educ Couns. 2005;59(1):38–45. https://doi.org/10.1016/j.pec.2004.09.006.
21. Amer M, Ateyah A, Hany R, Zohdy W. Prospective comparative study between microsurgical and conventional testicular sperm extraction in non-obstructive azoospermia: follow-up by serial ultrasound examinations. Hum Reprod. 2000;15(3):653–6. https://doi.org/10.1093/humrep/15.3.653.
22. Schlegel PN, Li PS. Microdissection TESE: sperm retrieval in non-obstructive azoospermia. Hum Reprod Update. 1998;4(4):439. https://doi.org/10.1093/humupd/4.4.439.
23. Awtani M, Kapoor GK, Kaur P, Saha J, Crasta D, Banker M. Anxiety and stress at different stages of treatment in women undergoing in vitro fertilization-intracytoplasmic sperm injection. J Hum Reprod Sci. 2019;12(1):47–52. https://doi.org/10.4103/jhrs.JHRS_23_18.
24. Chapter 8: Donation. Fertil Steril. 2007;87(4 Supplement 1):S28–32. https://doi.org/10.1016/j.fertnstert.2007.01.092
25. Benyamini Y, Gozlan M, Kokia E. On the self-regulation of a health threat:cognitions, coping, and emotions among women undergoing treatment for infertility. Cogn Ther Res. 2004;28(5):577–92. https://doi.org/10.1023/B:COTR.0000045566.97966.22.
26. Fekkes M, Buitendijk SE, Verrips GH, Braat DD, Brewaeys AM, Dolfing JG, et al. Health-related quality of life in relation to gender and age in couples planning IVF treatment. Hum Reprod. 2003;18(7):1536–43. https://doi.org/10.1093/humrep/deg276.
27. Boivin J, Shoog-Svanberg A, Andersson L, Hjelmstedt A, Bergh T, Collins A. Distress level in men undergoing intracytoplasmic sperm injection versus in-vitro fertilization. Hum Reprod. 1998;13(5):1403–6. https://doi.org/10.1093/humrep/13.5.1403.
28. Olivius C, Friden B, Borg G, Bergh C. Why do couples discontinue in vitro fertilization treatment? A cohort study. Fertil Steril. 2004;81(2):258–61. https://doi.org/10.1016/j.fertnstert.2003.06.029.

29. Lechner L, Bolman C, van Dalen A. Definite involuntary childlessness: associations between coping, social support and psychological distress. Hum Reprod. 2007;22(1):288–94. https://doi.org/10.1093/humrep/del327.
30. Ragni G, Mosconi P, Baldini MP, Somigliana E, Vegetti W, Caliari I, Nicolosi AE. Health-related quality of life and need for IVF in 1000 Italian infertile couples. Hum Reprod. 2005;20(5):1286–91. https://doi.org/10.1093/humrep/deh788.
31. Kowalcek I, Wihstutz N, Buhrow G, Diedrich K. Coping with male infertility. Gender differences. Arch Gynecol Obstet. 2001;265(3):131–6. https://doi.org/10.1007/s004040100187.
32. Peterson BD, Pirritano M, Christensen U, Schmidt L. The impact of partner coping in couples experiencing infertility. Hum Reprod. 2008;23(5):1128–37. https://doi.org/10.1093/humrep/den067.
33. Schmidt L, Christensen U, Holstein BE. The social epidemiology of coping with infertility. Hum Reprod. 2005;20(4):1044–52. https://doi.org/10.1093/humrep/deh687.
34. Peterson BD, Newton CR, Rosen KH, Skaggs GE. Gender differences in how men and women who are referred for IVF cope with infertility stress. Hum Reprod. 2006;21(9):2443–9. https://doi.org/10.1093/humrep/del145.
35. Verhaak C, Burns LH. 11-Behavioral medicine approaches to infertility counseling. 2006. p. 169–95.
36. Jordan C, Revenson TA. Gender differences in coping with infertility: a meta-analysis. J Behav Med. 1999;22(4):341–58. https://doi.org/10.1023/a:1018774019232.
37. Kenny DA, Kashy DA, Cook WL. Dyadic data analysis. Guilford; 2020.
38. Cook WL, Snyder DK. Analyzing nonindependent outcomes in couple therapy using the actor-partner interdependence model. J Fam Psychol. 2005;19(1):133–41. https://doi.org/10.1037/0893-3200.19.1.133.
39. Hammarberg K, Astbury J, Baker H. Women's experience of IVF: a follow-up study. Hum Reprod. 2001;16(2):374–83. https://doi.org/10.1093/humrep/16.2.374.
40. Schmidt L, Holstein B, Boivin J, Sångren H, Tjørnhøj-Thomsen T, Blaabjerg J, et al. Patients' attitudes to medical and psychosocial aspects of care in fertility clinics: findings from the Copenhagen Multi-centre Psychosocial Infertility (COMPI). Res Program. 2003;18(3):628–37.
41. Boivin J. A review of psychosocial interventions in infertility. Soc Sci Med. 2003;57(12):2325–41. https://doi.org/10.1016/s0277-9536(03)00138-2.
42. Daniluk JC. Reconstructing their lives: a longitudinal, qualitative analysis of the transition to biological childlessness for infertile couples. J Couns Dev. 2001;79:439–49.
43. Mindes EJ, Ingram KM, Kliewer W, James CA. Longitudinal analyses of the relationship between unsupportive social interactions and psychological adjustment among women with fertility problems. Soc Sci Med. 2003;56(10):2165–80.
44. Rosset CM. Infertility and reproductive psychology. Papeles del Psicologo; 2008.
45. Moreno-Rosset C. Final report on R+ D+ I Project: La infertilidad en la mujer: aspectos psicosociales y neurobiológicos [Infertility in women: psychosocial and neurobiological aspects]. J Madrid Ministerio de Trabajo y Asuntos Sociales Instituto de la Mujer Expte. 2007;28(03)
46. Domar AD, Clapp D, Slawsby EA, Dusek J, Kessel B, Freizinger M. Impact of group psychological interventions on pregnancy rates in infertile women. Fertil Steril. 2000;73(4):805–11. https://doi.org/10.1016/s0015-0282(99)00493-8.
47. Terzioglu F. Investigation into effectiveness of counseling on assisted reproductive techniques in Turkey. J Psychosom Obstet Gynaecol. 2001;22(3):133–41. https://doi.org/10.3109/01674820109049965.
48. Schmidt PJ, Nieman LK, Danaceau MA, Adams LF, Rubinow DR. Differential behavioral effects of gonadal steroids in women with and in those without premenstrual syndrome. N Engl J Med. 1998;338(4):209–16. https://doi.org/10.1056/nejm199801223380401.
49. Garcia-Velasco JA, Fatemi HM. To pill or not to pill in GnRH antagonist cycles: that is the question! Reprod Biomed Online. 2015;30(1):39–42. https://doi.org/10.1016/j.rbmo.2014.09.010.

50. Redmond GP. Thyroid dysfunction and women's reproductive health. Thyroid. 2004;14(Suppl 1):S5–15. https://doi.org/10.1089/105072504323024543.
51. Usadi RS, Merriam KS. On-label and off-label drug use in the treatment of female infertility. Fertil Steril. 2015;103(3):583–94. https://doi.org/10.1016/j.fertnstert.2015.01.011.
52. Thondam SK, Alusi S, O'Driscoll K, Gilkes CE, Cuthbertson DJ, Daousi C. Impulse control disorder in a patient on long-term treatment with bromocriptine for a macroprolactinoma. Clin Neuropharmacol. 2013;36(5):170–2. https://doi.org/10.1097/WNF.0b013e31829fc165.
53. Seeman MV. Transient psychosis in women on clomiphene, bromocriptine, domperidone and related endocrine drugs. J Gynecol Endocrinol. 2015;31(10):751–4.
54. Shibli-Rahhal A, Schlechte JAJD, Disorders MOP. Prolactinomas: diagnosis and~ management. 2008. p. 125–40.
55. Snellen M, Power J, Blankley G, Galbally M. Pharmacological lactation suppression with D2 receptor agonists and risk of postpartum psychosis: a systematic review. Aust N Z J Obstet Gynaecol. 2016;56(4):336–40. https://doi.org/10.1111/ajo.12479.
56. Burns LH. Psychiatric aspects of infertility and infertility treatments. Psychiatr Clin North Am. 2007;30(4):689–716. https://doi.org/10.1016/j.psc.2007.08.001.
57. Bloch M, Azem F, Aharonov I, Ben Avi I, Yagil Y, Schreiber S, et al. GnRH-agonist induced depressive and anxiety symptoms during in vitro fertilization-embryo transfer cycles. Fertil Steril. 2011;95(1):307–9. https://doi.org/10.1016/j.fertnstert.2010.07.1073.
58. Lolak S, Rashid N, Wise TN. Interface of women's mental and reproductive health. Curr Psychiatry Rep. 2005;7(3):220–7. https://doi.org/10.1007/s11920-005-0057-9.
59. Stenbæk DS, Toftager M, Hjordt LV, Jensen PS, Holst KK, Bryndorf T, et al. Mental distress and personality in women undergoing GnRH agonist versus GnRH antagonist protocols for assisted reproductive technology. Hum Reprod. 2015;30(1):103–10. https://doi.org/10.1093/humrep/deu294.
60. Harlow BL, Cohen LS, Otto MW, Spiegelman D, Cramer DWJ Ao GP. Prevalence and predictors of depressive symptoms in older premenopausal women: the Harvard Study of Moods and Cycles. 1999;56(5):418–24.
61. Harlow BL, Wise LA, Otto MW, Soares CN, Cohen LS. Depression and its influence on reproductive endocrine and menstrual cycle markers associated with perimenopause: the Harvard Study of Moods and Cycles. Arch Gen Psychiatry. 2003;60(1):29–36. https://doi.org/10.1001/archpsyc.60.1.29.
62. Singata-Madliki M, Hofmeyr GJ, Lawrie TA. The effect of depot medroxyprogesterone acetate on postnatal depression: a randomised controlled trial. J Fam Plann Reprod Health Care. 2016;42(3):171–6. https://doi.org/10.1136/jfprhc-2015-101334.
63. Aussedat M, Jean-Louis J, Djahangirian O, Brochet MS. Clomiphene for the treatment of male infertility: a case report of mood change and a literature overview. Curr Drug Saf. 2017;12(3):208–15. https://doi.org/10.2174/1574886312666170616092036.
64. Rambhatla A, Mills JN, Rajfer J. The role of estrogen modulators in male hypogonadism and infertility. Rev Urol. 2016;18(2):66–72. https://doi.org/10.3909/riu0711.
65. Siedentopf F, Horstkamp B, Stief G, Kentenich H. Clomiphene citrate as a possible cause of a psychotic reaction during infertility treatment. Hum Reprod. 1997;12(4):706–7. https://doi.org/10.1093/humrep/12.4.706.
66. Awwad JT, Ghazeeri GS, Hannoun A, Isaacson K, Abou-Abdallah M, Farra CG. An investigational ovarian stimulation protocol increased significantly the psychological burden in women with premature ovarian failure. Acta Obstet Gynecol Scand. 2012;91(11):1273–8. https://doi.org/10.1111/aogs.12004.
67. Mamata D, Ray SK, Pratap K, Firuza P, Birla AR, Manish B. Impact of different controlled ovarian stimulation protocols on the physical and psychological burdens in women undergoing in vitro fertilization/intra cytoplasmic sperm injection. J Hum Reprod Sci. 2015;8(2):86–92. https://doi.org/10.4103/0974-1208.158615.

68. Bhongade MB, Prasad S, Jiloha RC, Ray PC, Mohapatra S, Koner BC. Effect of psychological stress on fertility hormones and seminal quality in male partners of infertile couples. Andrologia. 2015;47(3):336–42. https://doi.org/10.1111/and.12268.
69. de Klerk C, Macklon NS, Heijnen EM, Eijkemans MJ, Fauser BC, Passchier J, Hunfeld JA. The psychological impact of IVF failure after two or more cycles of IVF with a mild versus standard treatment strategy. Hum Reprod. 2007;22(9):2554–8. https://doi.org/10.1093/humrep/dem171.
70. Bak CW, Seok HH, Song SH, Kim ES, Her YS, Yoon TK. Hormonal imbalances and psychological scars left behind in infertile men. J Androl. 2012;33(2):181–9. https://doi.org/10.2164/jandrol.110.012351. Epub 2011 May 5. PMID: 21546616.
71. Hendrick V, Gitlin M, Altshuler L, Korenman S. Antidepressant medications, mood and male fertility. Psychoneuroendocrinology. 2000;25(1):37–51. https://doi.org/10.1016/s0306-4530(99)00038-4.
72. Worly BL, Gur TL. The effect of mental illness and psychotropic medication on gametes and fertility: a systematic review. J Clin Psychiatry. 2015;76(7):974–85. https://doi.org/10.4088/JCP.14r09080.
73. Friedman BE, Rogers JL, Shahine LK, Westphal LM, Lathi RB. Effect of selective serotonin reuptake inhibitors on in vitro fertilization outcome. Fertil Steril. 2009 Oct;92(4):1312-1314. https://doi.org/10.1016/j.fertnstert.2009.03.060. Epub 2009 May 6. PMID: 19423105.
74. Serafini P, Lobo DS, Grosman A, Seibel D, Rocha AM, Motta EL. Fluoxetine treatment for anxiety in women undergoing in vitro fertilization. Int J Gynaecol Obstet. 2009 May;105(2):136–9. https://doi.org/10.1016/j.ijgo.2008.12.013. Epub 2009 Feb 7.PMID: 19201400.
75. Hernandez-Nieto C, Lee J, Nazem T, Gounko D, Copperman A, Sandler B. Embryo aneuploidy is not impacted by selective serotonin reuptake inhibitor exposure. Fertil Steril. 2017;108(6):973–9. https://doi.org/10.1016/j.fertnstert.2017.08.040.
76. Clayton AH, Valladares Juarez EM. Female sexual dysfunction. Psychiatr Clin North Am. 2017;40(2):267–84. https://doi.org/10.1016/j.psc.2017.01.004.
77. Olivier JD, Esquivel-Franco D, Waldinger M, Olivier BJSD. Sexual dysfunction, depression and antidepressants: a translational approach. 2017. p. 59–76.
78. Gotlib D, Ramaswamy R, Kurlander JE, DeRiggi A, Riba M. Valproic acid in women and girls of childbearing age. Curr Psychiatry Rep. 2017;19(9):58. https://doi.org/10.1007/s11920-017-0809-3.
79. Hasnain M, Vieweg WV. Weight considerations in psychotropic drug prescribing and switching. Postgrad Med. 2013;125(5):117–29. https://doi.org/10.3810/pgm.2013.09.2706.
80. Reimers A. Contraception for women with epilepsy: counseling, choices, and concerns. Open Access J Contracept. 2016;7:69–76. https://doi.org/10.2147/oajc.S85541.
81. Isojärvi J. Disorders of reproduction in patients with epilepsy: antiepileptic drug related mechanisms. Seizure. 2008;17(2):111–9. https://doi.org/10.1016/j.seizure.2007.11.007.
82. Joffe H. Reproductive biology and psychotropic treatments in premenopausal women with bipolar disorder. J Clin Psychiatry. 2007;68(Suppl 9):10–5.
83. Singhal H, Premkumar PS, Chandy A, Kunjummen AT, Kamath MS. Patient experience with conscious sedation as a method of pain relief for transvaginal oocyte retrieval: a cross sectional study. J Hum Reprod Sci. 2017;10(2):119–23. https://doi.org/10.4103/jhrs.JHRS_113_16.
84. Kwan I, Wang R, Pearce E, Bhattacharya S. Pain relief for women undergoing oocyte retrieval for assisted reproduction. Cochrane Database Syst Rev. 2018;5(5):Cd004829. https://doi.org/10.1002/14651858.CD004829.pub4.
85. Arvat E, Giordano R, Grottoli S, Ghigo E. Benzodiazepines and anterior pituitary function. J Endocrinol Investig. 2002;25(8):735–47. https://doi.org/10.1007/bf03345110.
86. Nillni YI, Wesselink AK, Gradus JL, Hatch EE, Rothman KJ, Mikkelsen EM, Wise LA. Depression, anxiety, and psychotropic medication use and fecundability. Am J Obstet Gynecol. 2016;215(4):453.e451–8. https://doi.org/10.1016/j.ajog.2016.04.022.

87. Bojesen A, Juul S, Birkebaek NH, Gravholt CH. Morbidity in Klinefelter syndrome: a Danish register study based on hospital discharge diagnoses. J Clin Endocrinol Metab. 2006;91(4):1254–60. https://doi.org/10.1210/jc.2005-0697.
88. Bruining H, Swaab H, Kas M, van Engeland H. Psychiatric characteristics in a self-selected sample of boys with Klinefelter syndrome. Pediatrics. 2009;123(5):e865–70. https://doi.org/10.1542/peds.2008-1954.
89. Turriff A, Levy HP, Biesecker B. Prevalence and psychosocial correlates of depressive symptoms among adolescents and adults with Klinefelter syndrome. Genet Med. 2011;13(11):966–72. https://doi.org/10.1097/GIM.0b013e3182227576.
90. van Rijn S, Aleman A, Swaab H, Kahn R. Klinefelter's syndrome (karyotype 47,XXY) and schizophrenia-spectrum pathology. Br J Psychiatry J Ment Sci. 2006;189:459–60. https://doi.org/10.1192/bjp.bp.105.008961.
91. Amen DG, Stubblefield M, Carmicheal B, Thisted R. Brain SPECT findings and aggressiveness. Ann Clin Psychiatry. 1996;8(3):129–37. https://doi.org/10.3109/10401239609147750.
92. Miyagawa Y, Tsujimura A, Fujita K, Matsuoka Y, Takahashi T, Takao T, et al. Differential brain processing of audiovisual sexual stimuli in men: comparative positron emission tomography study of the initiation and maintenance of penile erection during sexual arousal. NeuroImage. 2007;36(3):830–42.
93. Yığman M, Yığman F, Tangal S, Haliloğlu AH, Çağlar GS. Pre-test anxiety levels and postoperative pain in non-obstructive azoospermic patients: is klinefelter syndrome a predisposing factor? Urologia. 2022;89(2):280–4. https://doi.org/10.1177/03915603211025236.
94. Selye H. A syndrome produced by diverse nocuous agents. 1936. J Neuropsychiatry Clin Neurosci. 1998;10(2):230–1. https://doi.org/10.1176/jnp.10.2.230a.
95. Bendayan M, Sais E, Alter L, Fathallah K, Jaoul M, Bosset PO, et al. For patients with non-obstructive azoospermia, the outcome of testicular sperm extraction correlates with self-esteem, sexual health and the quality of the couple's relationship. Basic Clin Androl. 2022;32(1):3. https://doi.org/10.1186/s12610-022-00153-z.
96. Topuz B, Ebiloğlu T, Sarıkaya S, Coğuplugil AE, Bedir S, Karataş ÖF. Evaluation of depression, anxiety and quality of life in patients with non-obstructive azoospermia. Rev Int Androl. 2021;19(2):73–9. https://doi.org/10.1016/j.androl.2019.09.005. Epub 2019 Dec 24. PMID: 31879204
97. Eisenberg ML, Li S, Cullen MR, Baker LC. Increased risk of incident chronic medical conditions in infertile men: analysis of United States claims data. Fertil Steril. 2016;105(3):629–36. https://doi.org/10.1016/j.fertnstert.2015.11.011.
98. Akbal C, Mangir N, Tavukçu HH, Ozgür O, Simşek F. Effect of testicular sperm extraction outcome on sexual function in patients with male factor infertility. Urology. 2010;75(3):598–601. https://doi.org/10.1016/j.urology.2009.07.1330.
99. Eliveld J, van der Bles I, van Wely M, Meißner A, Soufan AT, Heijboer AC, et al. The risk of hypogonadism after testicular sperm extraction in men with various types of azoospermia: a prospective cohort study. Reprod Biomed Online. 2023;46(6):973–81. https://doi.org/10.1016/j.rbmo.2023.02.003.
100. Rosen RC, Cappelleri JC, Smith MD, Lipsky J, Peña BM. Development and evaluation of an abridged, 5-item version of the International Index of Erectile Function (IIEF-5) as a diagnostic tool for erectile dysfunction. Int J Impot Res. 1999;11(6):319–26. https://doi.org/10.1038/sj.ijir.3900472.
101. Brennan C, Worrall-Davies A, McMillan D, Gilbody S, House A. The hospital anxiety and depression scale: a diagnostic meta-analysis of case-finding ability. J Psychosom Res. 2010;69(4):371–8. https://doi.org/10.1016/j.jpsychores.2010.04.006.

Chapter 16
Summary of the Most Recent International Guidelines on Nonobstructive Azoospermia

Parviz K. Kavoussi, Halil Ibrahim Ivelik, and Murat Gül

Key Points

1. Diagnostic testicular biopsy is not routinely recommended for distinguishing obstructive azoospermia from non-obstructive azoospermia (NOA) according to guidelines from the American Urological Association/American Society for Reproductive Medicine (AUA/ASRM) and European Association of Urology (EAU).
2. Varicocele repair in men with clinical varicocele and NOA lacks definitive evidence of therapeutic benefit, according to expert opinion.
3. Microdissection testicular sperm extraction is recommended as the preferred method for sperm retrieval in men with NOA undergoing surgical intervention, based on a moderate recommendation from AUA/ASRM guidelines.
4. Both fresh and cryopreserved sperm retrieved through surgical procedures may be used for intracytoplasmic sperm injection in men with NOA, with no substantial differences observed in in vitro fertilization success rates.

P. K. Kavoussi (✉)
Austin Fertility & Reproductive Medicine/Westlake IVF, Austin, TX, USA

H. I. Ivelik
Faculty of Medicine, Department of Urology, Kutahya Health Sciences University, Kutahya, Turkey

M. Gül
Department of Urology, Selçuk University School of Medicine, Konya, Türkiye

Department of Andrology, Selçuk University School of Medicine, Konya, Türkiye

W. Zohdy et al. (eds.), *Non-Obstructive Azoospermia*,
https://doi.org/10.1007/978-3-031-99431-9_16

Introduction

Infertility affects a significant portion of couples worldwide, with male factors contributing to approximately 50% of cases [1]. Non-obstructive azoospermia (NOA), characterized by the absence of sperm in the ejaculate due to testicular dysfunction, presents a particularly challenging scenario in male infertility management. The American Urological Association/American Society for Reproductive Medicine (AUA/ASRM) and the European Association of Urology (EAU) provide guidelines to assist clinicians in navigating the diagnostic and therapeutic complexities associated with NOA. These guidelines serve as invaluable tools in standardizing care and optimizing outcomes for patients with NOA. This chapter aims to review the diagnostic approaches, treatment modalities, and recommendations outlined in the guidelines of AUA/ASRM and EAU regarding NOA. By synthesizing and analyzing the recommendations from these esteemed urological societies, clinicians can make informed decisions tailored to the individual needs of patients presenting with NOA.

Specific Society Guideline statements on NOA

The Number of Semen Analyses Required to Confirm the Diagnosis of NOA

As it is common in clinical practice to find variation between semen analysis parameters in the same individual at different times, it is important for the clinical to understand the ranges of semen parameter values to guide further evaluation and treatment. The definition of azoospermia is a complete absence of sperm from the ejaculate, diagnosed by at least two semen analyses revealing no sperm by high-power light microscopy with the additional finding of no sperm in the concentrated centrifuged pellet after 15 min of centrifugation at a speed of at least 3000 × g or greater [1]. NOA is defined as azoospermia secondary to testicular sperm production impairment [2]. Both the AUA/ASRM and EAU guidelines recommend two separate consecutive semen analyses [3, 4].

The Optimal Time Interval Between Semen Analyses to Confirm the Diagnosis of NOA

The AUA/ASRM guidelines recommend an interval of 1 month following the initial semen analysis to perform a confirmatory semen analysis if the first one revealed azoospermia [3]. The EAU guidelines do not offer guidance on the interval between the two semen analyses.

The Need for a Hormonal Panel in Men with NOA and Which Hormonal Results to Obtain

Men with NOA commonly present with elevated gonadotropins—follicle-stimulating hormone (FSH) and luteinizing hormone (LH)—as a feedback response of the hypothalamic–pituitary–gonadal axis to primary testicular cell dysfunction. The AUA/ASRM guidelines recommend obtaining a serum hormonal panel including total testosterone and an FSH level. When the initial testosterone level is low, it is recommended to obtain free testosterone, estradiol, LH, and prolactin levels [3]. The EAU guidelines recommend testing testosterone as part of the diagnostic evaluation of male infertility, primarily to detect hypogonadism for overall health impacts. The EAU guidelines suggest that, due to conflicting data, FSH levels cannot be used to predict the success of surgical sperm retrieval in men with NOA [4].

Genetic Testing in Patients with NOA

The AUA/ASRM and the EAU guidelines recommend genetic testing in men with NOA to rule out genetically identifiable etiologies and guide treatment options. The recommendation is to obtain a karyotype and a Y chromosome microdeletion assay in men presumed to have NOA, such as those with azoospermia, atrophic testicles, and elevated FSH levels [3].

With Which Genetic Disorders Should a Surgical Sperm Retrieval Be Performed in Patients with NOA

The EAU guidelines recommend against any form of surgical sperm retrieval in men with AZFa and AZFb deletions, while sperm retrieval can be attempted in men with AZFc Y chromosome microdeletions [4].

Testicular Biopsy to Differentiate Between OA and NOA

It is critical to understand if a man with azoospermia has OA or NOA to guide his treatment options. Although the use of diagnostic testicular biopsies to differentiate between OA and NOA was the norm in the past, with advancements in clinical diagnostic tools, currently the AUA/ASRM guidelines recommend against the routine use of diagnostic testicular biopsy for this purpose. In men with NOA, with testosterone deficiency, small volume testicles, and elevated FSH levels, a diagnostic biopsy provides little additional diagnostic value since the diagnosis is already clear. A diagnostic testicular biopsy may be considered in men with azoospermia, normal semen volume, normal testicular volumes, and normal serum FSH levels, with at least one palpable vas deferens. In such cases, the clinical diagnostic clues available make it challenging to differentiate between OA and NOA without a diagnostic biopsy [3]. The EAU guidelines go further to consider a biopsy outside of the use of retrieved sperm for assisted reproductive technology (ART) as inappropriate [4].

Clinical Findings/Tests That Help Differentiate Between OA and NOA

The clinical findings that are suggested to help differentiate between OA and NOA by the AUA/ASRM guidelines include semen volume, physical examination findings, and FSH levels [3]. The EAU guidelines discuss the role of scrotal ultrasound in determining the signs in patients with testicular dysgenesis and tumors and suggest that testicular volumes measured by ultrasound can be associated with spermatogenic function [4].

Predictors of Successful Surgical Sperm Retrieval in Men with NOA

As surgical sperm retrieval rates in men with NOA are far from 100%, useful predictors of success would be helpful in counseling patients on their odds, which would potentially assist in their decision-making. The EAU guidelines indicate that "no preoperative biochemical and clinical variables may be considered sufficient and reliable predictors of positive sperm retrieval at surgery in patients with NOA." They also state that the presence of hypospermatogenesis on histopathology is correlated with higher odds of retrieving sperm compared to men with maturation arrest and Sertoli cell-only patterns [4]. There is no statement on predictors of the success of surgical sperm retrieval in men with NOA in the AUA/ASRM guidelines.

Genetic Counseling for Patients with NOA

EAU guidelines mandate genetic counseling consultation in couples with genetic abnormalities prior to proceeding with any ART protocols [4].

Antioxidant Use Prior to Surgical Sperm Retrieval in Men with NOA

Although there is a large body of medical literature on the use of antioxidants in infertile men, there is no definitive data on its utility prior to surgical sperm retrieval in men with NOA. There are no specific statements on the use of antioxidants prior to surgical sperm retrieval in men with NOA by either the AUA/ASRM or the EAU guidelines.

Hormonal Therapy Prior to Surgical Sperm Retrieval in Men with NOA

The AUA/ASRM and EAU guidelines state that there are limited data on the beneficial effects of hormonal treatments using selective estrogen receptor modulators, gonadotropins, and aromatase inhibitors prior to surgical sperm retrieval in men with NOA. There is a lack of data to advocate for hormonal therapy as a standard of care prior to retrieval [4, 5].

Duration of Hormonal Therapy Prior to Surgical Sperm Retrieval in Men with NOA

Hypogonadotropic hypogonadism, also known as secondary hypogonadism, which presents with low levels of serum FSH and LH and low testosterone levels, is the exception in men with NOA, which allows for an opportunity to have sperm appear in the semen with medical treatment. Excluding men with NOA and hypogonadotropic hypogonadism, there is no mention of specific durations of hormonal treatment for men with NOA prior to surgical sperm retrieval in either the AUA/ASRM or EAU guidelines. However, the EAU guidelines comment on the optimization of testosterone levels to stimulate spermatogenesis, which may improve the odds of finding sperm during a surgical sperm retrieval in men with NOA [4].

Hormonal Therapy in Hypergonadotropic Men with NOA

The EAU guidelines indicate that human chorionic gonadotropin (hCG) and/or FSH may be given in men with elevated gonadotropins with the possibility of a "gonadotropin reset," which could improve Sertoli cell function [4]. The AUA/ASRM does not comment on this scenario.

NOA Due to Exogenous Testosterone

The EAU guidelines suggest that following spermatogenic suppression with exogenous testosterone therapy, administration of hCG in conjunction with clomiphene citrate or FSH can help with the resumption of spermatogenesis [4]. The AUA/ASRM guidelines state that men who desire current or future fertility potential should not be prescribed testosterone therapy as a monotherapy. There is also mention that it is appropriate to treat testosterone deficiency with selective estrogen receptor modulators, hCG, and/or aromatase inhibitors [5].

Overall Surgical Sperm Retrieval Rate in Men with NOA

The EAU guidelines report a 52% overall surgical sperm retrieval rate in men with NOA. This data was obtained from a meta-analysis of case–control studies [4]. The AUA/ASRM guidelines do not quote a surgical sperm retrieval rate in men with NOA.

Duration of Time Embryology Team Searches for Sperm Before Declaring an Absence of Sperm in MicroTESE Specimens

There is a great deal of variation on whether reproductive urologists have laboratory personnel in the operating room during surgical sperm retrievals, which most reproductive urologists would consider optimal, or if specimens are collected and sent to the laboratory for examination. Beyond that, there is no standard of care timeframe that is mandated for the laboratory team to search for sperm in the retrieved testicular tissue. There are no specific statements in either the AUA/ASRM or the EAU guidelines on the duration of time the laboratory team should take to search for surgically retrieved sperm prior to declaring an absence of sperm in the sample.

Use of Fresh Versus Frozen Sperm Retrieved from Men with NOA

The AUA/ASRM guidelines report that there is no significant difference in fertilization, clinical pregnancy, and live birth rates when comparing fresh versus cryopreserved surgically retrieved sperm from men with NOA for use with ART., There are different advantages to using fresh versus frozen sperm [5]. The use of fresh sperm eliminates the cellular stress from undergoing the freeze–thaw process and may be beneficial in cases with very low numbers of sperm due to sperm survival rates after freeze–thaw; however; in cases where sperm are not found, the female partner underwent unnecessary ovarian stimulation with the associated costs. It should be considered that the clinical outcomes appear to be similar with fresh versus frozen sperm.

Varicocele Repair in Men with NOA

Varicoceles are abnormal dilations of scrotal veins draining into the pampiniform plexus and are present in 15% of men in the general population, 40% of men presenting for primary infertility evaluations, and 80% of men presenting for secondary infertility evaluations, making it the most common diagnosis made in infertile men [6]. Varicoceles have been shown to have an adverse impact on testicular function by multiple mechanisms, including elevation of testicular temperatures, inducing DNA fragmentation, apoptosis, and oxidative stress [7–10]. The AUA/ASRM and EAU guidelines state that there should be consideration for varicocele repair in men with varicocele-associated NOA. The potential benefits include the possible appearance of sperm in the ejaculate following varicocele repair and improvement in surgical sperm retrieval rates in men who remain azoospermic following varicocele repair and require microdissection testicular sperm extraction (microTESE). The AUA/ASRM guidelines state that couples should be counseled that there is an absence of definitive evidence to support varicocele repair in men with NOA [4, 5].

Incidence of Clinically Significant Varicoceles in Men with NOA

As 15% of men in the general population are estimated to have a varicocele—and varicoceles are found in 40% of men presenting for a primary infertility evaluations—and given that 1% of men in the general population and 15% of men seeking fertility evaluation are azoospermic, some overlap between these two diagnoses is expected in certain individuals [6, 11, 12]. The AUA/ASRM guidelines report that there is an incidence of 4.3% to 13.3% of men with varicoceles with concomitant NOA [5].

Subclinical Varicocele Repair in Men with NOA

Both the AUA/ASRM and EAU guidelines generally recommend against the treatment of subclinical varicoceles [4, 5].

Varicocele Repair Resulting in the Appearance of Sperm in the Ejaculate in Men with NOA

Considering the incidence of men with NOA who are found to have a palpable clinical varicocele, the question arises whether it is beneficial to repair the varicocele. The EAU guidelines report an increase in surgical sperm retrieval rate (OR: 2.65) as well as a 44% incidence of the appearance of sperm in the ejaculate following varicocele repair in men with NOA. However, this is not based on a high level of quality evidence, and the recommendation is for shared decision-making with appropriate counseling [4].

Imaging-Guided Testicular Biopsies in Men with NOA

The EAU guidelines indicate that although there is inconsistent data for its routine use prior to performing surgical sperm retrieval, Doppler ultrasound assessment of the testicle for regions of higher levels of perfusion can direct targeted areas for retrievals [4].

FNA Testicular Mapping in Men with NOA

The EAU guidelines indicate that fine needle aspiration (FNA) testicular mapping should not currently be used as the technique of choice for surgical sperm retrieval in men with NOA and that "FNA mapping cannot be recommended as a primary therapeutic intervention in men with NOA until further randomized controlled trials are undertaken" [4].

Conventional TESE (cTESE) vs MicroTESE in Men with NOA

MicroTESE is the surgical sperm retrieval technique of choice in men with NOA advocated for by both the AUA/ASRM and EAU guidelines. MicroTESE offers the highest sperm retrieval rates in comparison to other techniques such as testicular sperm aspiration (TESA), FNA mapping, and cTESE [4, 5].

Duration to Wait Prior to Performing MicroTESE Following Failed cTESE in Men with NOA

The EAU guidelines recommend a duration of 3 to 6 months to perform microTESE following a failed cTESE, with a salvage microTESE surgical sperm retrieval rate of 46.5%. The complication rates include an intratesticular hematoma rate of 51.7% and a testicular fibrosis rate of 30% at 6 months following cTESE [4].

Odds of Success Performing Salvage MicroTESE Following Failed MicroTESE in Men with NOA

The EAU guidelines report a successful surgical sperm retrieval rate of 18.4% to 42.8% in men with NOA undergoing salvage microTESE after a failed microTESE [4].

Expert Opinion

The expert opinion emphasizes the cautious approach required in diagnosing and managing NOA. While diagnostic testicular biopsy may offer insights into the etiology of NOA, guidelines from the AUA/ASRM and the EAU advise against its routine use due to the predictive value of clinical and laboratory parameters. Furthermore, the expert opinion does not necessarily recommend against but does cast doubt on the therapeutic benefit of varicocele repair in men with NOA, highlighting the need for controlled studies to validate its efficacy. In terms of sperm retrieval, microTESE emerges as the preferred technique, supported by a moderate recommendation from AUA/ASRM guidelines. The expert opinion underscores the importance of evidence-based decision-making and the need for further research to elucidate optimal management strategies for NOA, as well as shared decision-making between the physician and patient.

Conclusions

In conclusion, the management of NOA requires a comprehensive approach guided by evidence-based recommendations from leading urological societies. The guidelines provided by the AUA/ASRM and the EAU offer valuable insights into diagnostic strategies, treatment options, and recommendations for NOA. Key conclusions drawn from these guidelines include the limited role of diagnostic testicular biopsy, the uncertain benefit of varicocele repair in NOA, and the preference for microTESE for sperm retrieval in surgical interventions. Moving forward, further research is warranted to validate these recommendations and refine management approaches for NOA, with the ultimate goal of improving outcomes for couples facing male infertility.

References

1. Jarow JP, Espeland MA, Lipshultz LI. Evaluation of the azoospermic patient. J Urol. 1989;142(1):62–5.
2. Mazzilli F, et al. Azoospermia: incidence, and biochemical evaluation of seminal plasma by the differential pH method. Panminerva Med. 2000;42(1):27–31.
3. Schlegel PN, et al. Diagnosis and treatment of infertility in men: AUA/ASRM guideline part I. Fertil Steril. 2021;115(1):54–61.
4. Minhas S, et al. European Association of Urology Guidelines on male sexual and reproductive health: 2021 update on male infertility. Eur Urol. 2021;80(5):603–20.
5. Schlegel PN, et al. Diagnosis and treatment of infertility in men: AUA/ASRM guideline PART II. J Urol. 2021;205(1):44–51.
6. Nagler HM, Luntz RK, Martinis FG. Varicocele. Infertility in the male. St. Louis: Mosby Year Book; 1997. p. 336–59.
7. Smith R, et al. Increased sperm DNA damage in patients with varicocele: relationship with seminal oxidative stress. Hum Reprod. 2006;21(4):986–93.
8. Agarwal A, Makker K, Sharma R. Clinical relevance of oxidative stress in male factor infertility: an update. Am J Reprod Immunol. 2008;59(1):2–11.
9. Hassan A, el-Nashar EM, Mostafa T. Programmed cell death in varicocele-bearing testes. Andrologia. 2009;41(1):39–45.
10. Wu GJ, et al. Apoptosis-related phenotype of ejaculated spermatozoa in patients with varicocele. Fertil Steril. 2009;91(3):831–7.
11. Willott GM. Frequency of azoospermia. Forensic Sci Int. 1982;20(1):9–10.
12. Jarow J, Sigman M, Kolettis PN, Lipshultz LR, McClure RD, Nangia AK, Naughton CK, Prins GS, Sandlow JI, Schlegel PN. The evaluaiton of the azoospermic male. American Urological Association Best Practices Statement. 2011.

Chapter 17
Future of Nonobstructive Azoospermia (NOA)

Ahmed Ragab, Murat Gül, and Rupin Shah

Key Points

- The integration of transcriptomics and proteomics in predicting surgical sperm retrieval (SSR) in nonobstructive azoospermia (NOA) patients could enhance decision-making and patient outcomes.
- New genetic tests (next-generation sequencing [NGS] and whole-exome sequencing [WES]) and improvements in data sharing among research consortia are important in discovering genetic defects causing male infertility and decreasing the number of idiopathic cases.
- Advances in epigenetic analysis techniques will enhance diagnostic and therapeutic strategies, improving fertility care.
- Emerging technologies such as predictive modeling, multiphoton microscopy, and metabolomic scanning hold promise for improving the diagnosis and management of NOA, despite application challenges.
- Technological advancements in micro-TESE should also be coupled with high levels of sample preparation and sperm selection in the laboratory.
- The integration of artificial intelligence (AI) and advanced sperm sorting technologies may enhance the identification and selection of viable sperm, thereby improving outcomes in assisted reproductive technology (ART).
- The advancements in round spermatid injection, stem cell therapy, and artificial gamete technology offer promising avenues for addressing cases with idiopathic

A. Ragab (✉)
Department of Andrology, Faculty of Medicine, Beni-Suef University, Beni-Suef, Egypt

M. Gül
Department of Urology, Selçuk University School of Medicine, Konya, Türkiye

Department of Andrology, Selçuk University School of Medicine, Konya, Türkiye

R. Shah
Department of Urology, Lilavati Hospital and Research Centre, Mumbai, Maharashtra, India
e-mail: drrupinshah@gmail.com

W. Zohdy et al. (eds.), *Non-Obstructive Azoospermia*,
https://doi.org/10.1007/978-3-031-99431-9_17

NOA; however, further research is crucial to ensure their safety, efficacy, and ethical application.
- Gene therapy for male infertility is still experimental but will play a major role in the management of cases with severe affection of spermatogenesis.

Introduction

Nonobstructive azoospermia (NOA) is a substantial challenge in the management of male infertility. Currently, the therapeutic approach primarily focuses on sperm retrieval by micro-dissection testicular sperm extraction (micro-TESE) [1]. However, the success rate of surgical sperm retrieval (SSR) is only around 50% [2, 3]. Thus, half of the men undergo a traumatic, potentially harmful, expensive surgery without gaining any benefit, and without any further therapeutic option [4]. Thus, there is still a need for major innovations in the evaluation and management of NOA.

We anticipate future advancements in several crucial domains related to the management of NOA. These include: (I) the prediction of sperm presence in the testes of men diagnosed with NOA (predicting SSR) using (a) proteomics, (b) transcriptomics, (c) single-cell RNA sequencing and multiomics, (d) seminal plasma (SP) circular-RNA, and (e) metabolomics; (II) the identification of genetic causes of NOA, including single gene defects and epigenetic problems, through next-generation sequencing (NGS) and whole-exome sequencing (WES); (III) the restoration of fertility by correction of gene defects; (IV) innovations in intraoperative techniques to identify sperm bearing tubules; and (V) progress in laboratory techniques for the identification and selection of spermatozoa within the extracted tissue, alongside the integration of artificial intelligence (AI) in these processes.

Prediction of Sperm Presence in the Testes of Men Diagnosed with NOA

Proteomics

The study of SP proteins has revealed significant biomarkers that can differentiate various forms of azoospermia [5]. ***L-Lactate Dehydrogenase C*** (LDHC) is vital for glycolysis and sperm motility, with its absence correlating to spermatogenesis intensity [6]. Another glycolytic enzyme, ***Phosphoglycerate kinase 2*** (PGK2), is essential for sperm development and is primarily expressed in elongated spermatids [7]. ***Transketolase-like protein 1*** (TKTL1) helps distinguish NOA subtypes, as its expression starts in spermatogonia [8]. ***Testis expressed 101*** (TEX101) serves as a germ cell-specific protein that plays a vital role during sperm capacitation and binding to the zona pellucida. Its levels in SP reflect spermatogenesis status, with high levels indicating normal spermatogenesis and low levels suggesting conditions such as Sertoli cell-only syndrome (SCOS) [9]. Additionally, ***Extracellular matrix***

protein 1 (ECM1) has emerged as a significant biomarker for diagnosing NOA and differentiating various forms of azoospermia. A study involving 119 SP samples from men with both normal spermatogenesis and azoospermia identified ECM1, along with TEX101, as key in differentiating between OA and NOA [10]. They found that a cutoff level of 2.3 μg/ml of ECM1 could distinguish OA from normal spermatogenesis with 100% specificity and OA from NOA with 73% specificity at 100% sensitivity. This suggests that ECM1 plays a critical role in the molecular processes underlying NOA [11, 12].

Despite the advancements in proteomic analysis for identifying male infertility biomarkers, further research is necessary to overcome challenges related to detection methods and sample sizes. This continued investigation is crucial for enhancing diagnostic accuracy and clinical applicability in the context of male infertility [5].

Transcriptomics

The exploration of gene expression during meiosis has identified various RNA molecules as potential biomarkers for NOA patients. These RNA types include microRNAs (miRNAs), messenger RNAs (mRNAs), circular RNAs (circRNAs), and long non-coding RNAs (lncRNAs), each playing distinct roles in gene regulation and spermatogenesis. Notably, miRNAs have been highlighted for their stability in SP, making them promising noninvasive markers for assessing spermatogenesis [5].

Li et al. [13] conducted a thorough analysis of 80 studies to determine the potential use of SP for biomarker detection in NOA patients. The biomarkers examined were diverse, including RNAs. The study has shown a different expression of specific miRNAs in NOA patients with both positive and negative TESE outcomes, suggesting their potential in predicting SSR, though further validation is needed. Additionally, the transfer RNA-derived small RNA (tsRNA), RF-Val-AAC-010, was significantly elevated in NOA patients with successful micro-TESE, indicating its promise as a biomarker and its role in spermatogenesis [14].

Despite the promising nature of these RNA molecules as noninvasive biomarkers, challenges remain in applying transcriptomics for predicting SSR in clinical settings. Issues such as moderate specificity and sensitivity of predictive models, the complexity of the SP transcriptome, and variability in miRNA expression complicate the landscape. Overall, larger and more comprehensive investigations are essential to validate the clinical applications of these biomarkers [5].

Single-Cell RNA Sequencing and Multiomics

Recent advancements in single-cell RNA sequencing (scRNA-seq) include techniques like cellular indexing of transcriptomes and epitopes by sequencing (CITE-seq) or RNA expression and protein sequencing (REAP-seq) [15, 16], which allow simultaneous measurement of surface markers and transcriptome data through oligonucleotide-conjugated antibodies [17]. Single-cell multiomics analyses have also emerged, enabling the study of transcriptomes and chromatin accessibility, particularly in spermatogenesis [18]. A limitation of scRNA-seq is its lack of spatial context, which spatial transcriptome analysis addresses by examining transcriptomes in specific tissue regions using techniques like immunohistochemistry. Although research on spatial transcriptomics in spermatogenesis is limited [19], future technological advancements will deepen our understanding of this process [17].

Seminal Plasma (SP) Circular-RNA

Circular RNA (CircRNA) has been studied for its potential role in regulating sperm production and its potential use in NOA diagnosis and treatment [20–22]. Different expression patterns have been found in the testes of NOA patients compared to OA patients, linking certain CircRNAs to NOA-related signaling pathways [23]. CircRNAs have been identified in SCOS patients, suggesting their involvement in spermatogenic cell proliferation and intercellular communication [20]. CircRNAs in SP have been identified as predictors of micro-TESE success in idiopathic NOA [24].

Metabolomics

Existing research suggests that metabolic fingerprinting of SP can be used as a useful diagnostic tool for men experiencing infertility [25, 26]. **Gilany et al.** [27] investigated metabolic profiling of SP of NOA men with successful and unsuccessful TESE and discovered 36 distinguishing metabolites as prognostic biomarkers for positive and negative TESE men. Furthermore, another study [28] revealed that the metabolic fingerprint, particularly the oxidative status, differed significantly between positive and negative TESE patients. These results indicate that SP metabolites have great potential as specific biomarkers for SSR prediction. The main shortcoming of these studies is that these metabolites lack effective validation and are not included in the Human Metabolome Database. Hence, more in-depth studies are required in the future [13].

Identification of Genetic Causes of NOA: Single Gene Defects and Epigenetic Problems

The exploration of genetic factors contributing to NOA has provided valuable insights, especially concerning maturation arrest (MA). This area of research is crucial, given that more than 40% of NOA cases remain unexplained, suggesting a significant genetic influence that is not yet fully understood [29].

Several genetic variants have been identified in NOA cases with MA at premeiotic, meiotic, and postmeiotic arrest stages, which could help develop a gene panel for each type [30]. The MA phenotype shows the highest rate of monogenic defects, involving 22 genes. Six genes involved in meiosis (MEI1, MEIOB, TEX11, SYCE1, STAG3, SETX) are directly linked to spermatocyte arrest, while four new recessive genes (ADAD2, TERB1, SHOC1, MSH4) have also been identified as responsible for MA [29, 31, 32]. Knockout mouse models for these genes replicate human phenotypes and have been validated in idiopathic NOA patients. ADAD2 is associated with incomplete spermatogenic arrest [29], while the other three genes are linked to complete spermatogenic arrest [33]. Besides these recurrently mutated candidate genes, another 13 genes have been reported only in single studies as causative for MA at different stages with the support of in vitro or in vivo experimental data [34].

The validation of numerous NOA-related genes, particularly those responsible for meiotic arrest, has been enhanced through collaborative data sharing among laboratories and members of the International Male Infertility Genomics Consortium (http://www.imigc.org) and the Genetics of Male Infertility Initiative (GEMINI) consortium (http://www.gemini.conradlab.org) [29, 35–37].

The shift from traditional low-resolution genetic testing methods (such as karyotyping and FISH) to single-gene testing represents a significant advancement in the diagnosis and treatment of male infertility, as supported by both mouse and emerging human studies [38, 39]. ***Next generation sequencing (NGS)-based whole exome sequencing (WES)*** or ***gene panel sequencing*** has allowed the identification of a growing number of novel monogenic causes of azoospermia [34]. However, these technologies are not yet established in clinical practice and are still limited to research purposes [38].

The genetic variability associated with NOA indicates a significant level of locus heterogeneity for its monogenic causes [40]. ***WES*** has reduced the incidence of idiopathic NOA, often linked to conditions like SCOS and MA [41], and led to the discovery of numerous genes associated with male infertility [42, 43]. Recent cohort studies or familial studies also demonstrated the relevance of WES and highlighted the involvement of additional genes in the etiology of NOA [29, 44, 45]. Given the extreme genetic heterogeneity of NOA and the declining costs of WES, experts advocate for its integration into genetic testing for infertility [46]. A recent study utilizing WES identified causative mutations in genes related to spermatogenesis in 23% of NOA cases through a targeted gene selection strategy [46]. WES has also identified novel pathogenic variants in five genes (CCDC155, NANOS2, SPO11, TEX14, and WNK3) affecting fertility in eight multiplex families [47]. Those examples were followed later by numerous studies that led to the identification of hundreds of genes now related to male infertility [38].

In addition to identifying single genes with mutations in infertile men, NGS technologies allow the detection of copy number and structural variants in patients. Not unlike a high-resolution microarray, NGS technologies can detect deletions and duplications that are as small as 50 base pairs, and this high resolution opens a window of discovery in the sub-250 kb range that was previously difficult to detect with traditional microarrays. As these technologies become more routine, it is expected that a growing number of microdeletions and microduplications will be observed in infertile men, and understanding their impact and heritability, as well as the pathways they disrupt, will enhance our understanding of this complex condition [38].

Moreover, NGS technologies provide advanced methods for studying the epigenome and understanding male infertility [48–51]. A key technique for detecting DNA methylation is bisulfite genomic sequencing, which converts unmethylated cytosines to uracil while preserving methylated ones, followed by PCR amplification and sequencing [52]. Other methods for assessing sperm epigenetics include the Methyl Flash Global DNA Methylation and Hydroxymethylation ELISA kits, which quantify 5-methylcytosine and 5-hydroxymethylcytosine levels [53]. Histone modification patterns are analyzed using chromatin immunoprecipitation (ChIP) with specific antibodies, applicable in ChIP-chip and ChIP-seq. Mass spectrometry can validate histone codes [54], and micrococcal nuclease aids in analyzing chromatin units (MNase-ChIP) [54, 55]. Also, high-throughput sequencing is relevant [55]. For protamine studies, sperm nuclear proteins are extracted and quantified using acetic acid–urea gel electrophoresis [56, 57], with arrays used for hybridizing protamine-associated DNA [55].

Ongoing basic and translational research, along with high-throughput technologies, will enhance epigenetic testing and our understanding of sperm epigenomics, improving diagnosis, prevention, and treatment of infertility [58].

Restoration of Fertility by Correction of Gene Defects

Gene editing techniques, specifically clustered regularly interspaced short palindromic repeats (CRISPR)/CRISPR-associated (Cas) protein 9 (CRISPR/Cas9), zinc-finger nucleases (ZFNs), and transcription activator-like effector nucleases (TALENs), offer promising opportunities to improve infertility treatments in men through targeted genetic modifications. These technologies can correct genetic defects in sperm precursor or testicular somatic cells, potentially restoring spermatogenesis. Current research focuses on using gene editing to address mutations causing testicular dysfunction in men with NOA [59–62].

Numerous candidate genes have been identified for potential future gene therapy in male infertility. Marker genes of Sertoli cells include anti-Müllerian hormone, aromatase, cytokeratin-18, GATA1, laminin 5, M2A antigen, p27kip1, vimentin, connexin 26, connexin 43, inhibin, sulfated glycoprotein 2, androgen receptor, and WT-1. Transcription factors include Pem (Rhox5), CREB, Sox3, and DAX1, which are essential for spermatogenesis and are expressed in Sertoli cells. Additionally, Leydig cells may also be target cells in KS, having insufficiency and distressed apoptosis regulation [63]. Marker genes, including P450 steroid hydroxylase, 3-HSD, androgen receptor, LHR, and Ad4BP/SF-1, are expressed in Leydig cells and are involved in steroidogenesis as well as spermatogenesis [64].

Despite the potential benefits, challenges such as the complex genetic nature of NOA, ethical concerns, high costs, and the need for rigorous safety assessments must be addressed before these techniques can be widely implemented in clinical practice [65–67].

Innovations in Intraoperative Techniques to Identify Sperm Bearing Tubules

The use of metabolite spectroscopy prior to micro-TESE shows promise in predicting SSR rates in men with NOA, particularly through the correlation of choline signal intensity with successful outcomes [68, 69]. The effectiveness of MRI in predicting SSR in NOA patients undergoing micro-TESE has also been evaluated. Larger testicular volumes correlated positively with SSR, while higher apparent diffusion coefficients (ADC) and magnetization transfer ratios (MTR) correlated negatively. However, the high cost of MRI may limit its use as a routine preoperative diagnostic tool [70].

The stepwise mini-incision micro-TESE technique appears to offer advantages in terms of reduced invasiveness and operative time [71], although further research is necessary to confirm its effectiveness in minimizing testicular parenchyma damage [70].

The integration of robotic assistance in micro-TESE procedures may enhance SSR outcomes through enhanced imaging capabilities; however, it currently serves more as a proof of concept rather than a definitive improvement in clinical outcomes [72].

Several technologies are currently being investigated for their potential to noninvasively identify areas of spermatogenesis in the testis. ***Multiphoton microscopy*** (MPM) demonstrates significant potential for enhancing the identification and selection of spermatozoa by allowing real-time visualization of spermatogenesis in testicular tissue without the need for exogenous labels or extensive processing [73, 74]. However, there are limits to this technology, including the narrow field of view, potential for motion artifact, and concern for the possible mutagenic potential of lasers on spermatozoa [75]. Further clinical studies are necessary to validate its application during micro-TESE procedures [70]. ***Raman spectroscopy*** has been used for distinguishing between seminiferous tubules with ongoing spermatogenesis and those with spermatogenic arrest, with high sensitivity and specificity in murine models [76]. However, further research is required to translate these findings into human clinical applications [77].

Full-field optical coherence tomography (FFOCT) [78] and ***confocal fluorescence microscopy*** [79, 80] are promising techniques for the identification and selection of spermatozoa-bearing tubules. These technologies offer significant advantages, such as the ability to analyze fresh tissue without processing or staining, but their efficacy in human subjects remains to be established [70]. Likewise, the introduction of the ***ORBEYE 4 K-3D microscope*** represents a significant advancement in microsurgical techniques by enhancing ergonomics and visualization during procedures like micro-TESE, but has limited accessibility due to high costs [81, 82]. This technology not only improves the identification and selection of tubules with spermatozoa but also addresses longstanding challenges associated with traditional operative microscopy [70].

Similarly, the integration of ***advanced ultrasound techniques***, including color Doppler [83], contrast-enhanced ultrasound [84], and the ultrasonographic measurement of seminiferous tubule dimensions [85] could enhance the identification and selection of favourable tubules in men with NOA, thereby improving the outcomes of micro-TESE procedures. These methodologies provide insights into testicular perfusion and seminiferous tubule characteristics, which are useful for optimizing SSR success rates [86].

Intraoperative ***Laser Doppler-Assisted TESE*** is another advanced technique in the field [70]. A study involving 12 patients with NOA analyzed 40 biopsies from 20 testicles using color Doppler ultrasound for perfusion mapping. Areas with varying perfusion were marked, and after testicular incision, a laser Doppler flowmeter assessed blood flow. Biopsies were collected for sperm retrieval and histological analysis. Results showed a positive correlation between sperm quality and quantity with higher perfusion levels. Larger studies are needed to confirm these findings [87].

Finally, ***narrow band-imaging*** [88] and ***ultrasonically actuated silicon microprobe*** [89] are new technologies that demonstrate potential for enhancing the identification and selection of spermatogenic areas, although further clinical studies are essential to validate their efficacy in human applications. These innovations could significantly improve surgical outcomes in assisted reproductive techniques by enabling more precise targeting of sperm-containing tubules [70].

The future directions of micro-TESE technology will include an improvement in surgical techniques and tissue processing [70]. High-resolution optics can enable higher precision, better visualization, and lower complications during micro-TESE [77]. A 4 K-3D videomicroscope may also be developed for the micro-TESE procedure. The 4 K-3D videomicroscope resulted in nonsignificantly shorter operative time and better ergonomics for operating room staff in varicocele repair [90]. More research on its efficacy for micro-TESE should be conducted. Technological advancements in surgery should also be coupled with better techniques of sample preparation and sperm selection in the laboratory [91].

Progress in Laboratory Techniques for the Identification and Selection of Spermatozoa Within the Extracted Tissue

Germ cell-specific proteins may serve as potential biomarkers for the detection of viable sperm in the semen of men diagnosed with NOA prior to proceeding with microTESE [92]. Whether such methods can be used to detect rare sperm in microTESE specimens is yet to be studied.

Use of Artificial Intelligence (AI) to Enhance Sperm Selection

Aside from the techniques that have been described, AI can be developed to assist in sperm identification and selection for better outcomes of ART [91]. AI is useful for interpreting large sets of data when a small margin of error is required. Parameters for the selection of sperm, such as motility and morphology, may be evaluated and characterized by AI. Although this technology holds promise, it is still in evolution [70, 77].

Wu et al. utilized a deep learning-based computer-aided sperm analysis (CASA) system to automate sperm identification in testicular biopsy samples. A total of 702 testicular biopsy samples were collected from 30 patients. The images were normalized, passed through glare filters, and subjected to diffraction correction. A deep object detection network was then trained on this dataset. The model was benchmarked against embryologists' performance on the detection task. The deep learning CASA system achieved a mean average precision (mAP) of 0.741. Moreover, the proposed method is capable of functioning in real time. These findings suggest that deep learning-based technologies can improve the efficiency of finding sperm in testicular biopsy samples [93].

Recently, ***Goss et al.*** explored the use of machine learning and AI to automate sperm detection in surgical sperm samples. A convolutional neural network was trained on over 10,000 sperm images from eight NOA patients to ensure diverse sperm morphology representation. In the first phase, the AI outperformed an embryologist in identifying spermatozoa, detecting 1997 sperm compared to 1937 by the embryologist, and did so more quickly. In the second phase, when integrated into an ICSI microscope, the AI-assisted embryologist reduced identification time, though the total sperm count remained similar to the embryologist alone. Overall, the findings indicate that AI can significantly enhance sperm detection efficiency in labs, potentially reducing extraction time from hours to minutes and improving fertility treatment success rates, showcasing AI's transformative role in reproductive medicine [94].

Advancements in Sperm Sorting and Identification Technologies

The advances in sperm sorting and identification technologies, particularly for micro-TESE specimens, significantly enhance the recovery of viable sperm, thereby improving the success rates of assisted reproductive technologies [70, 95]. Various methods, including enzymatic digestion, microfluidics, and advanced selection techniques, demonstrate promising results in isolating functional sperm, although further research is necessary to optimize these approaches and validate their efficacy in clinical settings [70].

Microfluidics technology has advanced significantly in sperm sorting, employing various techniques such as dielectrophoresis, spiral channels, and pinched flow fractionation to enhance the efficiency and effectiveness of isolating both motile and nonmotile sperm [96–100]. Continued research and optimization of these methods are essential to improve their application in clinical settings, particularly for patients with specific reproductive challenges [99].

Fluorescence-activated cell sorting (FACS) demonstrates potential for effectively sorting spermatozoa from micro-TESE testicular tissue, as evidenced by a pilot study [70, 101].

Although ***magnetic-activated cell sorting (MACS)*** shows an improvement in pregnancy rates over conventional sperm selection techniques, its effectiveness is restricted to uniform sperm samples [99]. Additional research is needed to confirm its efficacy and safety [102].

Advanced sperm selection techniques such as hyaluronic acid-based methods [103] and zeta sperm selection [104] also demonstrate promising potential in enhancing fertilization outcomes, yet further research is necessary to establish their efficacy [70, 105].

Future Directions, Challenges, Limitations

The advances in reproductive technologies, including ***round spermatid injection*** [106], ***stem cell therapy*** [107–109], and ***artificial gamete technology*** [110, 111], offer promising avenues for addressing severe male infertility, particularly in cases of idiopathic NOA; however, further research is crucial to ensure their safety, efficacy, and ethical application [75, 112, 113]**.** Establishment of approaches for further efficient and safer ***gene transfer*** could provide great benefit to male infertility patients. However, in comparison with other organs, testicular gene transfer needs caution and careful consideration of the biological and ethical issues involved [38]. Additionally, recent findings regarding the ***intratesticular microbiome*** [70, 114–118] **and *epigenetic factors*** [48–51] highlight the complexity of male infertility and the necessity for targeted approaches and innovative strategies. ***Histone modifications*** are important prognostic markers and potential therapeutic targets, with histone deacetylases (HDACs) being key in epigenetic therapy. While no epigenetic drugs are specifically aimed at infertility, existing treatments may provide benefits due to shared mechanisms [54, 119, 120]. Moreover, artificial intelligence (AI) has the potential to develop algorithms that enhance clinical decision-making and predict outcomes for men with NOA, thereby enhancing patient counseling and optimizing resource allocation [75].

Conclusions

Advances in genetic research, technology, and integrative approaches are changing the landscape of NOA. Transcriptomics, proteomics, and multiomics are anticipated to improve predictions of surgical sperm retrieval in males with NOA. New genetic tests (NGS and WES) and data sharing help discover genetic causes of NOA and decrease the number of idiopathic cases. Furthermore, epigenetic analysis techniques are expected to enhance diagnostic and therapeutic strategies. Innovations like predictive modeling and multiphoton microscopy show promise for NOA management. Future advancements in surgical technology, like high-resolution optics and robotic assistance, and sperm sorting and identification technologies are crucial for enhancing the recovery of viable sperm from testicular biopsy samples. Ultimately, a comprehensive approach, including artificial intelligence (AI) integration, is needed to enhance clinical outcomes in males with NOA.

References

1. Oka S, Shiraishi K, Matsuyama H. Effects of human chorionic gonadotropin on testicular interstitial tissues in men with non-obstructive azoospermia. Andrology. 2017;5(2):232–9. https://doi.org/10.1111/andr.12292. Epub 2016 Nov 16. PMID: 27860441
2. Tsujimura A, Matsumiya K, Miyagawa Y, Takao T, Fujita K, Koga M, et al. Prediction of successful outcome of microdissection testicular sperm extraction in men with idiopathic nonobstructive azoospermia. J Urol. 2004;172:1944–7. https://doi.org/10.1097/01.ju.0000142885.20116.60. PubMed PMID:15540761
3. Abdel Raheem A, Garaffa G, Rushwan N, De Luca F, Zacharakis E, Abdel Raheem T, et al. Testicular histopathology as a predictor of a positive sperm retrieval in men with non-obstructive azoospermia. BJU Int. 2013;111:492–9. https://doi.org/10.1111/j.1464-410X.2012.11203.x. PubMed PMID:22583840
4. Zohdy W, Shah R, Ho CC, Calik G, Malhotra V, Erkan BK, et al. Changes in testosterone levels following surgical sperm retrieval in men with non-obstructive azoospermia: systematic review and meta-analysis. World J Mens Health. 2024;42:e78. https://doi.org/10.5534/wjmh.240129.
5. Fontana L, Sirchia SM, Pesenti C, Colpi GM, Miozzo MR. Non-invasive biomarkers for sperm retrieval in non-obstructive patients: a comprehensive review. Front Endocrinol (Lausanne). 2024;15:1349000. https://doi.org/10.3389/fendo.2024.1349000. PMID: 38689732; PMCID: PMC11058837
6. Hamil KG, Sivashanmugam P, Richardson RT, Grossman G, Ruben SM, Mohler JL, et al. HE2beta and HE2gamma, new members of an epididymis-specific family of androgen-regulated proteins in the human. Endocrinology. 2000;141:1245–53. https://doi.org/10.1210/en.141.3.1245.

7. Ghanami Gashti N, Sadighi Gilani MA, Jabari A, Qasemi M, Feizollahi N, Abbasi M. The germ cell-specific markers ZPBP2 and PGK2 in testicular biopsies can predict the presence as well as the quality of sperm in non-obstructive Azoospermia patients. Reprod Sci. 2021;28:1466–75. https://doi.org/10.1007/s43032-020-00427-9.
8. Davalieva K, Rusevski A, Velkov M, Noveski P, Kubelka-Sabit K, Filipovski V, et al. Comparative proteomics analysis of human FFPE testicular tissues reveals new candidate biomarkers for distinction among azoospermia types and subtypes. J Proteome. 2022;267:104686. https://doi.org/10.1016/j.jprot.2022.104686.
9. Korbakis D, Schiza C, Brinc D, Soosaipillai A, Karakosta TD, Legare C, et al. Preclinical evaluation of a TEX101 protein ELISA test for the differential diagnosis of male infertility. BMC Med. 2017;15(1):60. https://doi.org/10.1186/s12916-017-0817-5.
10. Drabovich AP, Dimitromanolakis A, Saraon P, Soosaipillai A, Batruch I, Mullen B, et al. Differential diagnosis of azoospermia with proteomic biomarkers ECM1 and TEX101 quantified in seminal plasma. Sci Transl Med. 2013;5(212):212ra160. https://doi.org/10.1126/scitranslmed.3006260.
11. Andrade DL, Viana MC, Esteves SC. Differential diagnosis of azoospermia in men with infertility. J Clin Med. 2021;10(14):3144. https://doi.org/10.3390/jcm10143144. PMID: 34300309; PMCID: PMC8304267
12. Malcher A, Stokowy T, Berman A, Olszewska M, Jedrzejczak P, Sielski D, et al. Whole-genome sequencing identifies new candidate genes for nonobstructive azoospermia. Andrology. 2022;10(8):1605–24. https://doi.org/10.1111/andr.13269. Epub 2022 Sep 7. PMID: 36017582; PMCID: PMC9826517
13. Li J, Yang F, Dong L, Chang D, Yu X. Seminal plasma biomarkers for predicting successful sperm retrieval in patients with nonobstructive azoospermia: a narrative review of human studies. Basic Clin Androl. 2023;33(1):9. https://doi.org/10.1186/s12610-023-00184-0. PMID: 37076787; PMCID: PMC10116801
14. Tang XJ, Xiao QH, Wang XL, He Y, Tian YN, Xia BT, et al. Single-cell transcriptomics-based study of transcriptional regulatory features in the non-obstructive azoospermia testis. Front Genet. 2022;13:875762. https://doi.org/10.3389/fgene.2022.875762. PMID: 35669193; PMCID: PMC9163961
15. Stoeckius M, Hafemeister C, Stephenson W, Houck-Loomis B, Chattopadhyay PK, Swerdlow H, et al. Simultaneous epitope and transcriptome measurement in single cells. Nat Methods. 2017;14(9):865–8. https://doi.org/10.1038/nmeth.4380. Epub 2017 Jul 31. PMID: 28759029; PMCID: PMC5669064
16. Peterson VM, Zhang KX, Kumar N, Wong J, Li L, Wilson DC, et al. Multiplexed quantification of proteins and transcripts in single cells. Nat Biotechnol. 2017;35(10):936–9. https://doi.org/10.1038/nbt.3973. Epub 2017 Aug 30
17. Suzuki T. Overview of single-cell RNA sequencing analysis and its application to spermatogenesis research. Reprod Med Biol. 2023;22(1):e12502. https://doi.org/10.1002/rmb2.12502. PMID: 36726594; PMCID: PMC9884325
18. Lee J, Hyeon DY, Hwang D. Single-cell multiomics: technologies and data analysis methods. Exp Mol Med. 2020;52(9):1428–42. https://doi.org/10.1038/s12276-020-0420-2. Epub 2020 Sep 15. PMID: 32929225; PMCID: PMC8080692
19. Chen H, Murray E, Sinha A, Laumas A, Li J, Lesman D, et al. Dissecting mammalian spermatogenesis using spatial transcriptomics. Cell Rep. 2021;37(5):109915. https://doi.org/10.1016/j.celrep.2021.109915. PMID: 34731600; PMCID: PMC8606188
20. Zhu F, Luo Y, Bo H, Gong G, Tang R, Fan J, et al. Trace the profile and function of circular RNAs in Sertoli cell only syndrome. Genomics. 2021;113:1845–54. https://doi.org/10.1016/j.ygeno.2021.04.022.
21. Derakhshan Z, Bahmanpour S, Alaee S, Fallahi J, Tabei SMB. The role of circular RNAs in male infertility and reproductive cancers: a narrative review. Iran J Med Sci. 2023;48(6):527–41. https://doi.org/10.30476/IJMS.2022.95302.2661. PMID: 38094281; PMCID: PMC10715113

22. Ge P, Zhang J, Zhou L, Lv MQ, Li YX, Wang J, et al. CircRNA expression profile and functional analysis in testicular tissue of patients with non-obstructive azoospermia. Reprod Biol Endocrinol. 2019;17:100. https://doi.org/10.1186/s12958-019-0541-4. PubMed PMID: 31775841; PubMed Central PMCID: PMCPMC6880412
23. Bo H, Liu Z, Tang R, Gong G, Wang X, Zhang H, et al. Testicular biopsies microarray analysis reveals circRNAs are involved in the pathogenesis of non-obstructive azoospermia. Aging (Albany NY). 2020;12:2610–25. https://doi.org/10.18632/aging.102765. PubMedPMID: 32029690; PubMed Central PMCID: PMCPMC7041731
24. Ji C, Wang Y, Wei X, Zhang X, Cong R, Yao L, et al. Potential of testis-derived circular RNAs in seminal plasma to predict the outcome of microdissection testicular sperm extraction in patients with idiopathic non-obstructive azoospermia. Hum Reprod. 2021;36:2649–60. https://doi.org/10.1093/humrep/deab196.
25. Jafarzadeh N, Mani-Varnosfaderani A, Minai-Tehrani A, Savadi-Shiraz E, Sadeghi MR, Gilany K. Metabolomics fingerprinting of seminal plasma from unexplained infertile men: a need for novel diagnostic biomarkers. Mol Reprod Dev. 2015;82(3):150. https://doi.org/10.1002/mrd.22457. Epub 2015 Feb 10
26. Gilany K, Moazeni-Pourasil RS, Jafarzadeh N, Savadi-Shiraz E. Metabolomics fingerprinting of the human seminal plasma of asthenozoospermic patients. Mol Reprod Dev. 2014;81(1):84–6. https://doi.org/10.1002/mrd.22284.
27. Gilany K, Mani-Varnosfaderani A, Minai-Tehrani A, Mirzajani F, Ghassempour A, Sadeghi MR, et al. Untargeted metabolomic profiling of seminal plasma in nonobstructive azoospermia men: a noninvasive detection of spermatogenesis. Biomed Chromatogr. 2017;31(8) https://doi.org/10.1002/bmc.3931. Epub 2017 Feb 5
28. Gilany K, Jafarzadeh N, Mani-Varnosfaderani A, Minai-Tehrani A, Sadeghi MR, Darbandi M, Pahlevanzadeh Z, et al. Metabolic fingerprinting of seminal plasma from non-obstructive azoospermia patients: positive versus negative sperm retrieval. J Reprod Infertil. 2018;19(2):109–14. PMID: 30009145; PMCID: PMC6010822
29. Krausz C, Riera-Escamilla A, Moreno-Mendoza D, Holleman K, Cioppi F, Algaba F, et al. Genetic dissection of spermatogenic arrest through exome analysis: clinical implications for the management of azoospermic men. Genet Med. 2020;22(12):1956–66. https://doi.org/10.1038/s41436-020-0907-1. Epub 2020 Aug 3. PMID: 32741963; PMCID: PMC7710580
30. Ozturk S. Genetic variants underlying spermatogenic arrests in men with non-obstructive azoospermia. Cell Cycle. 2023;22(9):1021–61. https://doi.org/10.1080/15384101.2023.2171544. Epub 2023 Feb 5. PMID: 36740861; PMCID: PMC10081088
31. Salas-Huetos A, Tüttelmann F, Wyrwoll MJ, Kliesch S, Lopes AM, Goncalves J, et al. Disruption of human meiotic telomere complex genes TERB1, TERB2 and MAJIN in men with non-obstructive azoospermia. Hum Genet. 2021;140(1):217–27. https://doi.org/10.1007/s00439-020-02236-1. Epub 2020 Nov 19. Erratum in: Hum Genet. 2021 Jan;140(1):229. doi: 10.1007/s00439-020-02244-1. PMID: 33211200; PMCID: PMC7893731
32. Yao C, Yang C, Zhao L, Li P, Tian R, Chen H, et al. Bi-allelic SHOC1 loss-of-function mutations cause meiotic arrest and non-obstructive azoospermia. J Med Genet. 2021;58(10):679–86. https://doi.org/10.1136/jmedgenet-2020-107042. Epub 2020 Sep 8. PMID: 32900840; PMCID: PMC8479749
33. Wang Y, Chen Y, Chen J, Wang L, Nie L, Long J, et al. The meiotic TERB1-TERB2-MAJIN complex tethers telomeres to the nuclear envelope. Nat Commun. 2019;10(1):564. https://doi.org/10.1038/s41467-019-08437-1. PMID: 30718482; PMCID: PMC6361898
34. Cioppi F, Rosta V, Krausz C. Genetics of Azoospermia. Int J Mol Sci. 2021;22(6):3264. https://doi.org/10.3390/ijms22063264. PMID: 33806855; PMCID: PMC8004677
35. Kasak L, Laan M. Monogenic causes of non-obstructive azoospermia: challenges, established knowledge, limitations and perspectives. Hum Genet. 2021;140(1):135–54. https://doi.org/10.1007/s00439-020-02112-y. Epub 2020 Jan 18

36. Xavier MJ, Salas-Huetos A, Oud MS, Aston KI, Veltman JA. Disease gene discovery in male infertility: past, present and future. Hum Genet. 2021;140(1):7–19. https://doi.org/10.1007/s00439-020-02202-x. Epub 2020 Jul 7. PMID: 32638125; PMCID: PMC7864819
37. Capalbo A, Poli M, Riera-Escamilla A, Shukla V, Kudo Høffding M, Krausz C, et al. Preconception genome medicine: current state and future perspectives to improve infertility diagnosis and reproductive and health outcomes based on individual genomic data. Hum Reprod Update. 2021;27(2):254–79. https://doi.org/10.1093/humupd/dmaa044.
38. Mostafa T, Fakhro KA, Arafa M. Advances in genetics of male infertility. In: Agarwal A, Saleh R, Boitrelle F, Shah R, editors. Current and future advances in male infertility: a compendium for clinicians and researchers. Cham: Springer; 2024. p. 155–74. https://doi.org/10.1007/978-3-031-62648-7_8.
39. Okutman O, Rhouma MB, Benkhalifa M, Muller J, Viville S. Genetic evaluation of patients with non-syndromic male infertility. J Assist Reprod Genet. 2018;35(11):1939–51. https://doi.org/10.1007/s10815-018-1301-7. Epub 2018 Sep 26. PMID: 30259277; PMCID: PMC6240550
40. Krausz C. Editorial for the special issue on the molecular genetics of male infertility. Hum Genet. 2021;140(1):1–5. https://doi.org/10.1007/s00439-020-02245-0.
41. Krausz C, Riera-Escamilla A. Genetics of male infertility. Nat Rev Urol. 2018;15:369–84. https://doi.org/10.1038/s41585-018-0003-3. PMID: 29622783
42. Mitchell MJ, Metzler-Guillemain C, Toure A, Coutton C, Arnoult C, Ray PF. Single gene defects leading to sperm quantitative anomalies. Clin Genet. 2017;91(2):208–16. https://doi.org/10.1111/cge.12900. Epub 2016 Nov 22
43. Ray PF, Toure A, Metzler-Guillemain C, Mitchell MJ, Arnoult C, Coutton C. Genetic abnormalities leading to qualitative defects of sperm morphology or function. Clin Genet. 2017;91(2):217–32. https://doi.org/10.1111/cge.12905. Epub 2016 Dec 9
44. Fakhro KA, Elbardisi H, Arafa M, Robay A, Rodriguez-Flores JL, Al-Shakaki A, et al. Point-of-care whole-exome sequencing of idiopathic male infertility. Genet Med. 2018;20(11):1365–73. https://doi.org/10.1038/gim.2018.10. Epub 2018 Apr 12
45. Oud MS, Houston BJ, Volozonoka L, Mastrorosa FK, Holt GS, Alobaidi BKS, et al. Exome sequencing reveals variants in known and novel candidate genes for severe sperm motility disorders. Hum Reprod. 2021;36(9):2597–611. https://doi.org/10.1093/humrep/deab099. PMID: 34089056; PMCID: PMC8373475
46. Kherraf ZE, Cazin C, Bouker A, Fourati Ben Mustapha S, Hennebicq S, Septier A, et al. Whole-exome sequencing improves the diagnosis and care of men with non-obstructive azoospermia. Am J Hum Genet. 2022;109(3):508–17. https://doi.org/10.1016/j.ajhg.2022.01.011. Epub 2022 Feb 15. PMID: 35172124; PMCID: PMC8948161
47. Okutman O, Muller J, Skory V, Garnier JM, Gaucherot A, Baert Y, et al. A no-stop mutation in MAGEB4 is a possible cause of rare X-linked azoospermia and oligozoospermia in a consanguineous Turkish family. J Assist Reprod Genet. 2017;34(5):683–94. https://doi.org/10.1007/s10815-017-0900-z. Epub 2017 Apr 11. PMID: 28401488; PMCID: PMC5427651
48. Berger SL, Kouzarides T, Shiekhattar R, Shilatifard A. An operational definition of epigenetics. Genes Dev. 2009;23(7):781–3. https://doi.org/10.1101/gad.1787609. PMID: 19339683; PMCID: PMC3959995
49. Sinha A, Singh V, Yadav S. Multi-omics and male infertility: status, integration and future prospects. Front Biosci (Schol Ed). 2017;9(3):375–94. https://doi.org/10.2741/s493.
50. Krzastek SC, Smith RP, Kovac JR. Future diagnostics in male infertility: genomics, epigenetics, metabolomics and proteomics. Transl Androl Urol. 2020;9(Suppl 2):S195–205. https://doi.org/10.21037/tau.2019.10.20. PMID: 32257860; PMCID: PMC7108983
51. Alhathal N, Maddirevula S, Coskun S, Alali H, Assoum M, Morris T, et al. A genomics approach to male infertility. Genet Med [Internet]. 2020;22(12):1967–75. https://doi.org/10.1038/s41436-020-0916-0.

52. Li Y, Tollefsbol TO. DNA methylation detection: bisulfite genomic sequencing analysis. Methods Mol Biol. 2011;791:11–21. https://doi.org/10.1007/978-1-61779-316-5_2. PMID: 21913068; PMCID: PMC3233226
53. Cheng Y, Tang Q, Lu Y, Li M, Zhou Y, Wu P, et al. Semen quality and sperm DNA methylation in relation to long-term exposure to air pollution in fertile men: a cross-sectional study. Environ Pollut [Internet]. 2022;300:118994. https://doi.org/10.1016/j.envpol.2022.118994.
54. Lennartsson A, Ekwall K. Histone modification patterns and epigenetic codes. Biochim Biophys Acta. 2009;1790(9):863–8. https://doi.org/10.1016/j.bbagen.2008.12.006. Epub 2009 Jan 8
55. Hammoud SS, Nix DA, Hammoud AO, Gibson M, Cairns BR, Carrell DT. Genome-wide analysis identifies changes in histone retention and epigenetic modifications at developmental and imprinted gene loci in the sperm of infertile men. Hum Reprod. 2011;26(9):2558–69. https://doi.org/10.1093/humrep/der192. Epub 2011 Jun 17. PMID: 21685136; PMCID: PMC3157626
56. Aoki VW, Liu L, Carrell DT. Identification and evaluation of a novel sperm protamine abnormality in a population of infertile males. Hum Reprod. 2005;20(5):1298–306. https://doi.org/10.1093/humrep/deh798. Epub 2005 Feb 10
57. Aoki VW, Liu L, Jones KP, Hatasaka HH, Gibson M, Peterson CM, Carrell DT. Sperm protamine 1/protamine 2 ratios are related to in vitro fertilization pregnancy rates and predictive of fertilization ability. Fertil Steril. 2006;86(5):1408–15. https://doi.org/10.1016/j.fertnstert.2006.04.024. Epub 2006 Sep 29
58. Navarro-Gomezlechon A, Garrido N. Epigenetic alterations in male infertility. In: Agarwal A, Saleh R, Boitrelle F, Shah R, editors. Current and future advances in male infertility: a compendium for clinicians and researchers. Cham: Springer; 2024. p. 175–95. https://doi.org/10.1007/978-3-031-62648-7_9.
59. Mittal RD. Gene editing in clinical practice: where are we? Indian J Clin Biochem. 2019;34(1):19–25. https://doi.org/10.1007/s12291-018-0804-4. Epub 2019 Jan 1. PMID: 30728669; PMCID: PMC6346614
60. Li X, Sun T, Wang X, Tang J, Liu Y. Restore natural fertility of Kitw/Kitwv mouse with nonobstructive azoospermia through gene editing on SSCs mediated by CRISPR-Cas9. Stem Cell Res Ther. 2019;10(1):271. https://doi.org/10.1186/s13287-019-1386-7. PMID: 31445521; PMCID: PMC6708192
61. Doroftei B, Ilie OD, Puiu M, Ciobica A, Ilea C. Mini-review regarding the applicability of genome editing techniques developed for studying infertility. Diagnostics (Basel). 2021;11(2):246. https://doi.org/10.3390/diagnostics11020246. PMID: 33562517; PMCID: PMC7915733
62. Wang HQ, Wang T, Gao F, Ren WZ. Application of CRISPR/Cas technology in spermatogenesis research and male infertility treatment. Genes (Basel). 2022;13(6):1000. https://doi.org/10.3390/genes13061000. PMID: 35741761; PMCID: PMC9223233
63. Aksglaede L, Wikström AM, Rajpert-De Meyts E, Dunkel L, Skakkebaek NE, Juul A. Natural history of seminiferous tubule degeneration in Klinefelter syndrome. Hum Reprod Update. 2006;12(1):39–48. https://doi.org/10.1093/humupd/dmi039. Epub 2005 Sep 19
64. Parrington J, Coward K, Gadea J. Sperm and testis mediated DNA transfer as a means of gene therapy. Syst Biol Reprod Med. 2011;57(1–2):35–42. https://doi.org/10.3109/19396368.2010.514022.
65. Ormond KE, Bombard Y, Bonham VL, Hoffman-Andrews L, Howard H, Isasi R, Musunuru K, Riggan KA, Michie M, Allyse M. The clinical application of gene editing: ethical and social issues. Per Med. 2019;16(4):337–50. https://doi.org/10.2217/pme-2018-0155. Epub 2019 Jul 23
66. Doudna JA. The promise and challenge of therapeutic genome editing. Nature. 2020;578(7794):229–36. https://doi.org/10.1038/s41586-020-1978-5. Epub 2020 Feb 12. PMID: 32051598; PMCID: PMC8992613

67. Sikiru AB, Truong MN, Zohdy W. Future prospects for the advancement of treatment of men with NOA: focus on gene editing, artificial sperm, stem cells, and use of imaging. Asian J Androl. 2024; https://doi.org/10.4103/aja202486. Epub ahead of print
68. Karakus C, Ozyurt R. Correlation between high Choline metabolite signal in spectroscopy and sperm retrieval chance at micro-TESE. Eur Rev Med Pharmacol Sci. 2022;26(4):1125–30. https://doi.org/10.26355/eurrev_202202_28102.
69. Hesham Said A, Ragab A, Zohdy W, Ibrahim AS, Abd El Basset AS. Diffusion-weighted magnetic resonance imaging and magnetic resonance spectroscopy for non-invasive characterization of azoospermia: a prospective comparative single-center study. Andrology. 2023;11(6):1096–106. https://doi.org/10.1111/andr.13392. Epub 2023 Feb 6
70. Kavoussi PK, Atmoko W, Pinggera GM. Technologies to improve sperm retrieval in men undergoing micro-TESE for NOA. Asian J Androl. 2024; https://doi.org/10.4103/aja202450. Epub ahead of print
71. Zhang YX, Yao CC, Huang YH, Li P, Zhi EL, Zhu ZJ, et al. Efficacy of stepwise mini-incision microdissection testicular sperm extraction for nonobstructive azoospermia with varied etiologies. Asian J Androl. 2023;25(5):621–6. https://doi.org/10.4103/aja2022125. Epub 2023 Feb 24. PMID: 36861503; PMCID: PMC10521958
72. Parekattil SJ, Gudeloglu A. Robotic assisted andrological surgery. Asian J Androl. 2013;15(1):67–74. https://doi.org/10.1038/aja.2012.131. Epub 2012 Dec 17. PMID: 23241637; PMCID: PMC3739118
73. Ramasamy R, Sterling J, Fisher ES, Li PS, Jain M, Robinson BD, et al. Identification of spermatogenesis with multiphoton microscopy: an evaluation in a rodent model. J Urol. 2011;186(6):2487–92. https://doi.org/10.1016/j.juro.2011.07.081. Epub 2011 Oct 21. PMID: 22019169
74. Najari BB, Ramasamy R, Sterling J, Aggarwal A, Sheth S, Li PS, et al. Pilot study of the correlation of multiphoton tomography of ex vivo human testis with histology. J Urol. 2012;188(2):538–43. https://doi.org/10.1016/j.juro.2012.03.124. Epub 2012 Jun 15. PMID: 22704107
75. Tharakan T, Luo R, Jayasena CN, Minhas S. Non-obstructive azoospermia: current and future perspectives. Fac Rev. 2021;10:7. https://doi.org/10.12703/r/10-7. PMID: 33659925; PMCID: PMC7894261
76. Liu YF, Di L, Osterberg EC, He L, Li PS, Li Z. Use of Raman spectroscopy to identify active spermatogenesis and Sertoli-cell-only tubules in mice. Andrologia. 2016;48(10):1086–91. https://doi.org/10.1111/and.12542. Epub 2016 Jan 25. PMID: 26804545
77. Diaz P, Dullea A, Chu KY, Zizzo J, Loloi J, Reddy R, et al. Future of male infertility evaluation and treatment: brief review of emerging technology. Urology. 2022;169:9–16. https://doi.org/10.1016/j.urology.2022.06.036. Epub 2022 Jul 26. PMID: 35905774
78. Ramasamy R, Sterling J, Manzoor M, Salamoon B, Jain M, Fisher E, et al. Full field optical coherence tomography can identify spermatogenesis in a rodent sertoli-cell only model. J Pathol Inform. 2012;3:4. https://doi.org/10.4103/2153-3539.93401. Epub 2012 Feb 29. PMID: 22439124; PMCID: PMC3307228
79. Greenhalgh JR, Griffith TS, Wald M. The use of immunofluorescence in microdissection testicular sperm extraction. J Androl. 2009;30(5):548–51. https://doi.org/10.2164/jandrol.108.006049. Epub 2009 Feb 19. PMID: 19234316
80. Smith RP, Lowe GJ, Kavoussi PK, Steers WD, Costabile RA, Herr JC, et al. Confocal fluorescence microscopy in a murine model of microdissection testicular sperm extraction to improve sperm retrieval. J Urol. 2012;187(5):1918–23. https://doi.org/10.1016/j.juro.2011.12.053. Epub 2012 Mar 16. PMID: 22425054
81. Ahmad FI, Mericli AF, DeFazio MV, Chang EI, Hanasono MM, Pederson WC, et al. Application of the ORBEYE three-dimensional exoscope for microsurgical procedures. Microsurgery. 2020;40(4):468–72. https://doi.org/10.1002/micr.30547. Epub 2019 Dec 19. PMID: 31855291

82. Weinstock RJ, Ainslie-Garcia MH, Ferko NC, Qadeer RA, Morris LP, Cheng H, et al. Comparative assessment of ergonomic experience with heads-up display and conventional surgical microscope in the operating room. Clin Ophthalmol. 2021;15:347–56. https://doi.org/10.2147/OPTH.S292152. PMID: 33542618; PMCID: PMC7854362
83. Pinggera GM, Mitterberger M, Bartsch G, Strasser H, Gradl J, Aigner F, et al. Assessment of the intratesticular resistive index by colour Doppler ultrasonography measurements as a predictor of spermatogenesis. BJU Int. 2008;101(6):722–6. https://doi.org/10.1111/j.1464-410X.2007.07343.x. Epub 2008 Jan 8. PMID: 18190642
84. Zhang S, Du J, Tian R, Xie S, Li F, Li Z. Assessment of the use of contrast enhanced ultrasound in guiding microdissection testicular sperm extraction in nonobstructive azoospermia. BMC Urol. 2018;18(1):48. https://doi.org/10.1186/s12894-018-0367-y. PMID: 29792185; PMCID: PMC5966902
85. Nariyoshi S, Nakano K, Sukegawa G, Sho T, Tsuji Y. Ultrasonographically determined size of seminiferous tubules predicts sperm retrieval by microdissection testicular sperm extraction in men with nonobstructive azoospermia. Fertil Steril. 2020;113(1):97–104.e2. https://doi.org/10.1016/j.fertnstert.2019.08.061. PMID: 32033740
86. Najari BB. Ultrasound evaluation of seminiferous tubules: a promising prognostic tool for men with nonobstructive azoospermia undergoing microsurgical testicular sperm extraction. Fertil Steril. 2020;113(1):73–4. https://doi.org/10.1016/j.fertnstert.2019.09.015. Epub 2019 Nov 11. PMID: 31727416
87. Herwig R, Tosun K, Schuster A, Rehder P, Glodny B, Wildt L, et al. Tissue perfusion-controlled guided biopsies are essential for the outcome of testicular sperm extraction. Fertil Steril. 2007;87(5):1071–6. https://doi.org/10.1016/j.fertnstert.2006.10.010. Epub 2006 Dec 14. PMID: 17173898
88. Enatsu N, Miyake H, Chiba K, Fujisawa M. Identification of spermatogenically active regions in rat testes by using narrow-band imaging system. Urology. 2015;86(5):929–35. https://doi.org/10.1016/j.urology.2015.08.021. Epub 2015 Sep 8. PMID: 26362950
89. Ramkumar A, Lal A, Paduch DA, Schlegel PN. An ultrasonically actuated silicon-microprobe-based testicular tubule assay. IEEE Trans Biomed Eng. 2009;56(11):2666–74. https://doi.org/10.1109/TBME.2009.2026910. Epub 2009 Jul 21. PMID: 19628447
90. Best JC, Gonzalez D, Alawamlh OAH, Li PS, Ramasamy R. Use of 4K3D video microscope in male infertility microsurgery. Urol Video J. 2020;7:100046. https://doi.org/10.1016/j.urolvj.2020.100046. Epub 2020 Jun 15. PMID: 32661513; PMCID: PMC7357899
91. Kresch E, Efimenko I, Gonzalez D, Rizk PJ, Ramasamy R. Novel methods to enhance surgical sperm retrieval: a systematic review. Arab J Urol. 2021;19(3):227–37. https://doi.org/10.1080/2090598X.2021.1926752. PMID: 34552774; PMCID: PMC8451700
92. Zhang J, Kanoatov M, Jarvi K, Gauthier-Fisher A, Moskovtsev SI, Librach C, et al. Germ cell-specific proteins AKAP4 and ASPX facilitate identification of rare spermatozoa in non-obstructive azoospermia. Mol Cell Proteomics. 2023;22(6):100556. https://doi.org/10.1016/j.mcpro.2023.100556. Epub 2023 Apr 21. PMID: 37087050; PMCID: PMC10209038
93. Wu DJ, Badamjav O, Reddy VV, Eisenberg M, Behr B. A preliminary study of sperm identification in microdissection testicular sperm extraction samples with deep convolutional neural networks. Asian J Androl. 2021;23(2):135–9. https://doi.org/10.4103/aja.aja_66_20. PMID: 33106465; PMCID: PMC7991821
94. Goss DM, Vasilescu SA, Vasilescu PA, Cooke S, Kim SH, Sacks GP, et al. Evaluation of an artificial intelligence-facilitated sperm detection tool in azoospermic samples for use in ICSI. Reprod Biomed Online. 2024;49(1):103910. https://doi.org/10.1016/j.rbmo.2024.103910. Epub 2024 Feb 22. PMID: 38652944
95. World Health Organization. WHO laboratory manual for the examination and processing of human semen. 6th ed. Geneva: World Health Organization; 2021.
96. Son J, Samuel R, Gale BK, Carrell DT, Hotaling JM. Separation of sperm cells from samples containing high concentrations of white blood cells using a spiral channel. Biomicrofluidics. 2017;11(5):054106. https://doi.org/10.1063/1.4994548. PMID: 29034050; PMCID: PMC5617737

97. Shuchat S, Park S, Kol S, Yossifon G. Distinct and independent dielectrophoretic behavior of the head and tail of sperm and its potential for the safe sorting and isolation of rare spermatozoa. Electrophoresis. 2019;40(11):1606–14. https://doi.org/10.1002/elps.201800437. Epub 2019 Apr 15. PMID: 30892707
98. Huang HY, Lai YL, Yao DJ. Dielectrophoretic microfluidic device for in vitro fertilization. Micromachines (Basel). 2018;9(3):135. https://doi.org/10.3390/mi9030135. PMID: 30424069; PMCID: PMC6187277
99. Mangum CL, Patel DP, Jafek AR, Samuel R, Jenkins TG, Aston KI, et al. Towards a better testicular sperm extraction: novel sperm sorting technologies for non-motile sperm extracted by microdissection TESE. Transl Androl Urol. 2020;9(Suppl 2):S206–14. https://doi.org/10.21037/tau.2019.08.36. PMID: 32257861; PMCID: PMC7108989
100. Samuel R, Son J, Jenkins TG, Jafek A, Feng H, Gale BK, et al. Microfluidic system for rapid isolation of sperm from microdissection TESE Specimens. Urology. 2020;140:70–6. https://doi.org/10.1016/j.urology.2019.12.053. Epub 2020 Feb 26. PMID: 32112776
101. Mittal S, Mielnik A, Bolyakov A, Schlegel P, Paduch D, et al. Pd68-01 pilot study results using fluorescence activated cell sorting of spermatozoa from testis tissue: a novel method for sperm isolation after TESE. J Urol. 2017;197(4S):e1339.
102. Garrido N, Gil Juliá M. The use of non-apoptotic sperm selected by magnetic activated cell sorting (MACS) to enhance reproductive outcomes: what the evidence says. Biology (Basel). 2024;13(1):30. https://doi.org/10.3390/biology13010030. PMID: 38248461; PMCID: PMC10813240
103. Parmegiani L, Cognigni GE, Bernardi S, Troilo E, Taraborrelli S, Arnone A, et al. Comparison of two ready-to-use systems designed for sperm-hyaluronic acid binding selection before intracytoplasmic sperm injection: PICSI vs. sperm slow: a prospective, randomized trial. Fertil Steril. 2012;98(3):632–7. https://doi.org/10.1016/j.fertnstert.2012.05.043. Epub 2012 Jun 29. PMID: 22749221
104. Ghorbani-Sini R, Izadi T, Tavalaee M, Azadi L, Hajian M, Rahimi Zamani M, et al. Comparison of sperm telomere length between two sperm selection procedures: density gradient centrifugation and zeta potential. Int J Fertil Steril. 2020;14(1):51–6. https://doi.org/10.22074/ijfs.2020.5981. Epub 2020 Feb 25. PMID: 32112636; PMCID: PMC7139234
105. Lepine S, McDowell S, Searle LM, Kroon B, Glujovsky D, Yazdani A. Advanced sperm selection techniques for assisted reproduction. Cochrane Database Syst Rev. 2019;7(7):CD010461. https://doi.org/10.1002/14651858.CD010461.pub3. PMID: 31425620; PMCID: PMC6699650
106. Tanaka A, Suzuki K, Nagayoshi M, Tanaka A, Takemoto Y, Watanabe S, et al. Ninety babies born after round spermatid injection into oocytes: survey of their development from fertilization to 2 years of age. Fertil Steril. 2018;110(3):443–51. https://doi.org/10.1016/j.fertnstert.2018.04.033. PMID: 30098696
107. Crane GM, Jeffery E, Morrison SJ. Adult haematopoietic stem cell niches. Nat Rev Immunol. 2017;17(9):573–90. https://doi.org/10.1038/nri.2017.53. Epub 2017 Jun 12. PMID: 28604734
108. Wang J, Liu C, Fujino M, Tong G, Zhang Q, Li XK, Yan H. Stem cells as a resource for treatment of infertility-related diseases. Curr Mol Med. 2019;19(8):539–46. https://doi.org/10.2174/1566524019666190709172636. PMID: 31288721; PMCID: PMC6806537
109. Tachibana M, Amato P, Sparman M, Gutierrez NM, Tippner-Hedges R, Ma H, et al. Human embryonic stem cells derived by somatic cell nuclear transfer. Cell. 2013;153(6):1228–38. https://doi.org/10.1016/j.cell.2013.05.006. Epub 2013 May 15. PMID: 23683578; PMCID: PMC3772789
110. Achermann AP, Esteves SC. Clinical Management of men with nonobstructive azoospermia due to spermatogenic failure. In: Parekattil S, Esteves S, Agarwal A, editors. Male infertility: contemporary clinical approaches, andrology, ART and antioxidants. Cham: Springer; 2020. p. 283–95. https://doi.org/10.1007/978-3-030-32300-4_23.

111. Hendriks S, Dancet EA, van Pelt AM, Hamer G, Repping S. Artificial gametes: a systematic review of biological progress towards clinical application. Hum Reprod Update. 2015;21(3):285–96. https://doi.org/10.1093/humupd/dmv001. Epub 2015 Jan 21. PMID: 25609401
112. Tharakan T, Luo R, Foran D, Smith M, Jayasena CN, Minhas S. Strategies in infertile azoospermic patients with negative microdissection testicular sperm extraction surgery. Turk J Urol. 2020; https://doi.org/10.5152/tud.2020.20435.
113. Arafa MM, Elbardisi HT. Fertility preservation for boys and adolescents. In: Parekattil S, Esteves S, Agarwal A, editors. Male infertility: contemporary clinical approaches, andrology, ART and antioxidants. Cham: Springer; 2020. p. 819–29. https://doi.org/10.1007/978-3-030-32300-4_65.
114. Chen H, Luo T, Chen T, Wang G. Seminal bacterial composition in patients with obstructive and non-obstructive azoospermia. Exp Ther Med. 2018;15(3):2884–90. https://doi.org/10.3892/etm.2018.5778. Epub 2018 Jan 19. PMID: 29456693; PMCID: PMC5795641.
115. Campbell K, Suarez Arbelaez MC, Ghomeshi A, Ibrahim E, Roy S, Singh P, et al. Next-generation sequencing analysis of semen microbiome taxonomy in men with nonobstructive azoospermia vs. fertile controls: a pilot study. F S Sci. 2023;4(3):257–64. https://doi.org/10.1016/j.xfss.2023.06.001. Epub 2023 Jun 13. PMID: 37321541; PMCID: PMC10527663
116. Alfano M, Ferrarese R, Locatelli I, Ventimiglia E, Ippolito S, Gallina P, et al. Testicular microbiome in azoospermic men-first evidence of the impact of an altered microenvironment. Hum Reprod. 2018;33(7):1212–7. https://doi.org/10.1093/humrep/dey116. PMID: 29850857; PMCID: PMC6012977
117. Cai H, Cao X, Qin D, Liu Y, Liu Y, Hua J, et al. Gut microbiota supports male reproduction *via* nutrition, immunity, and signaling. Front Microbiol. 2022;13:977574. https://doi.org/10.3389/fmicb.2022.977574. PMID: 36060736; PMCID: PMC9434149
118. Chen P, Li Y, Zhu X, Ma M, Chen H, He J, et al. Interaction between host and microbes in the semen of patients with idiopathic nonobstructive azoospermia. Microbiol Spectr. 2023;11(1):e0436522. https://doi.org/10.1128/spectrum.04365-22. Epub 2023 Jan 12. PMID: 36633411; PMCID: PMC9927269
119. Quina AS, Buschbeck M, Di Croce L. Chromatin structure and epigenetics. Biochem Pharmacol. 2006;72(11):1563–9. https://doi.org/10.1016/j.bcp.2006.06.016. Epub 2006 Jul 11. PMID: 16836980
120. Yahaya TO, Bashar DM, Oladele EO, Umar J, Anyebe D, Izuafa A. Epigenetics in the etiology and management of infertility. World J Med Genet. 2022;10(2):7–21. https://doi.org/10.5496/wjmg.v10.i2.7.

Index

W. Zohdy et al. (eds.), *Non-Obstructive Azoospermia*,
https://doi.org/10.1007/978-3-031-99431-9

O

T

MIX
Papier aus verantwortungsvollen Quellen
Paper from responsible sources
FSC® C105338

If you have any concerns about our products,
you can contact us on
ProductSafety@springernature.com

In case Publisher is established outside the EU,
the EU authorized representative is:
Springer Nature Customer Service Center GmbH
Europaplatz 3, 69115 Heidelberg, Germany

Printed by Libri Plureos GmbH
in Hamburg, Germany